BOONE COUNTY LIBRARY
2040 9100 771 555 0

D1405864

Praise for *The Jennifer Nicole Lee Fitness Model Diet*

"As publishers and owners of a company which publishes several top fitness and bodybuilding magazines, we have had the privilege of working with some of the most iconic personalities in this industry. JNL is beautiful in spirit as well as body, and is always ready to share her knowledge, energy and insights, making her one of the top fitness celebrities today. We are proud to call her a dear friend in the fitness world, and of all of her accomplishments, most importantly this book. It's a must-read for anyone looking to get a real look into the world of a super fitness model."

—**STEVE & ELYSE BLECHMAN**, Owners of Advanced Research Press, Publisher, Editor in Chief of *Fitness RX* and *Muscular Development*

"In a career as one of the chief photographers in the fitness industry, I have had the pleasure of working with the biggest names. However, shooting with JNL is always an experience. She is funny, sexy, approachable, and such a professional to work with, time and time again. The first time I photographed her was in 2004 for her first magazine cover, Fitness RX. *And with every photo shoot, she just gets better and better. She has been able to master the art form of fitness modeling, and is indeed a living legend. This book is a must-read for anyone who wants to really get inside of 'La Tigra's' head and learn a lot about fitness modeling and how to live like one."*

—**PER BERNAL**, Celebrity Photographer for *Fitness RX/Muscular Development*, and Chief Photographer of Advanced Research Press, Inc.

"Being a top photographer, I have worked with some of the world's most beautiful women. My photography focuses on fashion, fitness, glamour and beauty - and it's amazing to see that JNL has the ability to cross over to all of these fields. She is not only a fitness model, but a super fitness model, with the ability to transform in front of my lens like a chameleon. She has mastered the art of being a top fitness model, and this book is essential to read if you too want to look like a fitness model, or become one."

—**MIKE BROCHU**, Top Beauty & Fashion Photographer, www.MikeBrochu.com

"Super fitness model Jennifer Nicole Lee has raised the bar in the industry. Her extensive knowledge, experience, and the time and energy she has placed into her career and the fitness industry, is unmatchable. As the President and owner of the hottest fitness federation to date, the World Bodybuilding and Fitness Federation, we are proud to have JNL as W.B.F.F. Miss Bikini Diva World Champion from 2008-2009."

—**PAUL DILLETT**, President and CEO of the W.B.F.F. and Legendary Professional Bodybuilder www.wbffshows.com

"Shooting JNL for the 2009 December issue of Iron Man *was an experience. Her upbeat personality and professionalism shown through on the magazine cover and entire editorial layout."*
–**MICHAEL NEVUEX**, Chief Photographer of *Iron Man*

"Jennifer Nicole Lee is one of those people that leave a mark and make an impact in your life. I have yet to meet anyone as passionate and driven to change people's lives. She is an outstanding trainer, model, businesswoman and mother."
–**AURELIO USECHE**, Owner of *MMA Authority Magazine*

"Jennifer Nicole Lee continues to rock the fitness industry worldwide. From 200#'s to $10,000 Diva Bikini Star, 'ZIPCODE' defines 'celebrity and top fitness model!' My camera loves her energy and the images are always destined for publication. Personally, I smile inside and out at the mention or thought of her name or latest endeavor. Shooting JNL is the definition of KOOL!"
–**JOHN "COACH A" ATHERTON, PHD**, www.jwathertonimages.com

"Jennifer Nicole was a great subject to work with when I interviewed her for the cover story that ran in the December, 2009 issue of Iron Man Magazine. *Whether it be by phone or e-mail, Jennifer would get back to me immediately regarding any questions I had as I was putting the piece together. In addition to being prompt, she was always in high spirits, full of energy–and funny as hell, too. Quite an all-around talent, to say the least."*
–**LONNIE TEPER**, Editor-at-Large, *Iron Man Magazine*

"As one of the industry's leading designers, I have the pleasure of dressing some of the world's fittest and beautiful women-and JNL is on the top of my list! JNL's Fitness Model Book is a quintessential read if anyone wants to break into the fitness modeling industry, or just follow the diets and exercise programs of a fitness model–to get that fitness magazine-cover-worthy look."
–**BERNADETTE BEDARD** of PassionFruitDesigns, www.PassionFruitDesigns.com

"I have had the pleasure of working with JNL on some major fitness modeling projects and appearances. And, being a highly sought-after celebrity hair and makeup artist with my own line, I have been around many very talented and extremely gorgeous women. However, JNL has always been special as she exudes genuine passion for her profession. This book is the official blueprint to becoming a fitness model, or following the lifestyle program to look like one."
–**KATIE B**, Celebrity Makeup Artist, www.katiebcosmetics.com

"JNL's book captures the spirit of the fitness industry. Heading the worlds most successful and largest supplement company, BSN, with the goal of providing our consumers the best that money can buy, it's our mission to help millions achieve their fitness goals. JNL's book shows how you can accomplish your goals with the right information, products and supplements. This book is a must-read for anyone who wants to become a fitness model, or benefit from the healthy lifestyle and enjoy looking like one."
—**CHRIS FERGUSON**, CEO of BSN, the World Leader in Cutting-Edge Physique & Performance Products, www.BSNOnline.net

"JNL is a true natural talent who always seems to get better with every project we work on. From working with her on the 007 production, Thump Gym photo shoots, and also her 2011 calendar and Behind the Scenes DVD, I have seen her evolve from a super fitness model to a juggernaut mega brand."
—**MIKEY V**, Celebrity & Top Fitness Model Photographer, www.MikeyVegas.com

"Jennifer Nicole Lee is Status Fitness Magazine's *first-ever cover model. JNL's cover helped build Status into a fitness industry favorite. Keep on changing people's lives. This book is a wellspring of information from one of the world's super fitness models. Thank you, Jennifer!"*
—**RODNEY JANG**, Editor-in Chief of *Status Fitness Magazine*, www.StatusFitness.com

"Being one of the industries leading celebrity photographers and videographers, I pride myself by working only with the best. JNL tops my list, and she is a joy to be around."
—**STEWART VOLLAND**, Celebrity Photographer and Videographer, www.StewartVolland.com

"Working with JNL is an experience in itself. Her book is a must-read for anyone wanting to transform their life and live a healthy one, just as JNL does—as a super fitness model."
—**WILLIAM DEL SOL**, founder of Willie's Boot Camp for Charity, www.williesbootcamp.com

"Being a top photographer for over 20 years, and shooting some of the world's most beautiful and talented people, I have seen many fit and gorgeous women. JNL definitely is one of our industry's most experienced super fitness models. Her book is a must-read for anyone who wants to break into the fitness modeling world."
—**RICHARD HUME**, Top Beauty and Fashion Photographer, www.HumePhoto.com

"Jennifer Nicole Lee is a vision of beauty. Her presence and personality exude positive energy. Jennifer is one of the most professional and creative talents in the fitness industry. She continues to set new standards in fitness, while inspiring fans around the world."
—**T.C. CHANG**, Top Beauty, Fashion, Physique and Fitness Model Photographer

Published by Advantage, Charleston, South Carolina.
Member of Advantage Media Group.

ADVANTAGE is a registered trademark and the Advantage colophon is a trademark of Advantage Media Group, Inc.

Printed in China.

ISBN: 978-1-59932-178-3
LCCN: 2010904622

The Jennifer Nicole Lee Fitness Model™ Diet

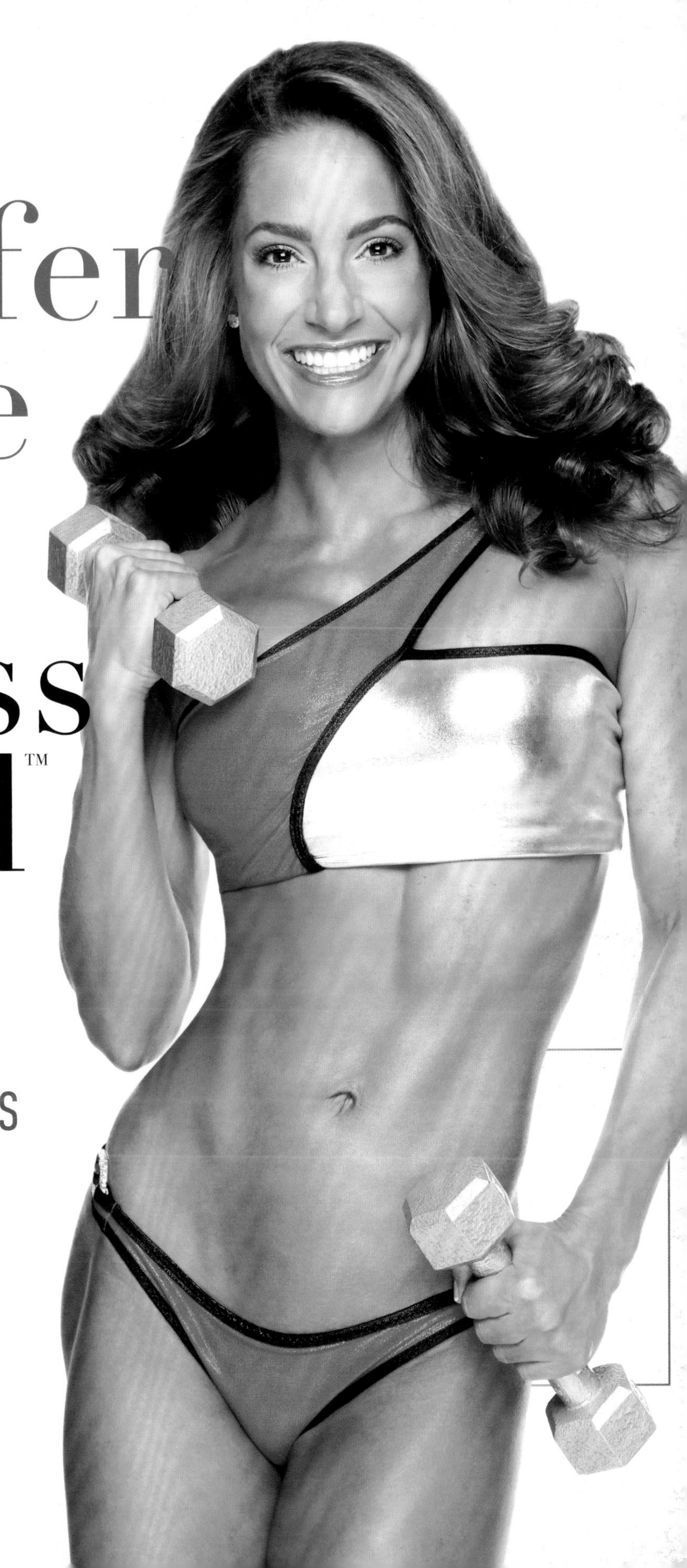

JNL'S SUPER FITNESS MODEL SECRETS TO A SEXY, STRONG, SLEEK PHYSIQUE

Advantage®

Medical Disclaimer

This book is written as a course of information only. The information in this book should by no means be considered a substitute for the advice of a qualified medial professional, who should always be consulted before beginning any new diet, exercise, or other health program.

This book is intended to be used by healthy adults, age 18 and over, as a means towards incorporating healthy habits for a fit lifestyle. This book is solely for informational and educational purposes and is not medical advice. Please consult a medical or health professional before you begin any new exercise, nutrition or supplementation program or if you have questions about your health. Please keep in mind that results may differ for each individual, even when using the same program.

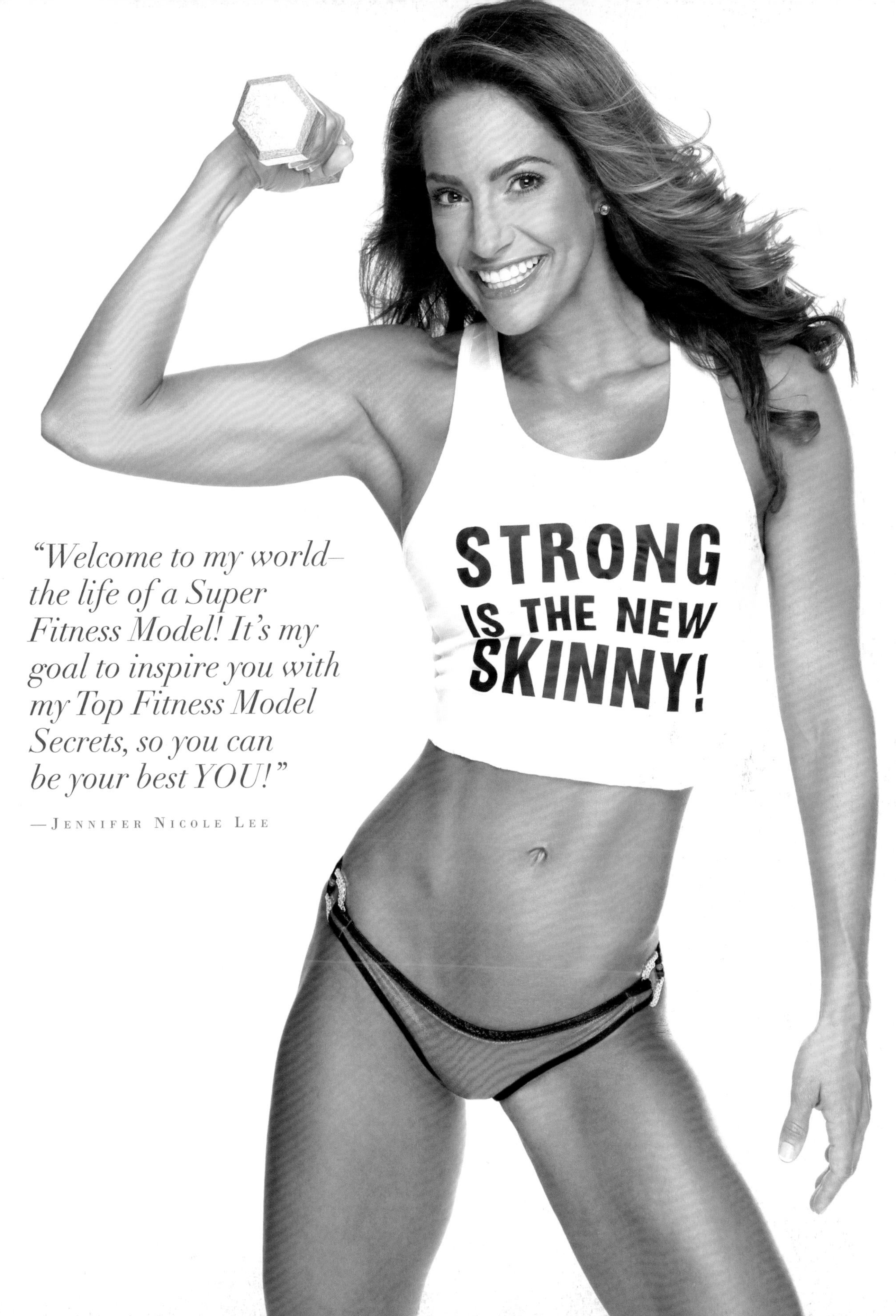

"Welcome to my world– the life of a Super Fitness Model! It's my goal to inspire you with my Top Fitness Model Secrets, so you can be your best YOU!"

—Jennifer Nicole Lee

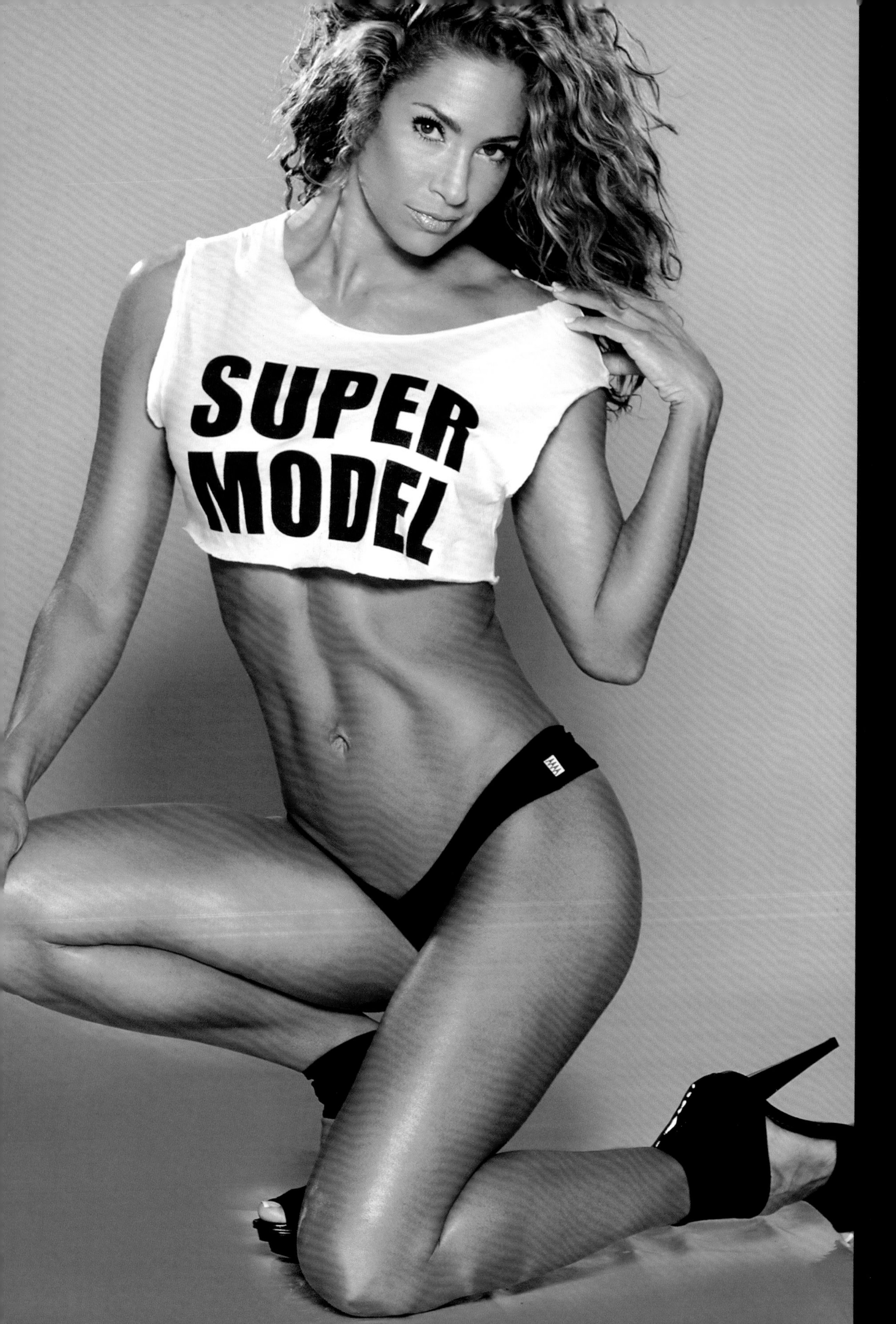
SUPER
MODEL

"Inside my book, you will learn my super fitness model secrets, to help you start your own fitness modeling career, or to at least enjoy the health benefits of living your life like one!"

—Jennifer Nicole Lee

FOR MORE HEALTHY LIFESTYLE PROGRAMS, BOOKS, PRODUCTS, AND MATERIALS BY JENNIFER NICOLE LEE, PLEASE VISIT:

www.**JenniferNicoleLee**.com

www.**TheFitnessModelDiet**.com

www.**TheFitnessModelBook**.com

www.**JNLAbCirclePro**.com

www.**FitnessModelProgram**.com

www.**BikiniModelProgram**.com

www.**TheSexyBodyDiet**.com

www.**JNLCrackTheCode**.com

www.**GetFitNowWithJNL**.com

www.**101ThingsNotToDo**.com

www.**ShopJNL**.com

www.**MindBodyandSoulDiet**.com

www.**MindBodyandSoulProgram**.com

www.**TrainWithJNL**.com

www.**TextMeJNL**.com

www.**JNLFusion**.com

www.**ChestMagic**.tv

DEDICATIONS

This book is dedicated to the millions of my "JNL fans and fitness friends" around the world. You all simply amaze me! The energy you all give me is a big sign that what I do day in and day out really does matter, and that my books, programs, and fitness products really have helped you not only to achieve your fitness goals, but to exceed them. Being a super fitness model, it is my duty to fill the void left wide open by of the wellness industry. My niche market is the woman who wants to look like a fitness model even if she isn't one. For the busy college student, the real-life working mom, the 9-5'er, the CEO, and the office executive — now you hold in your hands the blueprint for achieving that coveted fitness model physique! Your never-ending emails, phone calls, and letters of love, light, and encouragement telling me how I helped you achieve your fitness goals are the fuel to my fitness fire. I am successful, because YOU are successful. I know in my mind, body and soul that if I am able to motivate just one person to be better, then I have succeeded in life. To know that I am impacting millions on a global level gives me sheer joy that is priceless. So I thank you, and I dedicate this book to YOU!

I believe that we all share a common goal; to increase the quality of our lives through living a healthy and fit life. Your desires for greater well-being have provided me with a continued source of motivation. May my Fitness Model Book awaken the dormant athlete in you and strengthen you mentally, physical, and spiritually. May my fitness expertise, insight, and my motivation help you to achieve your life's goals and your fitness goals, while bringing health, healing, and happiness into your life.

I thank my entire book and management team who helped me create and design this book as a key to unlock the unlimited potential of my fitness friends.

Also, I dedicate this book to my foundation, my three kings: my soul-mate husband, Edward, and our two strong and handsome princes, Jaden and Dylan. I would like to also thank my husband for taking my infamous "Before" photo, which helped me to start my weight loss journey. And thank you, Eddie, for loving me then, loving me now, and loving me all through my different shapes, weights, and sizes. You have taught me what real, unconditional love is all about.

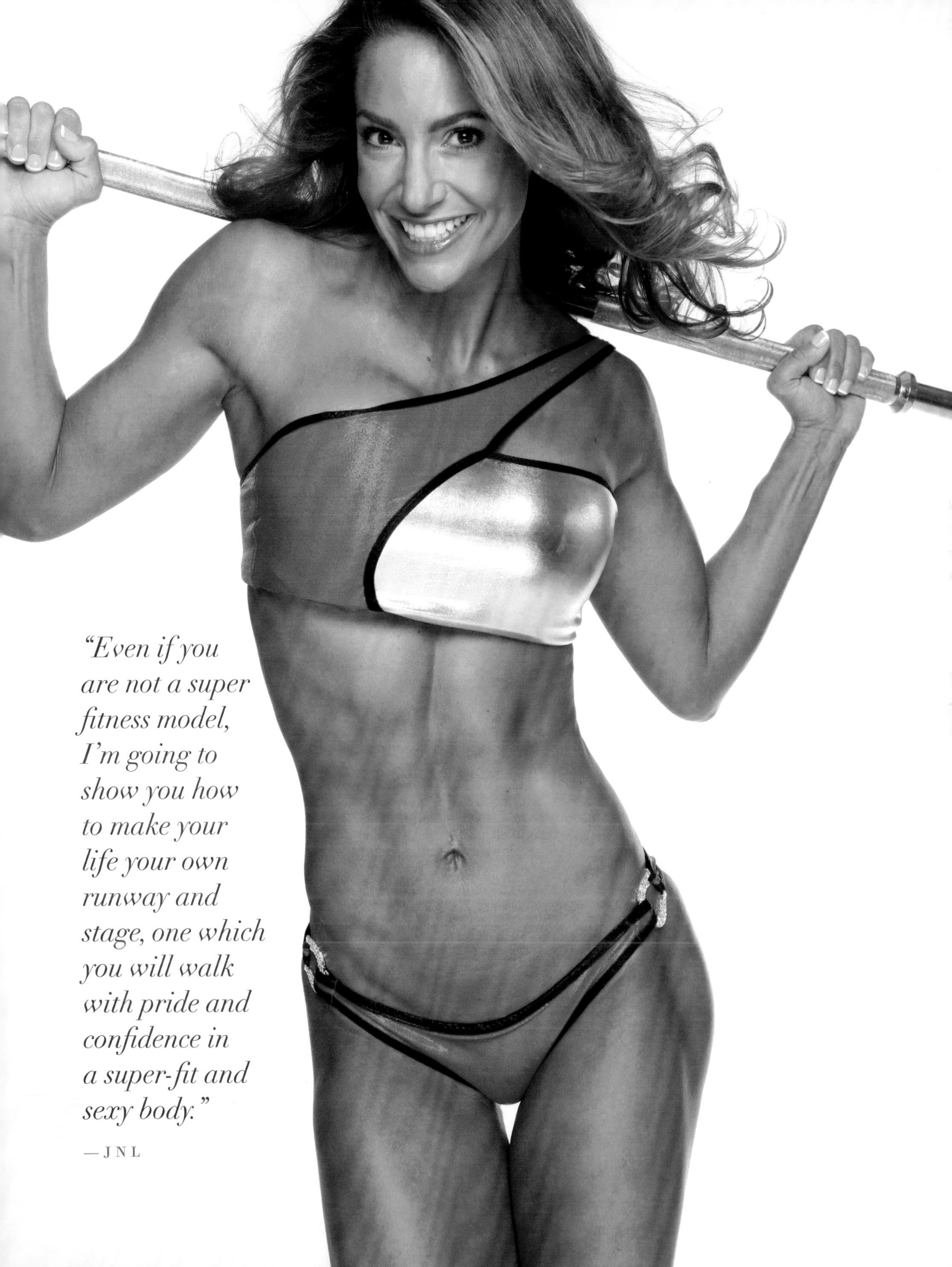

"Even if you are not a super fitness model, I'm going to show you how to make your life your own runway and stage, one which you will walk with pride and confidence in a super-fit and sexy body."

—JNL

And to my coach and personal trainer, "Wicked Willie," for always taking my training sessions seriously, and pushing my body to the next level. Thank you for taking my dream of crafting my "temple" – my body – to the ultimate vision of what a Top Fitness Model should look like! Also, thank you for spending countless hours training me for my important magazine photo shoots, fitness competitions, events, and appearances. Thanks to Unni, my coach's lovely girlfriend, for believing in me!

This dedication would not be complete without mentioning Queen Tara of Tara Productions. I admire you for your passion in life, your sweet spirit, being a mentor to me, and also mastering the art form of the ultimate infomercial. You are a true talent and genius! And to Princess Skye Madison, who is such a regal, royal, poised little angel. You are so blessed to have Tara as your mother and heartbeat to the world, and we are so lucky to have you in our lives.

And to The Dream Team, Michael and David, who are the brain and heart of the FBI. Thank you for believing in me, and allowing me to express my true genius as a master hypnotic presenter, marketer, and official spokesmodel of your global fitness empire.

And thank you to my best friend, Marli, for believing in me. You are my "life coach," always there to listen to me, support me, and help me find my way. Every day, you make my life richer, better, and worth living. You are an angel to me, and I appreciate you! Words cannot express my gratitude for all that you have done to help me and support me.

Thanks to my entire JNL Fusion Workout team, for helping me motivate millions by getting them max results in minimum time!

Smile,

J N L

SPECIAL NOTE TO YOU:

Please note that no ghost writer was involved in the writing of this book, thus maintaining my true voice and not allowing my expertise to be diluted. This book is a sincere gift from me to you. I have too much respect for all of my fitness friends to publish some regurgitated materials simply repackaged to be sold to you. I could never put my name on a book that I hadn't written, as I value you, my reader, and you deserve much more than that. In reading this book, know that it comes from my true experiences of becoming a super fitness model, and from my mind, body and soul! Enjoy!

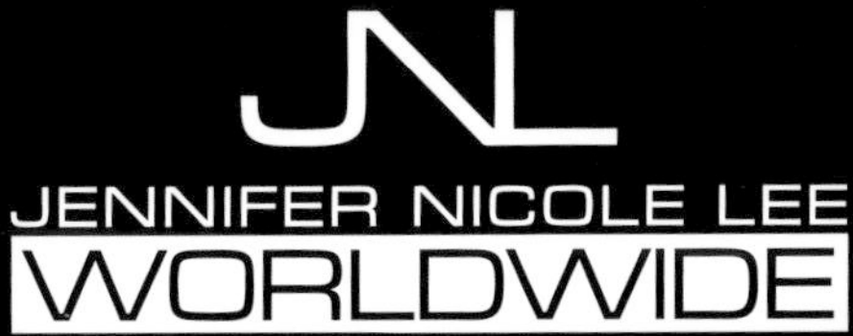

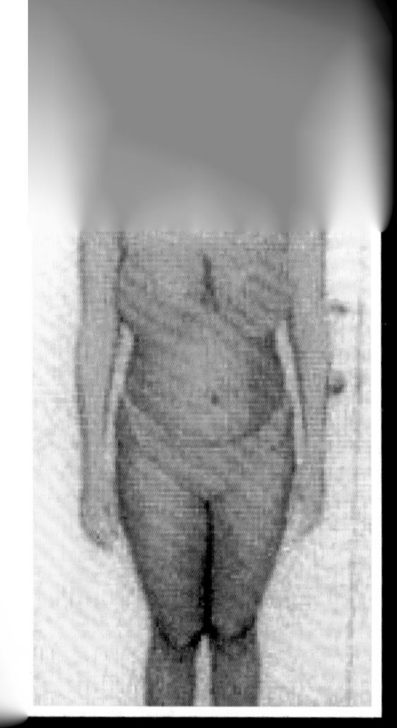

"I went from eing an ordinary overweight mom, to becoming an extraordinary ega super model ogul. My point is this: Anyone can become a super fitness model, or at least enjoy the health benefits of living like one. If I did it, you can do it too!"

—JNL

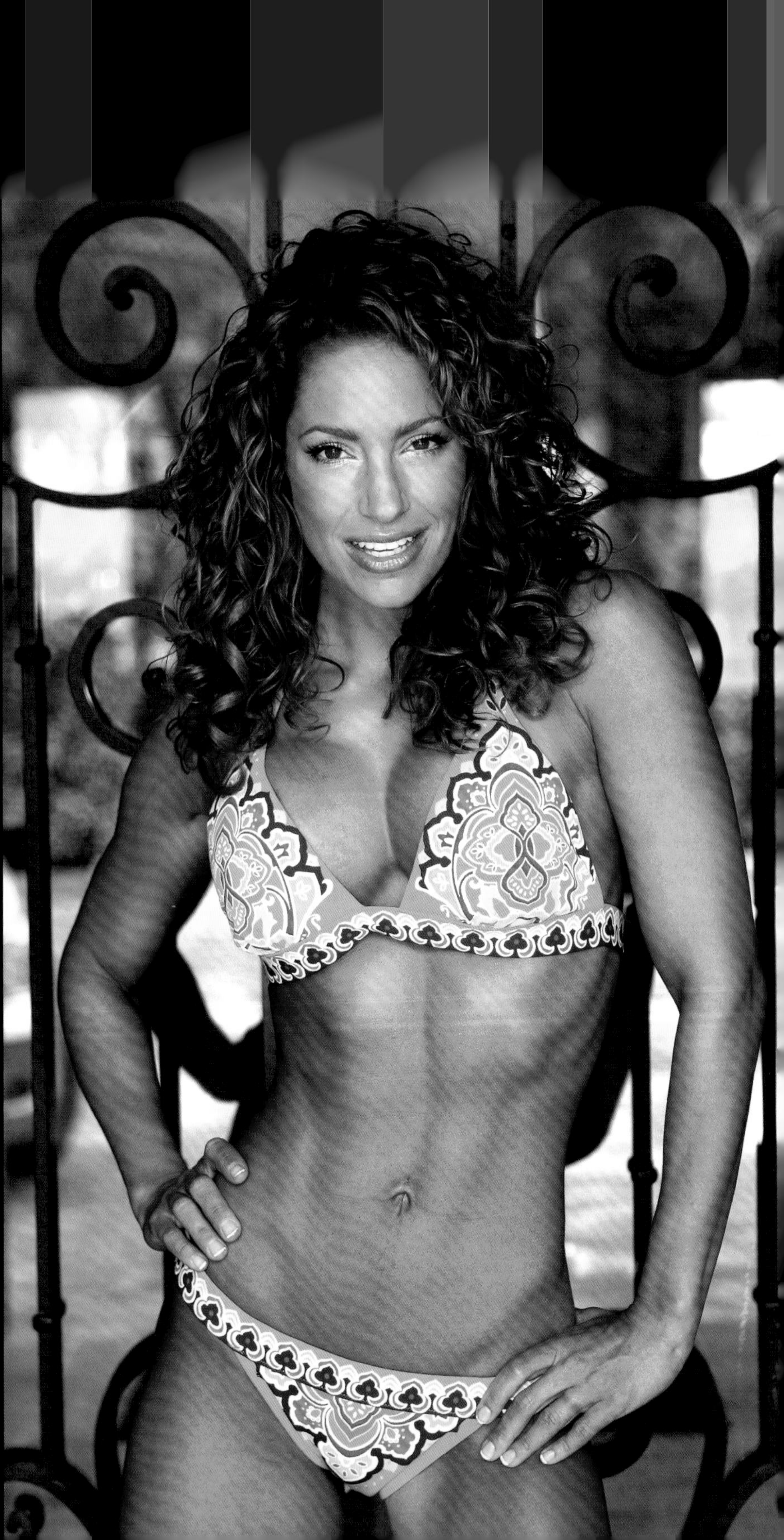

ACKNOWLEDGEMENTS

First of all, I thank God for giving me the desire, strength, and determination to achieve what I have thus far, and keeping me fueled for the rest of my successful journey!

And I would not be successful without the love and support from my husband Edward, who is the best father and husband, ever. Also, much eternal love to my two God-blessed sons, Jaden and Dylan. Thank you, boys, for being the best, funniest, smartest and most intelligent little angels a mother could ask for.

And to my Coach and personal Celebrity Trainer, "Wicked" Willie: you are the one who day in and day out keeps my mind, body and soul moving in the right, positive direction. You never allow me to give up or give in during my intense workouts. Words can't ever express my gratitude. I'm thankful to have you as my ever-reliable and faithful Coach.

To Thump Gym, the Gym of the Champions — thank you for allowing me to enjoy my workouts in peace, and providing a facility where the best of the best can train and achieve their fitness goals in privacy and comfort. Thank you Steve, for running such an exceptional gym! And thank you to my fellow hard working, super focused athletes and fellow champions and coaches who every day and every workout made it so worthwhile!

To "Mama Bear" Nadine, for believing in me, and taking my career to the next level. I believe in YOU, TOO!

To Leslie, my entertainment lawyer: not only are you super-intelligent and kind, you are patient. And when I found out that you also represent Dwayne "The Rock" Johnson, I knew that my career was in really good hands.

AND TO THE INDUSTRY! I would like to acknowledge all the wonderful, loving, and highly gifted individuals with whom I have had the pleasure of working during my journey. Every one of you has helped me "master" the art of being a top fitness model. So I thank you for giving me time and expertise in your specific fields.

To all of the photographers who have ever photographed me: you have each helped me become a master at fitness modeling, teaching me all the little tricks of how to pose, how to work with the lights, and how to really emphasize my strong points, while playing down the weak points of my body and face. In particular, I would like to thank Mike Brochu, Mikey Vegas, Richard Hume, John Cruz, Per Bernal of *Fitness RX* and *Muscular Development*, Andy McFarland, Irvin J. Gelb who gave me my nickname of "La Tigra" during my *MuscleMag Intl* cover photo shoot, Paul Buceta of *Oxygen* magazine, David Ford of *Status Fitness Magazine,* Stewart Volland, Kike San Martin of Iceberg Studios of Miami, Alfonso Moreno who shot me for my *MMA Authority Magazine* cover, and Michael Nouveau, and Lonnie Tepper of *Iron Man Magazine* for my December 2009 cover, and editorial spread, and allowing me to join the true legends of our fitness world with this historical issue and cover.

To all the Editors-in-Chief of all the magazines who have been PRO—JNL! Specifically Jeff O'Connell when you headed *Muscle & Fitness* - hi! Thank you, Jeff, for believing in me, and for your amazing write-up on me in the February 2006 issue of *Muscle & Fitness*,in your "Letter from the Editor". I thank you for comparing my passion for fitness to that of Schwarzenegger's.

To all the stylists, who have ever dressed me for a photo shoot, and/or event — thank you! I loved being your "Barbie doll" to dress up. Especially my best friend, executive assistant, and the best personal shopper and stylist all wrapped up in one amazing woman, Marli Resende.

To all the amazing hair and makeup artists who have dolled me up. It is thrilling to watch the most talented artists work their magic on me, turning me from "so-so" to so, so WOW! Thanks to all of you who have taken the time to transform my "morning face and bed hair" to something worth photographing. Katie B, you are at the top of my list!

To all the innovative videographers who have captured me on film, thank you for shining your video cameras on me. Thank you, Stewart Volland, for shooting my first-ever video for my first calendar shoot! Rob Riches, you are a genius, doing the work of ten people in half the time. Special thanks to Marianna Rodriguez and Christopher Michaels, Media team at BSN, for making me look good in post-production. And Mikey Vegas, for teaching me that my gift of motivating others to be their best is my strongest point.

Thanks to the Art Department at BSN, for designing some of the most amazing ad campaigns for BSN featuring me. Your vision, artistic graphic design, and tremendous work ethic show up in every print campaign that you have published.

To all of the magazines who have given me the pleasure to either be featured on their cover, or inside in an editorial, *specifically Ocean Drive Magazine, Oxygen, Fitness RX, Iron Man, Status Fitness, Natural Body Building, MuscleMag International, Max Sports & Fitness, American Curves, Muscle & Fitness Hers, Muscle & Fitness His, Muscle & Body, Natural Muscle, Best Body,* and *MMA Authority magazine.*

To all the interviewers, journalists, radio talk show hosts, and editorial writers who have ever done an article on me, thank you for taking the time to allow me to share my passions, views, and motivational stories of my personal struggles to inspire others to never give up in life.

Thank you to the number one at-home, interactive shopping channel, HSN, for allowing me to showcase my enthusiasm for increasing the quality of so many lives with wonderful products that I love. I so enjoy my live TV time, giving me the rare opportunity to empower, enlighten, educate and entertain people in over 100 million households to be their very best. I am honored to help so many improve their lives through my appearances on this amazing channel.

To "Queen Tara" of Tara Productions for being such a positive light in our industry, a great friend, a fabulous mom, and a go-to guru when I need direction! You are priceless. And to Princess Skye Madison, you are a true gift from heaven Your sweet little spirit touches everyone who comes in contact with you. And to the Princess of Production, Elisa, who always is super fun to have on set. Not only are you an amazing production guru, you are a true friend!

To Michael Casey and David Brodess of Fitness Brands, Inc. Thank you for believing in me and making me part of the global hit-making "Dream Team"! Your 20 years-plus combined experience in the DRTV is unmatchable, and I love working with all of you.

To the *Status Fitness* magazine team, such as Rodney Jang, David Ford, Ocean Bloom—thank you all for opening the door for me with your magazine, and putting me on the cover of your premiere issue. Thank you!

And to T.C. Chang, a true visionary and talent, from photography, to "digital painting," to graphic designing. My 2010 Status Fitness Calendar cover was the biggest gift you could have ever given me. You are a genius!

To my entire book team, my group of editors, and my publisher, I'm grateful to have such a marvelous group of people to work with. Thank you for listening to me when I said NO to a ghost writer, thus allowing me to let my true voice shine through in my book. Even though it would have made the process easier, the journey of authoring this book would not have made me stronger or better, and the book's content would not have resonated with my true spirit, had I used a ghost writer. A special thanks to Amy Ropp, the head designer of this book! She is not only truly talented, but a joy to work with!

To Paul and Allison Dillett of the World Bodybuilding & Fitness Federation; being crowned the *WBFF Miss Bikini Diva*, more than once, has been a sheer pleasure. Your WBFF Federation is light-years ahead of the fitness competition. The way you treat your athletes, fitness models and competitors is remarkable.

I applaud the female fitness pioneers and fitness models before me who led the way and blazed the trail, allowing me to follow through on my own journey. To name a few of my all -time favorites who truly are my icons and my heroes: Jane Fonda, who single-handedly ignited the fitness craze and whose role in *Barbarella* will never be forgotten; Sophia Loren, for proving that women only get more beautiful with age; Raquel Welch, for striking that iconic pose in an animal-print bikini in *One Million Years B.C.*

Also, thank you to the multi-tasking and multi-dimensional modern-day women and legendary super models who have become "masters of the art of modeling" and crossed over to being CEO's of their own empires. You inspire me every day: Kathy Ireland, Cindy Crawford, Christie Brinkley, Iman, and Tyra Banks. Thank you for showing me that we can be much more than just a pretty face, but also a "tour de force" in our own industry.

Thank you, Mom, for teaching me that it only takes the faith of a mustard seed to make mountains move and to have our dreams come true.

And lastly to all the haters, for teaching me what NOT to be, how NOT to act, what NOT to believe, and what NOT to become. If I didn't have you all telling me that I could not do it, while I was doing it, accomplishing what I have would not be so sweet and rewarding. Proving you all wrong was a nice little extra bonus and reward to my amazing journey of becoming a top fitness model and mega-model mogul.

And to all of my loyal, loving, super dedicated JNL fans from around the world! Your constant emails, letters of support, phone calls, and reaching out to me show me that what I am doing is making a BIG difference in your lives. I love each and every one of you, and I admire and respect you as my true fitness friends.

Believe,

JNL

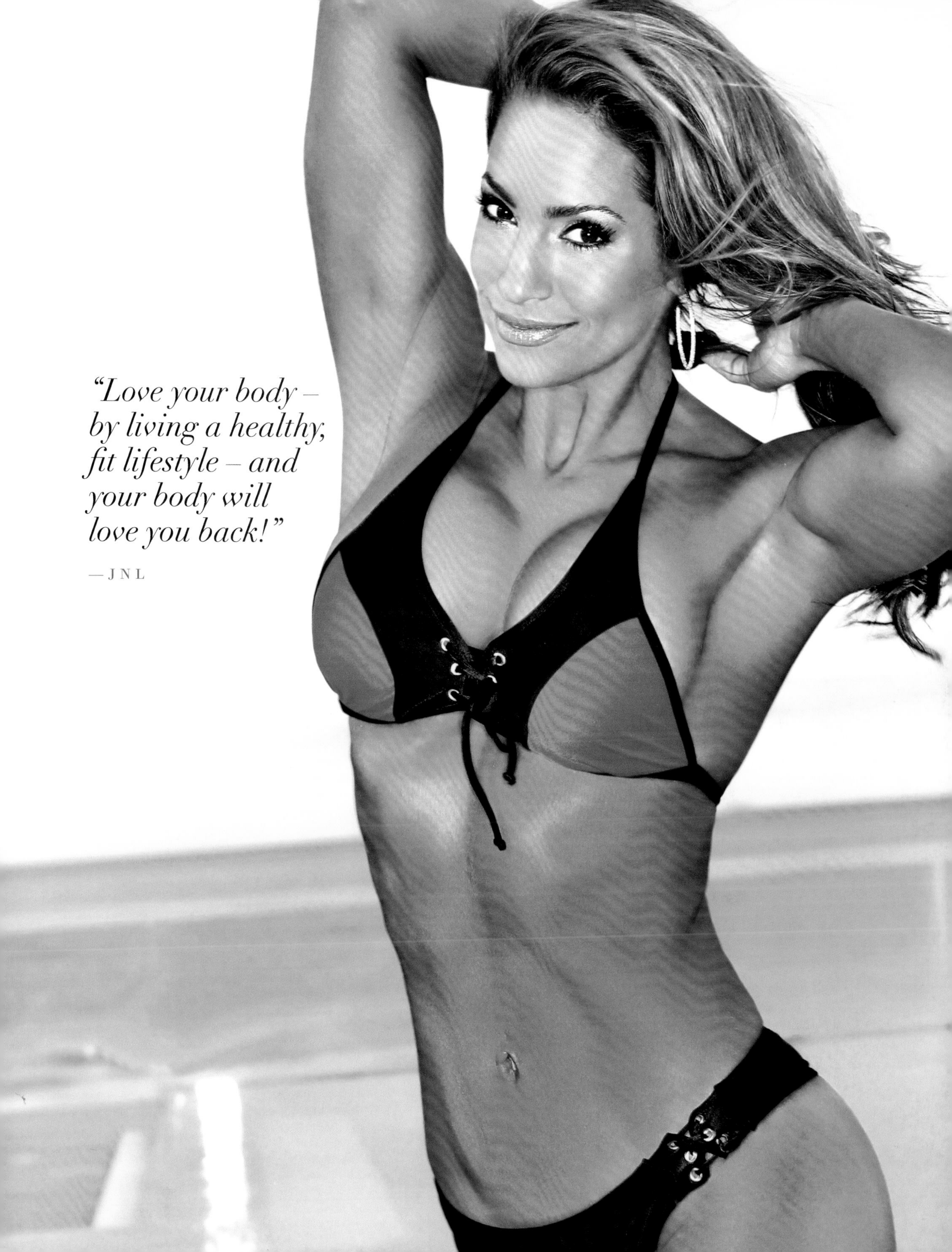
"Love your body –
by living a healthy,
fit lifestyle – and
your body will
love you back!"
—JNL

TABLE OF CONTENTS

FOREWORD

By Elsye Blechman

The first time I saw Jennifer Nicole Lee was at the Ms. Bikini Universe in 2004. To say she absolutely *"wowed"* me is an understatement. This long and lanky beauty stepped onstage and blew the competition away. At that time I had no idea that just one year before she had given birth to her second child and was 70 pounds overweight. In meeting with her after the show she told me that it was only two months before that she had decided to enter the show. What was her motivation I wondered? How on earth could someone get into competition shape so quickly? Having been in the fitness industry for some 30 years, I have seen a lot of "heavenly" bodies parade across the stage. But when you're in Jennifer's company, you can appreciate how her physical beauty, combined with her inner beauty, wrapped up in a passionate, optimistic and energetic aura, translates into a wonderful, cyclonic "tour de force."

After marrying and starting a family (Jennifer has two beautiful boys), a role she absolutely adores, she set out to redefine what a wife and mother *should* and *could* do. Indeed it was her wonderful family who gave her the motivation to succeed.

The focus that this first-generation Italian "ball of fire" has when she puts her mind to something is incredible and unstoppable. Jennifer went on to win the Ms. Bikini America contest in 2005 and the rest is history. She has established an incredible following not only in the highly competitive fitness world, but also among everyday women who are concerned about living a healthy lifestyle. Her down-to-earth practical advice when it comes to training, nutrition, diet and general philosophy regarding positive thinking has made her a most sought-after fitness and wellness celebrity.

Jennifer is a true entrepreneur. She is the CEO of a multi-million dollar empire having developed a swimsuit and fitness clothing line, running fitness boot camps, authoring bestselling books, and partnering with various supplement and fitness-minded exercise companies. Her Ab Circle Pro is a worldwide phenomenon and she makes monthly appearances to over 90 million households on the #1 interactive Home Shopping Network (HSN).

Jennifer had first graced the cover of *FitnessRx for Women* in the October 2004 issue and was featured in "Beauty– the Goddess Factor" She has been on numerous covers of ours since and has been featured doing many various high-intensity workouts, which are easy to follow and achieve amazing results. She will tell you that *FitnessRx for Women* was where she got her start– but I can tell you that she was destined for greatness all along. Our paths just crossed at the right time, and I feel extremely fortunate that they did! I can always count on Jennifer to exhibit the utmost professionalism and bring with her an abundance of uplifting confidence, which consistently comes through to her audience and readers.

In *The Jennifer Nicole Lee Fitness Model Diet*, Jennifer brings her years of knowledge, insight and experience in an easy-to-read, beautifully illustrated and photographed book, filled with a multitude of great ideas, fat-burning workouts, yummy low-fat recipes and a philosophy that will keep you on track. As if that isn't enough, Jennifer also offers tips on tanning, waxing, the war against cellulite, skincare, cosmetics, and the little adjustments that will give your workout better results and have you look your best. There's even a personal meal planning section. I don't think there's an area of interest she doesn't cover! This is a complete *tell-all* book that should be your *go-to* bible for anything fitness and healthy lifestyle living!

In conclusion, I am very proud to have been asked to write the forward to this book– but even more proud of Jennifer, for all of her ongoing accomplishments as she continues to enlighten and motivate her ever-expanding audience, and move the fitness and wellness industries forward in a positive and inspirational direction.

You rock, girlfriend!

ELYSE BLECHMAN
Co-owner and Vice President/Advanced Research Press, Inc.
Publisher of FitnessRx for Women *and* FitnessRx for Men

WELCOME TO A TOP FITNESS MODEL'S WORLD:

—INTRODUCTION

From Top Fitness Model & Author Jennifer Nicole Lee

> *"I have crossed global barriers by being a super fitness model, because living a fit lifestyle and being healthy is a universal language that the entire world understands."*
>
> —JNL

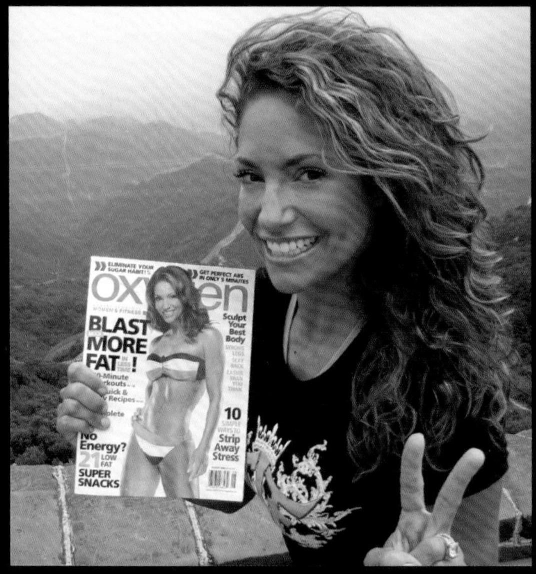

JNL in Bejing, China on the Great Wall ▲

HELLO, FITNESS FRIEND!

I am a Super Fitness Model. That's what I do. Some people are great at math, or at architecture, at writing poetry, or at gardening. I just happen to be excellent at fitness modeling. It's my passion. I love what I do, and I never get bored with it. After being on over 30 fitness magazine covers, in countless editorials, being featured in key media appearances, wildly successful global infomercial hits, and on TV for my fitness level and athletic-yet-feminine physique, it's kind of sunk in that this is my "thing".

I wasn't born into money or a prominent family, and I didn't have much growing up. But one thing is for sure: God gave me many gifts. Among them are being good in front of a camera, which I have worked on very hard, as it is a true craft and art form. I also have been able to fall in love with working out and living a super-fit healthy lifestyle. And I really do owe it to my parents for blessing me with photogenic facial features. It's not that I'm a narcissist, or self-absorbed, but rather that I have found my passion in fitness modeling, as well as in being a positive role model, a gifted communicator, and a hell of a fitness program developer. Everyone has her own "thing," and this happens to be mine.

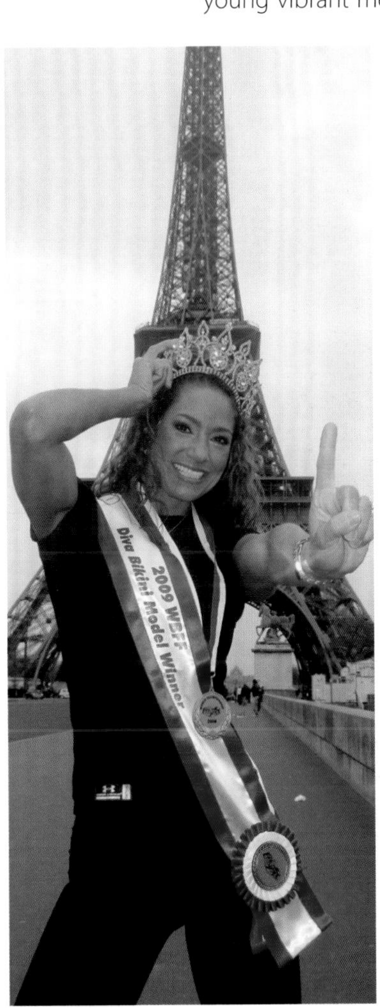

▲ JNL in Paris, France in front of the Eiffel Tower

But don't get me wrong. Becoming one of the world's leading fitness icons didn't happen overnight. Hard work and dedication are what got me to where I am today.

It's almost unbelievable that, just a short time ago, I was a fat and frumpy housewife with no get-up-and-go, no direction, and no true passions or goals in my life. That all changed when I fell in love with working out. When I actually connected with my inner strength through working out, is when I discovered my true self, the real me; the person who God intended me to be. Through living a healthy lifestyle, I shed my fat suit and said goodbye to the old me, revealing the new, fresh, young vibrant me who'd been lying dormant inside. I began my fitness journey because of the two most precious gifts God gave me – my sons. I knew that I not only had to get fit to keep up with the hectic demands of life, but also to be the best mom and wife that I could be. I wanted to prove to myself, my sons, and the rest of the world, that women can be their very best, even after motherhood – and that dreams really do come true!

Countless hours of working out, millions of "clicks" in front of a camera, and hundreds of bookings and events gave me priceless experience as one of the industry's leading fitness sensations. In this book, you'll find numerous "JNL" tools, tips and techniques that I learned along my journey to the success I enjoy today. Thanks to the urging of my fans around the world, my team and I have created this book to answer all of your questions about my personal methods for achieving and maintaining a top fitness model body.

I am delighted to be sharing with you my Fitness Model Diet, which is dedicated to you, helping you achieve

> *"I am delighted to be sharing with you my **Fitness Model Diet,** which is dedicated to you, helping you **achieve your fitness, weight loss, and lifestyle goals,** with the added benefit of looking like a coveted cover girl!"*

your fitness, weight loss, and lifestyle goals, with the added benefit of looking like a coveted cover girl! With twenty years of experience in the modeling business, the last six of which were focused intensively in the fitness industry, I pride myself on knowing how to help others look and feel their very best with the least amount of effort, by providing them with the secrets it took me so long to uncover. I am delighted that YOU don't have to go through all of the trials and errors that I did, and I invite you to get as much as you can out of this innovative program, which is laid out as simply as possible here for your benefit. It is my mission to continue to share and shine the light that my Higher Power has blessed me with, to help others realize and achieve their lifestyle goals. My mission is to help you better the quality of your life. I know that if you apply the Fitness Model Principles found in this program, the quality of your life will increase with joy, health, wellness, and beauty, from the inside out.

Now let me be clear. I want you to know what you will not find in my book. I am not a bully. I don't pride myself on forcing overweight people who have never worked out before to engage in any full-on super-athletic drills or workouts. That is dangerous. I am not out to intimidate those who suffer from chronic emotional eating by forcing them to work out 4 hours a day while living on lettuce and carrots. I don't get off on my image being glorified by scaring those who are severely out of shape, or belittling them, or being condescending to them. I can't even fathom cursing at or freaking out on anybody, as some "experts" do. To me that is not how a professional life coach, weight loss expert, or trainer should ever act. It's emotional abuse, and overweight people have suffered enough.

What you will find in my book is the successful and safe method of weight loss that I followed to help me lose over 80 pounds after the birth of my children. I did it, not through torture, torment, or overtraining and under-eating, but rather though practicing self-love and self-respect.

I'm not out to hurt you, but to help you, I don't want you to ever go through what I did, losing weight in a short period of time only to gain it all back. It's my goal to empower, enlighten, educate, and lead you, by passing you the torch of wisdom, courage, and power to create the same miracle in your life, the healthy, safe, and long-lasting way.

Believe,

JENNIFER NICOLE LEE

"Sexy, healthy, fit bodies come in all shapes and sizes. Celebrate YOUR body by loving it through fitness!"

—JNL

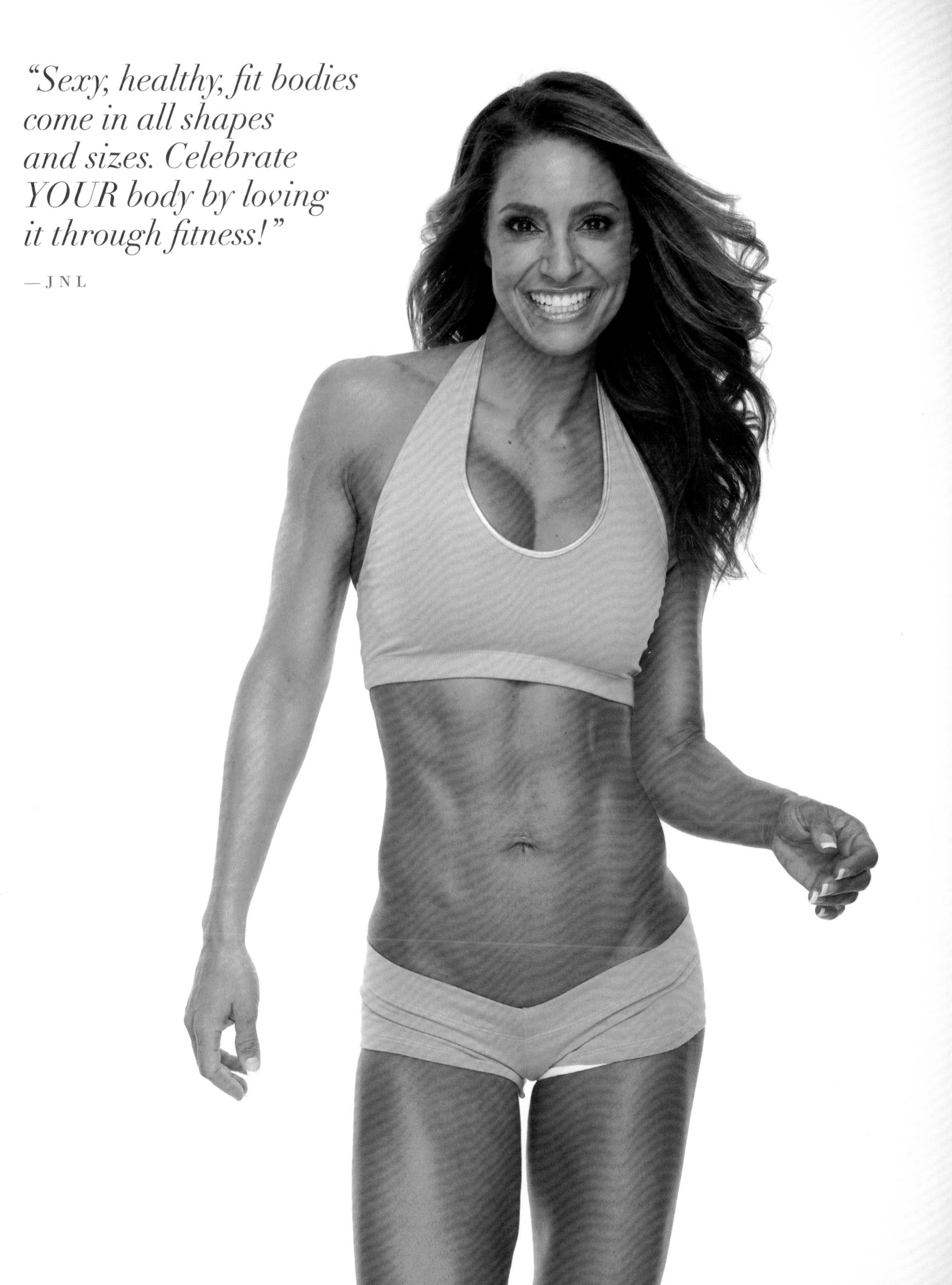

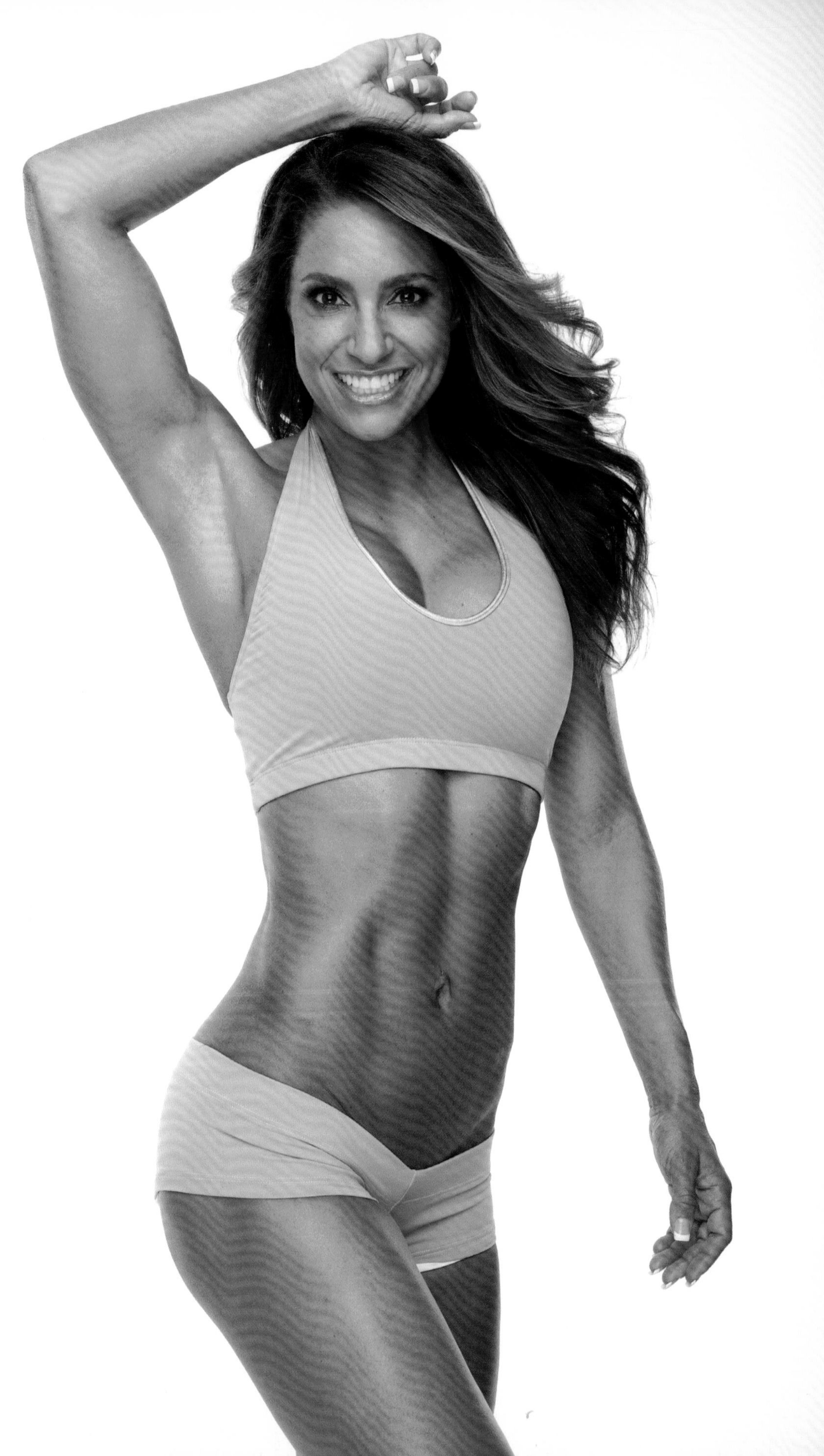

"Fitness models have more fun, because life is more fun when you are fit!!"

—JNL

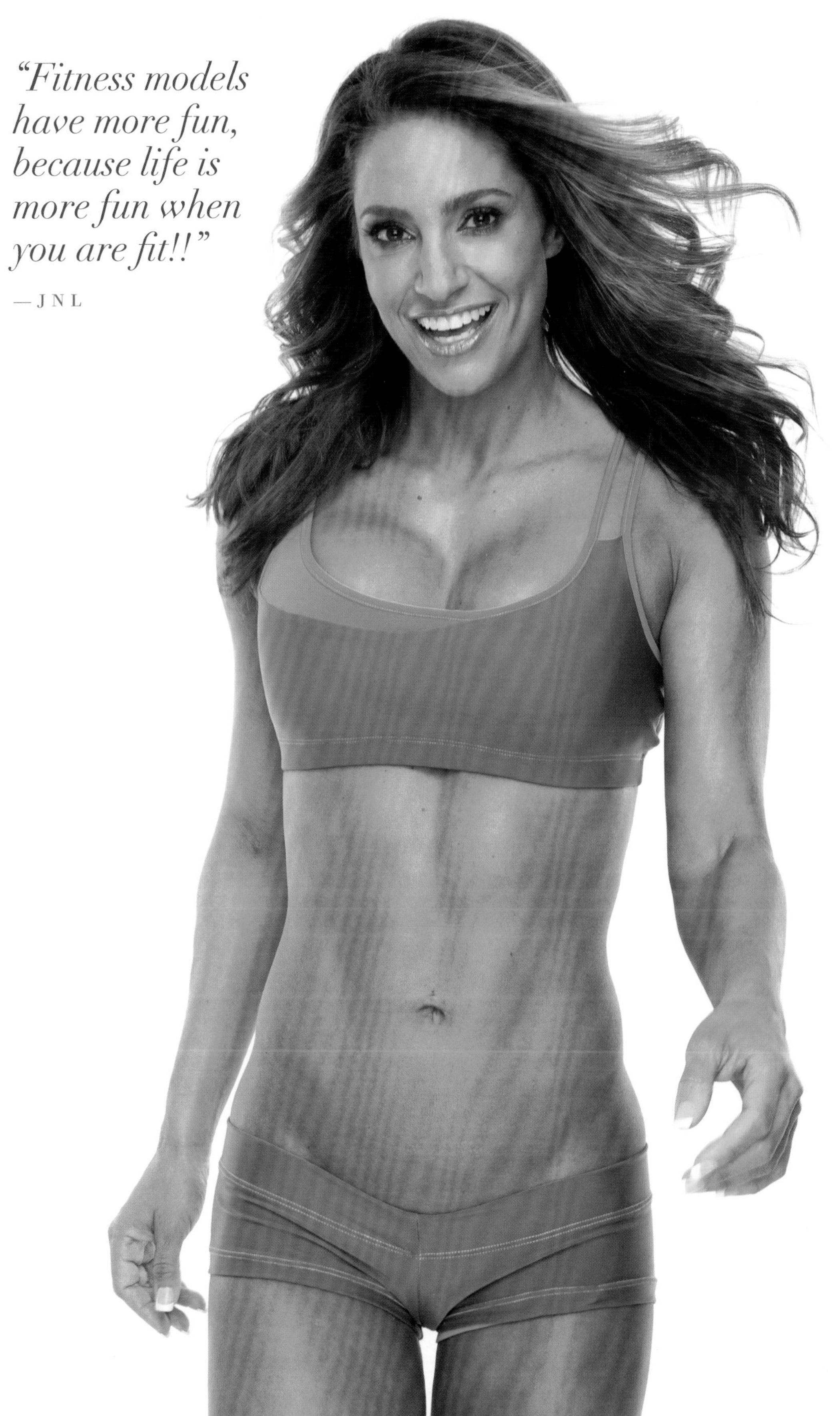

LIGHTS, CAMERA— ACTION!

Are You Really Ready to Become a Fitness Model – Or Just Enjoy Looking Like One?

PRE-FITNESS MODEL DIET CONSULTATION FROM JNL

"Celebrate, honor and love YOUR life— by being fit."

—JNL

> *"Being a super model, either in the business of fitness or beyond, is not as easy as it looks. There is a lot that goes behind a full production, from preparing for a photo shoot, to 'acting' in front of the camera or video lens. It's definitely an art form that I made it my goal to become excellent at."*
>
> —JENNIFER NICOLE LEE

> *"In the studio, I do try to have a thought in my head, so that its not like a bland, blank stare."*
>
> —CINDY CRAWFORD, *Top Model and Actress*

The life of a super fitness model is very rewarding and exciting, full of adventure and travel. But it can also be tremendously challenging and demanding. Thanks to personal experience, I know first-hand what it takes to become a fitness model, or even just to look like one. You must be committed and ready. So, my book is only intended for those who are dedicated to living out the journey of becoming their best possible selves, as challenging as it may be. And if, like me, you're someone who loves to live a superfit healthy lifestyle, then you're going to love this book!

Here's the funny part: I wasn't always fit, strong and healthy. And I didn't know anything about fitness modeling when I started. I wish that I could have had this blueprint that you are holding in your hands, because I would have been able to accomplish so much more in even less time. So use my book! Learn from my top fitness model secrets so you too, can achieve your dreams.

One of the most important aspects to address before starting my JNL Fitness model diet is preparing yourself for the life-improving miracles that are about to come your way. As a life coach, I spend an immense amount of time with my personal clients, prepping them and getting them ready for the amazing journey ahead.. I have found from my countless hours of experience that the number one principle to guarantee magical results is making sure that my clients are mentally committed to making these improvements in their lives.

You see, being "interested" in something, and being committed to it, are two totally different mindsets. In order for you to create positive transformations, you must be committed to making the necessary changes in your life that will yield success. How do we get you prepared? By making sure you are fully focused, dedicated, and ready to take on your brand-new life.

I get you to that point by taking you through an exercise I call the "Pre-Fitness Model Diet Consultation." In this exercise, I want you to take some quiet time to fully examine your past, and also your present state. Ask yourself these empowering questions:

1. *If I continue with my current lifestyle,* ***where will I be in one year? Two years? Five years? Ten years?***

2. *Is what I am doing currently working for me, or against me? Am I living my life to my utmost potential?*

3. ***If I don't start today making the necessary changes*** *in my life, where will my life end up?*

4. *Am I totally,* ***fully happy*** *with my life now?*

5. *Am I ready to prove to myself, my family, and to the world just how amazing and brilliant I am?*

6. *Do I fully understand that to be an example of personal excellence, I must go above and beyond my own expectations, and also the expectations of others?*

7. *Up until now, have I truly amazed myself and those closest to me with my own abilities?*

8. *Do I realize that, to be a winner, I must learn from other winners?*

9. *Do I accept that, during my journey to become my best, there will be times of frustration and growing pains, and that I must be persistent through them in order to achieve my desired results? Am I willing to press and push through these trying times?*

10. *Am I ready to jump-start my fitness level, and possibly even start a fitness modeling career?*

11. *Do I have a strong desire to become a fitness model, or to at least look like one?*

12. *Do I want to know the ins and outs of the fitness modeling industry?*

13. *Am I ready to master the secrets that JNL has learned firsthand in the fitness modeling industry?*

14. *Am I ready to implement the techniques in this book that can help me to get tons of exposure, ads in major magazines, even become a fitness magazine cover girl with big endorsement deals and contracts?*

If you answered YES all or most of these questions, then you are ready!

While reading my book, you'll discover a sense of excitement about your new-found lifestyle and fitness freedom. You'll be blessed with a new energy of health, healing and happiness. But you may also experience down times, difficulties and challenges. Keep steadfast! This is when you must be fully committed to stick with it, and to stay focused on your goals. Keeping your eyes on the prize is a "must" for you to be victorious. Many will try to distract you and deter you. As you'll see, when you aim at making your dreams come true, it's not about the destination, but the journey! You don't have to be perfect, but you do have to persist.

And this is when you must revisit your Fitness Model Book, and rededicate yourself to your goals.

You may feel that you are moving too slowly towards your goals, that your desired outcomes are not happening as fast as you would like. You may ask yourself "Why haven't I lost weight yet? Why isn't this working faster? Why don't I have the body of my dreams now?" When these negative feelings boil up, you must remember that success doesn't happen overnight. Striving to be your fittest best takes time, patience, and constant effort. So don't give up, and enjoy the ride!

Just sit back, relax, take a big deep breath in and then exhale. You are about to embark on one of the most magical and miraculous times of your life. Just know that you will reach your goals, if you just use all of the priceless information in my book. Just like my own personal transformation of going from a fat and frumpy housewife to a super fitness model, it didn't happen overnight – but it did happen! Because I wouldn't give up or give in, I am now able to give you the gift of motivation to help you realize your own dream life. I proudly pass the torch of wisdom to you, so that you, too, can succeed in all areas of your life – through health, healing, and happiness.

ASK JNL

"So JNL, what do I do if I hit a plateau? Or feel at times that I am not getting results?"

—Jamie, mother of 4, Columbus, Ohio

JAMIE, THAT'S AN EXCELLENT QUESTION! If you start out getting results, but then hit a plateau, I urge you to keep at it. This happens to me, but I choose to work through it, instead of allowing this "downtime" to get the best of me. It's only natural to hit plateaus. It's part of the journey. Consider this your "relaxation station," where you rest and recover to ramp up for the future amazing benefits to come.

It's like when you are at the spa, enjoying a much-needed break to reflect on your journey thus far, and planning how you can do better for the next chapter. You need that breather to rest up for the future. The same concept is at work here. Don't waste your energy getting frustrated. Actually use this time to get re-energized! Plateaus happen to everyone in every aspect of life, especially when you are learning something new. Success comes in waves, just like the ocean. So when a wave of success is on its way out, use the quiet downtime to strategize, mastermind, and prepare for your continued success.

Learning fitness model secrets is like learning any new skill. For anyone who has ever studied the piano, or tried to play a new sport, or attended a university to learn a new subject; there is always a learning curve, and plateaus along the way. It's in this moment that the losers are separated from the winners. It's in this moment, in which you decide to continue and carry on, that you become a winner. A winner is the loser who picks herself up one last time and goes on! So keep plugging through. This is where you must be committed to your success, not just "interested."

CHAPTER 1

WHY YOU MUST BELIEVE TO BECOME A FITNESS MODEL

–Or Enjoy Looking Like One!

"If you are focused, dedicated, passionate, and willing to never give up –then I believe in you!"

—JNL

You all know that I am famous for my catchphrase, "Believe". It's my signature saying. It's how I sum up all that is possible into one single, simple, yet super-strong word. When I started my weight loss journey going from fat to fit, from frumpy to fabulous, no one believed in me. So I had to believe in myself. Use the acronym below to remind yourself of what it takes to stand out from the crowd, to be a cut above the rest, and to be a true champion in life as a fitness model.

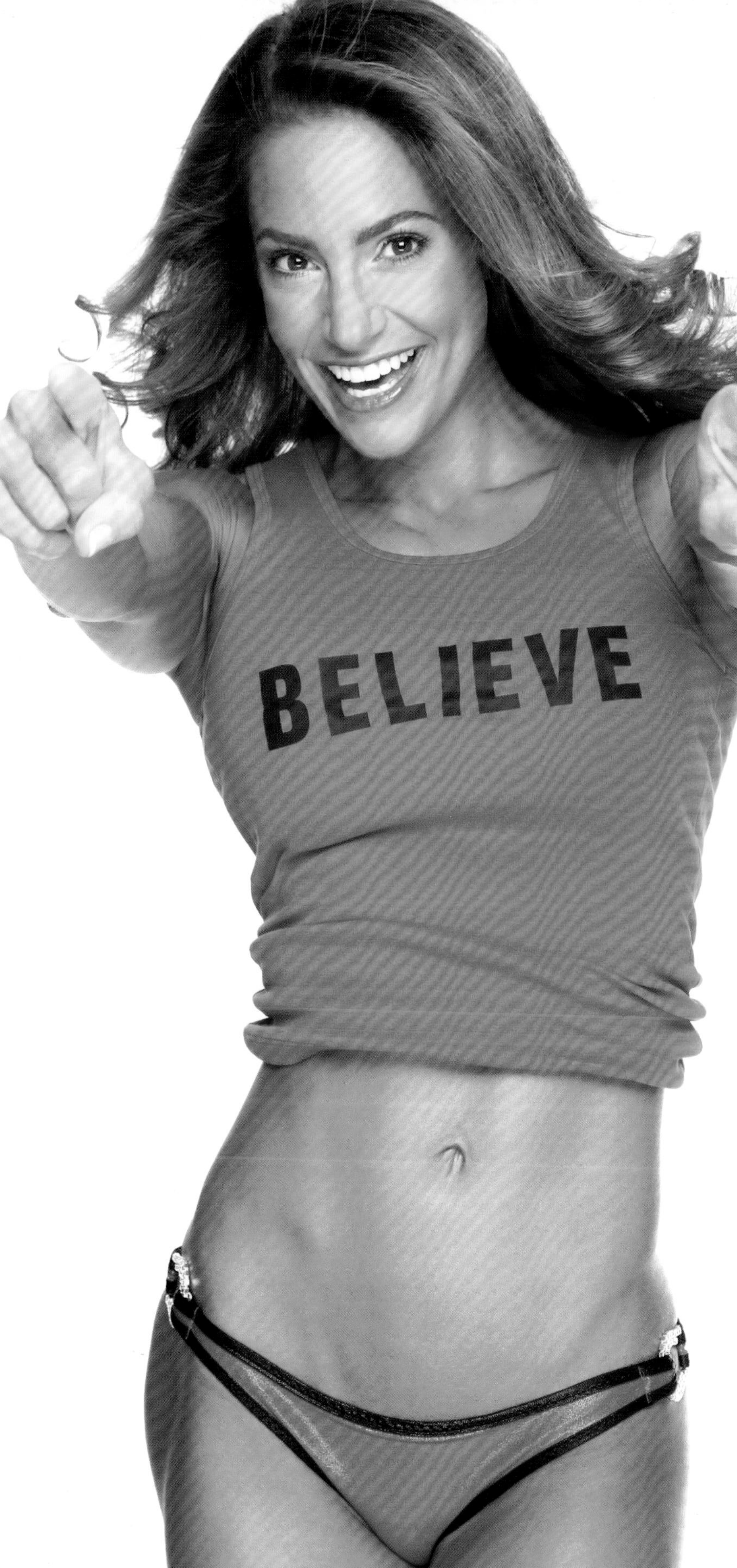

"Believe that you can, and YOU WILL!"

—JNL

B IS FOR BEAUTY: World-class fitness models are beautiful both inside and out. From all of my years modeling, I have met so many fitness models who were beautiful on the outside, but ugly, rude, and mean on the inside. And most of these rude, nasty models today are not being booked and have created a negative reputation for themselves in the industry. You see, the camera does not lie. When an outwardly beautiful fitness model is photographed, her bitterness and inner ugliness shine through her shell. You meet some horrible people in my industry, people who are out to get you. But I've also met so many loving, kind, openhearted and sweet fitness models with no motive but to be my friends. They are still a part of my life today and, yes, they are getting work and have super-busy, blessed and abundant careers.

So my advice to you, if you really want to make it in the fitness modeling industry, is to cultivate your inner beauty. Because there is a lot of "young, fit, and pretty" out there, you will and can be replaced easily if you are too hard to work with, have a difficult personality, or are just plain miserable. But when you are both beautiful on the inside and out, you become a powerhouse to be reckoned with!

E IS FOR EXERCISE: The foundation for a top fitness model is exercise! Working out is one of her deepest passions, and she loves to physically, mentally and emotionally challenge herself. She is not afraid of the "guys' side" of the weight room. She loves the feel of iron in her hands, and the sounds of the weights banging around. She's thinking about her next workout almost before she's finished the one she's doing. But one thing's for sure: you've got to allow for some downtime between your workouts. It's very important that you learn how to work out smarter, not harder, to get max results in minimum time.

There's a specific science to working out to get that fitness model body. If you want to get the sleek, sexy, strong look of a fitness model, you won't run for hours on end, or do a bunch of aerobics. That will get you nowhere, fast. Follow my workout plan, outlined for you further on in this book.

And yes, you have to make it fun! Since working out and exercising will become a solid part of your everyday routine, you must learn how to enjoy it. Whether it's working out with a super-positive fitness buddy, or listening to your favorite play list on your iPod, or rewarding yourself with a new hot outfit after you have reached your goal, I will teach you the tricks to making your workout feel like playtime.

L IS FOR LEARN: In this book you will LEARN a lot! Be ready to enjoy new fitness tips, great "JNL-Approved" recipes, how to eat more protein to maintain your muscle tone, and how to really quantum-leap your results. Be ready and willing to learn. An open mind is a very important key to your success.

I IS FOR IMAGINE: For you to truly realize your fitness potential, you must imagine yourself living life right now in your dream body. It's my job as your coach and mentor to awaken the inner athlete lying dormant inside of you, and to help you see and achieve your utmost potential. So have fun dreaming about how your life could be, and will be!

E IS FOR ENERGY: Having the energy to live the life of a top fitness model is extremely important. You must maintain your energy for what is important in your fit life. Planning out your meals, being ready for a photo shoot, preparing for a fitness competition, can all be very demanding. So save your time and energy for things, events, and activities that matter. Cut down on mindless television watching, and forget about wasting time on gossiping or sitting at the bar during happy hour. Instead, focus on getting your workouts in, grocery shopping for your healthy meals, and getting your beauty sleep. Your body will thank you!

V IS FOR VISUALIZE: Look around you. Everything you see started out as a thought! The word for making thoughts into reality is "materialize." In order to make your dreams materialize, you must first visualize them. My weight-loss journey all started with a horrible, unflattering photo of me that kicked my tail into high gear. That is the power of visualization. Seeing myself in that awful photo frustrated me so much that it turned on my inner fitness fire to full throttle. That's when I created my "fitness vision board" — torn-off covers of fitness magazines featuring the world's fittest and most beautiful women. Those positive visuals worked for me! My "Before" photo pushed me away from what I didn't want, while the positive, healthy "After" photos of top fitness models pulled me towards my goals just like magnets.

Try it yourself. Take your "Before" photo now, then choose some "After" photos that show how you'd like to look. This technique works!

E IS FOR EVOLVE: Don't make resolutions; they are too weak! Rather, create your own evolution. Don't resolve, but evolve. Make it your goal to evolve into the real, new, fit you! Enjoy the process of the transformation. Allow your identity to shift from "someone who wants to look like a fitness model" to that of "being a fitness model!" Take on the mindset of a fitness model, and your body will follow. Start living your life as though you are already a fitness model, and you will start your evolution.

CHAPTER 2:

BE BEAUTIFUL FROM THE INSIDE OUT!

"True beauty starts in the inside, from your spirit and soul, and shines through your body by what you say, how you think, how you behave, and through your personality."

—JNL

"A self-esteem issue doesn't change whether you're considered beautiful or not, because it's about what's inside of you."

— IMAN,
CEO, Mega Model turn Mogul, and Actress

"When you possess true beauty, it begins from the inside, and radiates out."

—JNL

"True inner beauty is timeless—standing the test of time."

—JNL

INTRODUCTION: WHY THE JNL FITNESS MODEL DIET TRUMPS ALL!

Let's face it. We all have been on some kind of diet or fitness program before. And yes, we did the exercises, and ate the food, but maybe found ourselves still unsatisfied with the way our bodies looked in the mirror, or how we felt in a bikini, or how our jeans fit and, more importantly, not happy with our fitness level.

Well, this is where my JNL Fitness Model Diet trumps all! With my JNL Fitness Model Diet, you will be able to achieve your fitness goals. If the idea of a lean, toned, fit, athletic, symmetrical and aesthetically-pleasing body appeals to you, then you are reading the right book.

And why does my Fitness Model Diet work? Well, because of its unique, yet simple, balance between cardio and resistance training combined, my fitness formula will give you maximum results in minimum time. When you see results from working out smarter, not harder, you will enjoy the process that much more. And when you see your body transforming into that super-fit, athletic body of a top fitness model, you will stick with it! It will never fail you as your results will have stickability, as muscle has memory. You will enjoy lifelong results that will never diminish.

> *"Don't be bitter; choose to be better! Don't be sour; choose to be sweet! Don't be jaded; choose to be joyful!"*
>
> —JNL

Another major reason why my Fitness Model Diet works is that it is motivating and will boost your confidence. When you are inspired to work out, and are also coached to build your confidence, you will experience fitness results like no other. You will get motivated from my own personal story of weight loss. You will gain more energy, stamina and endurance from your new, sexy, strong and sleek physique and your confidence level will soar to new, fresh, positive heights.

YOUR REAL INNER BEAUTY IS YOUR TRUE PERSONALITY WHICH ALWAYS SHINES THROUGH.

Joy, happiness, love, light, and that inner glow of energy that shines through your personality are what really make you beautiful and memorable. I have met so many fitness models who were beautiful on the outside, but ugly on in the inside. And many of them are not working today, because their true personalities caught up with them. Your true inner beauty shines through when you meet someone, work on a job, are photographed, or even when you are working out in the gym. Other people notice your aura, the real "you" inside, more than your outer shell. And when you have both inner beauty and outer beauty, you are a force to be reckoned with.

I believe that the key reasons why I am still working today as a top fitness model are my character, my friendly personality, and that I have worked hard at protecting, nurturing and cultivating my inner beauty. Real inner beauty matters so much more than we all are led to believe. Your personal energy is projected through interviews, photographs, and in ad campaigns. Everyone picks up on it. I know that this is equally important to your success as is your outer beauty. So ask yourself honestly, "How rich am I in inner beauty?"

JNL'S GUIDE TO CULTIVATING AN UNDENIABLY MAGNETIC INNER GLOW

"Magnetism, or having the 'it' factor can not be bought-as you must create this positive super charged energy which lights up any room you walk into. Follow my steps, and you too will increase your inner glow which radiates out, attracting all things that you desire."

—JNL

At times, life can come at you from all angles and leave you feeling defeated, and it's easy to take a negative attitude. But you must stop yourself in your own tracks when this happens. In order to banish all negativity, you must practice my top tips to cultivating a positive attitude and an inner beauty that projects straight through.

THINK POSITIVE THOUGHTS: Always be in control of your own mind, and catch yourself when you start thinking negatively.

BE GRATEFUL: It's impossible to be depressed or miserable when you are living your life in a constant state of gratitude. When you are grateful for your blessings, you radiate an upbeat aura that is contagious and beautiful. So count your blessings and name them one by one!

LOOK AT YOUR PAST SUCCESSES: If you start feeling down, take a moment to remember your past victories and successes. Sometimes we can't see the forest for the trees, so it's important to take a moment and step back to see just how beautiful we are in our own right. Take time to pat yourself on the back for the accomplishments that you have achieved thus far. This will refuel you, get you recharged and refocused, and ready to stay on your track to success.

TRACK YOUR PROGRESS: Another great way to insure that you keep your inner glow and happiness is to keep track of your progress. How do you ever really know what a success you are and how far you have come, if you don't take stock of your accomplishments? Set aside time every week to revisit your "before" photos. Reflect upon where you were in your life just a short time ago. Look at how far you have come, and imagine just how much further you will go!

PLAN YOUR FUTURE SUCCESSES: Success is not handed to us, but must be worked for and earned. So make time your best friend by using it to plan out your future successes. Make sure you put yourself on your "to do" list, and don't let anyone take you off of it!

KEEP YOURSELF ENGAGED: Beating the blues of life can be easy, if you keep yourself engaged in positive activities. Surround yourself with like-minded people, work out with a favorite fitness buddy, or spend quality time with your loved ones. Sitting alone sulking only makes you feel more miserable. So get up and go, keep yourself moving, and get out of that funk. Life is too short to waste on being bitter.

WRITE IN YOUR JOURNAL: Don't keep your anger and resentments all bottled up. Vent your frustrations in a positive way by writing in your journal. This is a daily practice of mine, and I find that there is something about expressing my feelings by writing them down that is positively therapeutic. When you let go and express yourself, you are much more likely not to fall back on emotional eating. So, when you feel a bit overwhelmed, find a quiet place, grab your journal, and get writing. And always remember to end your journal entry with a positive saying, to reinforce your determination to overcome all of life's challenges and finish on top.

CREATE YOUR FUTURE: Yes, it is true! You can actually be the captain of your own destiny, by being aware and mindful of how your personal choices create certain outcomes. Tell yourself that today will be a great day – that you will get your workout in, that you will eat for optimal health, and that you are in tune with your desires. By aligning your actions with your goals, you will create them, flow though life more smoothly, and achieve your dreams.

DON'T LET ANYONE OR ANYTHING STEAL YOUR INNER JOY FROM YOU: Your joy is yours to enjoy. It's your property, your gift, and you're entitled to have it. Many times there are people, situations or events in our lives that steal our joy. But the funny thing is that sometimes, it is we ourselves who create our own misery, and steal our own joy. When you feel that dark cloud of negativity seeping into your day, scare it away by declaring this positive affirmation. Say it loud and proud:

"My joy is mine! Nobody and nothing will steal my joy away from me! I won't allow even myself to destroy my own joy. I create my own joy in my life – and I am too blessed to be stressed."

By practicing these simple yet profound daily rituals, you will be "growing" your own inner joy that will add so much inner beauty to you! Aim to be a better person, and you will naturally be more beautiful.

Use this space below to write your name, write your signature, and the date to make your personal commitment to cultivating your inner glow, by aiming to practicing these simple yet profound daily rituals.

I ______________________(name) promise myself to stick to this guide to increase the quality of my lifestyle, to grow my inner positive spirit, and to not let anybody or anything steal my joy-including myself.

NAME____

SIGNATURE:____________________________ DATE:________________

THE JNL FITNESS MODEL DIET WILL BRING OUT YOUR INNER GLOW

"Dieting down, exercising obsessively, and eating little to nothing is not going to make you healthy and won't give you the results that you truly desire and deserve. My Fitness Model Diet will give you an undeniable healthy glow, making you seem as if your body jumped off of a major fitness magazine."

—JNL

Have you ever seen anyone lose weight, but look worse than they did before? They may have lost weight, but they also lost precious muscle tone, color in their face and cheeks, and also that little energetic bounce in their step. From dieting, overtraining, and severe deprivation, they became overly thin, frail, and weak. Their faces began to look drawn, turning to a shade close to gray, with dark circles under their eyes.

To me, that is NOT the picture of health. When someone is healthy, you can see it! My JNL Fitness Model Diet will give you that radiating inner glow.

"Strong is the new skinny!"

—JNL

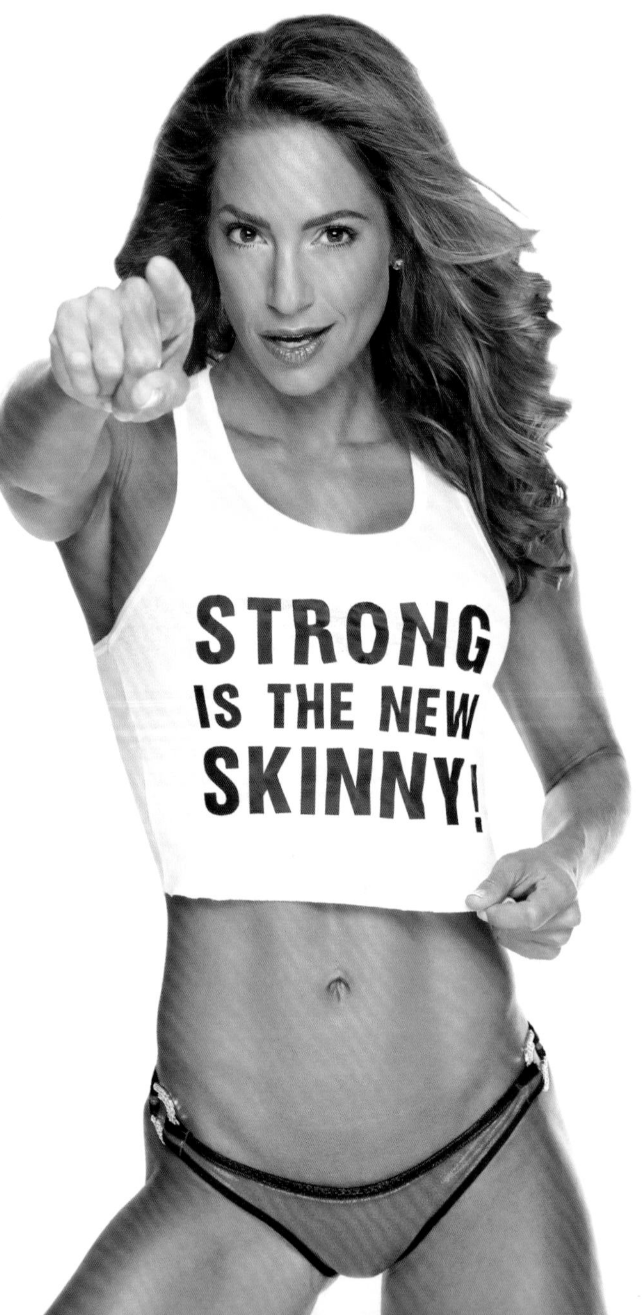

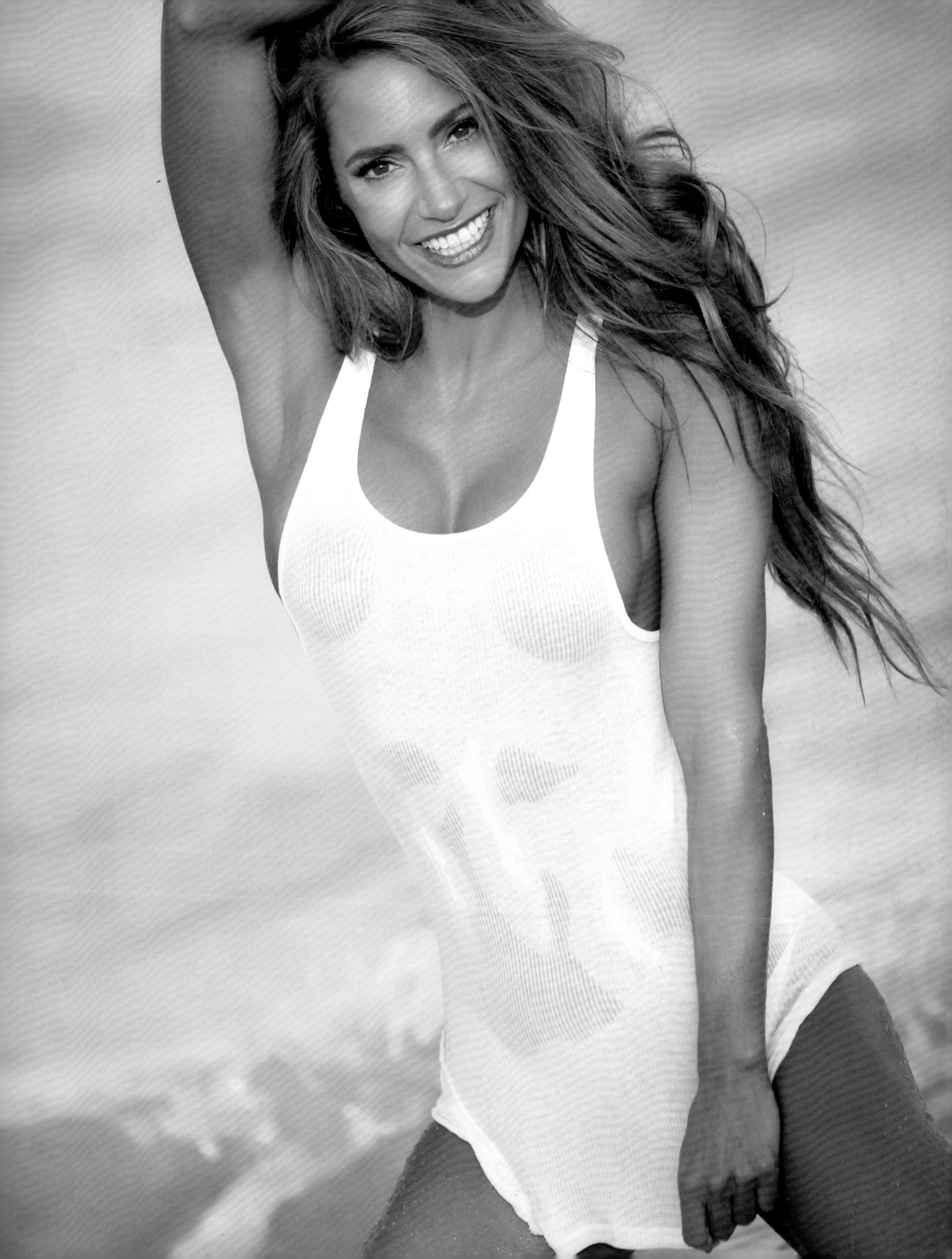

CHAPTER 3:

The JNL Fitness Model Beauty Program

YOUR EXTERNAL BEAUTY GUIDE

"Life is full of beauty. Take the time to notice it, appreciate it and create it."

—JNL

"Beauty comes in all ages, colors, shapes, and forms. God never makes junk."

—KATHY IRELAND,

Living legend Super-Model turned Mega-Mogul and CEO of Kathy Ireland World Wide

WHAT DOES THE JNL FITNESS MODEL DIET BODY LOOK LIKE?

I believe that a healthy body comes in many different body types. Being a size 0, or a "skinny fat person" does not necessarily equate with being healthy. I believe that being strong is not only beautiful, but essential to living a full, robust, fulfilling life worth celebrating.

What are the tale-tell signs of a fitness model physique created by the JNL Fitness Model Diet? Well, what do you see when you look at a top fitness model on the cover of a magazine? The model's abs are tight, her waistline whittled, and her shoulders are perfectly rounded off with muscular mushroom caps. Her teeth are bright white with a smile exuding unbreakable confidence. Her hair is full, healthy and shiny. She stands tall upon solid strong legs with sexy sweeping quads, with impressive "upright" glutes that lead up to a strong, feminine back.

She is poised, polished and statuesque with an athletic, yet feminine, build. Wearing a workout outfit or a bikini, she is the epitome of health, wellness, and fitness. And her image commands respect, as she represents all things healthy. She is a Fitness Model — the picture of strength and beauty that so many women strive to attain.

By following my JNL Fitness Model Diet, you will transform your body into your own version of a fitness model's body! Congratulations, because you hold in your hands your ticket to your very own sexy, strong, sleek and toned physique.

FITNESS MODEL BEAUTY ESSENTIALS

"Super fitness models are not born. They are made. Practice my JNL-approved beauty rituals, and you too can become and or look like a top fitness model."

— JNL

There are certain essential beauty rituals that all Fitness Model do religiously. Whether it's bronzing their skin to the perfect golden glow, whitening their teeth, or working out with weights to create beautiful lines in their body and physique, there's one thing for sure: these are principles and staples of every and all fitness models' beauty routine.

In this chapter you will discover the JNL Fitness Model Beauty Essentials. Here are the tools, tips and techniques that most fitness models rely upon to look and feel their absolute best!

THE FITNESS MODEL PROGRAM TANNING GUIDE

"Don't Bake it! Fake It!"

—JNL

There is an exact science to achieving the perfect golden glow! When I began fitness modeling, I didn't know all the sequential steps that went into achieving that "sun-kissed" skin tone to show off all of the body's lines, symmetry, and feminine muscle tone. You may be asking yourself WHY fake a tan? Well, first of all, when you bake in the tanning bed, you are actually speeding up the aging process, adding years to your skin and face. Far away are the days of the endless hours of sunbathing with no sun block. Welcome to the new era of beautiful, glowing healthy skin!

BENEFITS TO FAKING A TAN, AS OPPOSED TO BAKING A TAN

- Sunbathing and tanning beds pre-age you.
- Skin damage occurs when you bake in the sun and tanning beds.
- You can actually "tan off" about 5 good pounds! All fitness models and those in the fitness industry rely upon this trade secret. They know that the body looks leaner and more toned with a darker skin color.
- Your teeth appear whiter when you fake a tan.
- Your skin appears blemish-free when you are tanned, thus smoothing out acne, discolorations, stretch marks and the appearance of cellulite.

There's no doubt that faking a tan makes you feel thinner, sexier and healthier, and will help you look more like a Fitness Model. These days, baking in the sun is increasingly unpopular as more women realize the sun's UV rays age skin faster than anything (not to mention increasing your chance of developing the deadliest form of skin cancer, melanoma).

If you're ready to skip laying out but don't want to give up radiant glowing skin, self-tanners are a fitness model's best friend. Self-tanners can darken skin for up to a week, thanks to dihydroxyacetone, or DHA, the magical ingredient!

LIST OF FITNESS MODEL TANNING TOOLS YOU NEED

- Exfoliating gloves
- Shaving essentials (shaving cream and razors)
- "Tanning" Pajamas (black, long sleeved and long pants)
- "Tanning" bed sheets (that you can stain and not worry about it)

Two things you must do before you tan:

- Exfoliate your entire body and face.
- Shave and/or wax your legs, underarms, and your bikini line.

JNL FIT TIP:

First of all, in order to truly have beautiful skin, you must honor it and cherish it by property hydrating it both from the inside out by drinking lots of water, and also from the outside in, by moisturizing it daily with lotion. It's your largest organ, so go out of your way to show it some love with lots of water and lotion.

JNL'S TIPS FOR SELF-TANNING YOUR FACE AND BODY:

FITNESS MODEL™ TIP #1:

SAFETY FIRST! Forgo the Beds, and Go to a Tanning Salon for a Professional Application

If you want a goof-free, professionally applied tan, and have the budget to afford it, head to a spa or salon. For upwards of $60.00, you can get one of many options: Full body exfoliation and professional application of self-tanner, airbrush bronzing (where an aesthetician sprays a fine mist of tanner over your entire body), or your least expensive option, spray tanning. You can step into a booth and get sprayed on all sides for around $20.00 a session. Check out Boca Tanning, Hollywood Tans and Mystic Tans, three popular spray-tan chains.

FITNESS MODEL™ TIP #2:

TANNING OF THE FACE (How to NOT Look Like a Freak!)

This is a four-step process. Pull hair up in a ponytail before you start so you don't miss any parts.

STEP ONE: Prep skin by gently cleansing and exfoliating. Skip moisturizer, which may interfere with the tanner. Again, apply no creams on the face.

STEP TWO: Apply under-eye cream. According to major make up artists, you want the color of your skin to be lighter under the eyes; it makes you look younger.

STEP THREE: Blend a few drops of self-tanner and equal parts moisturizer in the palm of your hand then apply over face and neck. You only want to go one shade darker than your natural color.

STEP FOUR: Let color develop for three hours then follow up with a sweep of bronzer on forehead, cheeks and nose areas where the sun naturally shines.

Don't forget: Smooth remaining tanner over earlobes and upper ears. You don't want white ears and a dark face! Wash hands thoroughly and most importantly, don't skip the sunscreen! You don't want to bake it, just fake it!

FITNESS MODEL™ TIP #3:

HOW TO SELF-TAN YOUR BODY

I have simplified this tasking procedure into a simple four step process.

1. Start by exfoliating skin with a body scrub in the shower, paying special attention to rough areas including knees and elbows (dry skin absorbs higher concentrations of tanner). Shave before you tan!
2. Rub Vaseline on cuticles and nails. This protects your manicure and keeps fingertips and nails from staining. Or even better, you can use latex surgical gloves that you can find at your local pharmacy to stain-proof your hands.
3. Apply tanner starting with your legs. Apply over the shin and calf, sweeping tanner down over your ankle, foot and toes. Then apply tanner to your thigh from front to back, using the excess to cover your knee; repeat on your other leg.
4. For the final step, apply tanner to your hips, stomach and torso, following with your shoulders and arms. Wait 10 minutes to dry before dressing and avoid any excessive activity that will make you sweat for at least a few hours. If your tan hasn't set, sweat could cause streaking.

FITNESS MODEL™ TIP #4:

PICK THE RIGHT TANNER

There are several types of tanners: Tanners created just for the face, airbrush tanners, cream tans, bronzing gel, tinted tans and tan enhancers. There's body shimmer and bronzing powder. You can layer tanners as colors fade. How? Apply a lotion, then follow with bronzing powder or shimmer; just be careful not to go too dark.

Here is a list of my TOP Self Tanners:

- Jan Tana On Stage Competition Color
- Jan Tana Fast Tan-Use this if you need a fast, natural-looking immediate tan
- Jergen's Natural Glow Face Daily Moisturizer
- Jergen's Natural Glow Express — it's a body moisturizer as well!

JNL FIT TIP:

To laser or not to laser — that is the question

I WAS SOLD! Moving from waxing to laser was the best thing I did for my underarm and bikini line area. I would always get in-grown hairs in these delicate areas. Secondly, I would have to make frequent visits, as the hair would grow back FAST! Laser is JNL-approved because of the following reasons:

• Less visits due to hair not growing back as fast
• No more ingrown hairs-Yahoo!
• Softer skin because it will not need to recover from hot wax or painful yanking out of hair in the delicate areas.

If you do get laser, numbing gel is a MUST! Purchase a small tube from your med-spa, and ask your aesthetician to apply it to your bikini area before your laser treatment. Even though I love my laser treatments, you can't get them on your lip or brows. Choose waxing instead for these delicate facial areas.

FITNESS MODEL™ TIP #5:

HELP! I MESSED UP MY SELF TAN!

Don't fret if your tan ended up being streaky. It happens to the best of us, especially on our first few tries. You can fix this by exfoliating to even the color out. If you are not happy with the depth of the color, and need to be a bit darker, then re-apply the tanning solution, allowing yourself enough time for the color to show.

JNL TANNING TIP

A big obstacle for me was to not wash off the tanning solution from the top of my hands, while also not getting it onto my palms. I suggest you use an old wet towel. Again, I highly recommend simply wearing latex surgical gloves, and then blotting the tops of your hands at the end.

To top off your newly sun-kissed tan, give arms, legs and décolletage a subtle glow with a body shimmer.

We can accentuate our abs by contouring the abdominal muscles with our tanning solution. Get in front of your bathroom mirror and study your mid-section. If you need to do a few crunches before, so you can better see where your ab lines are, then do so. Then take some tanner on your finger (wearing a surgical glove) and "draw" on the shadows of your abdominal muscles. Let these contour lines dry a bit. Last step is to apply a light top coat to your entire midsection. Voilà–Instant Abs!

If you have any more questions, please feel free to take advantage of my super informative Audio Seminar entitled *"Don't Bake it, Fake It! Learn How to Achieve that Sexy Golden Bronze Glow Without the Harmful and Aging Side Effects of the Tanning Bed or Sun."* It's instantly downloadable and can be accessed at www.SHOPJNL.com under my *Audio Seminar* Section. So go visit www.SHOPJNL.com, and listen and learn!

THE FITNESS MODEL PROGRAM TEETH WHITENING GUIDE

"Let your inner goddess shine through your smile"

—JNL

"There is one physical feature that instantly makes someone more attractive when they use it-their smile!"

—JNL

"The eyes may be the windows to the soul, but the smile is the soul's door."

—JNL

I have learned many things from my fitness modeling experiences, but among the most important is the power of a smile. A smile is the number one feature that makes people attractive. It's like a door to your soul! Your smile's doormat can instantly say "WELCOME," or "GO AWAY;" it's all in how you use it. A smile is what makes someone approachable. And those with great smiles radiate warmth that draws others to them instantly, Your smile can tell others that you truly love your life, by radiating that energy. A to-die-for smile can light up a room, win you friends instantly, and also land you a big fitness modeling job. One main quality that all fitness models share is a killer smile worthy to grace a top fitness magazine cover.

When I prepare for a magazine cover photo shoot, it's my job to look like a million bucks. And yes, the clothes, shoes, and your body all help in the production. But that million-dollar look can only be found in something you already have – your smile.

So here is my top fitness model guide to getting your grill to look like a million-dollar smile!

At first thought, teeth whitening may not seem that important in the overall scheme of looking like a fitness model. But when you really think about it, all the top fitness models and cover girls have one feature in common: bright white smiles. To get your teeth looking their best, there are several methods you can consider to whiten and brighten them.

In selecting the method best for you, there are two major options to choose between:

- Over-the-counter Methods (or OTC for short)
- Professionally-done whitening treatments performed by a Dentist or Dental Assistant

OVER-THE-COUNTER:

Girls, if you are on a budget, this is your best bet for teeth whitening. The store bought whitening package includes a bleaching gel with a low concentrate. The teeth trays are one size fits all, or are paint-on gels or whitening strips. The cost is very low compared to what you will have to pay at your dentist office.

Cost: $20.00 to $100.00.

MY FAVORITE OVER-THE-COUNTER TAKE-HOME KIT: My all time favorite choice is the Crest WhiteStrips. They are tried and true! I give them a 10 out of 10 because they really make my teeth white and are easy to use. Plus they are so inexpensive!

JNL TIP FOR APPLYING CREST WHITE-STRIPS®: Many have complained that they can't get the strips to stick. But if you follow these simply rules, it will be a cinch! Brush your teeth, and floss. Be sure to dry the front of your teeth. A hand towel works well. Apply the strip to your top teeth first. Then move to the bottom. Lay down and relax. Don't talk because you will move the strips from their place.

DENTIST'S OFFICE VISITS

There are many benefits to in-office whitening. In-office whitening ensures significant, fast results. The tech or dentist (while carefully avoiding the gum area), applies the peroxide solution. Typically it stays on for about an hour, but it is checked every fifteen minutes. If the stains are severe, you might need multiple treatments. For maintenance, use an at-home whitener periodically.

JNL FAVORITE IN-OFFICE TEETH WHITENING METHOD: BRITESMILE:
The Britesmile advertisements got me really interested in brightening up my smile. This was the beginning of my teeth whitening love affair! At first, I was happy with the end result as I truly saw my stains disappear. The whiteness of my teeth got about 5-6 shades lighter. It can be expensive, but it was well worth it. Some others who have tried it complain of pain or sensitivity. I experienced only slight discomfort after my treatment, which quickly subsided. And here is a JNL tip – eat foods free of artificial coloring for about a week after the procedure.

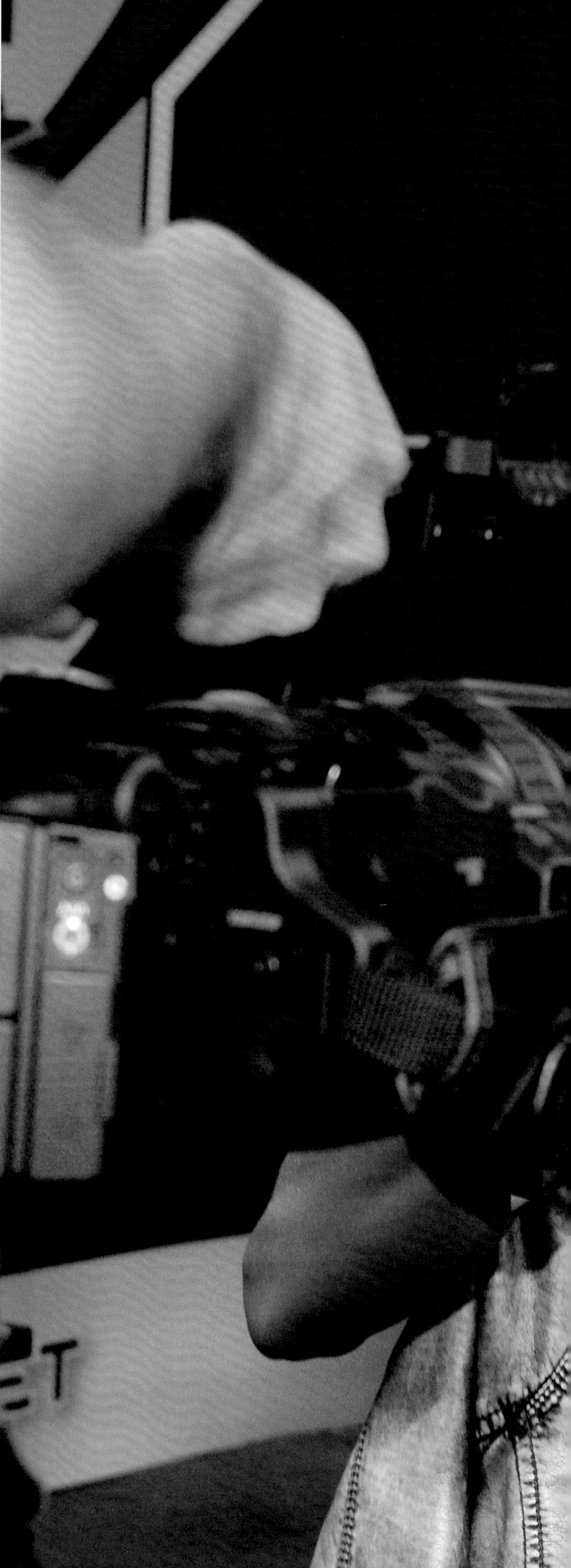

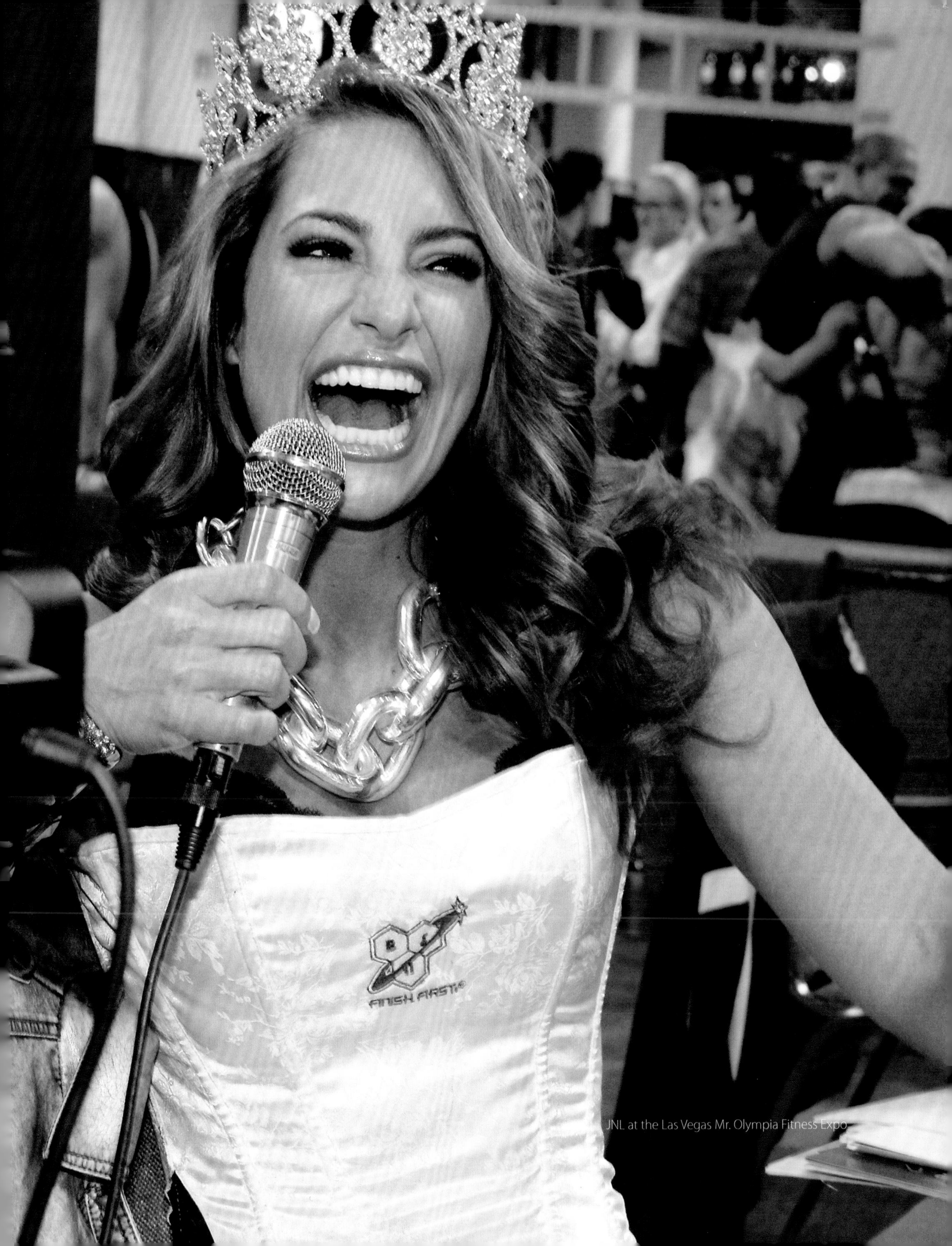

JNL at the Las Vegas Mr. Olympia Fitness Expo

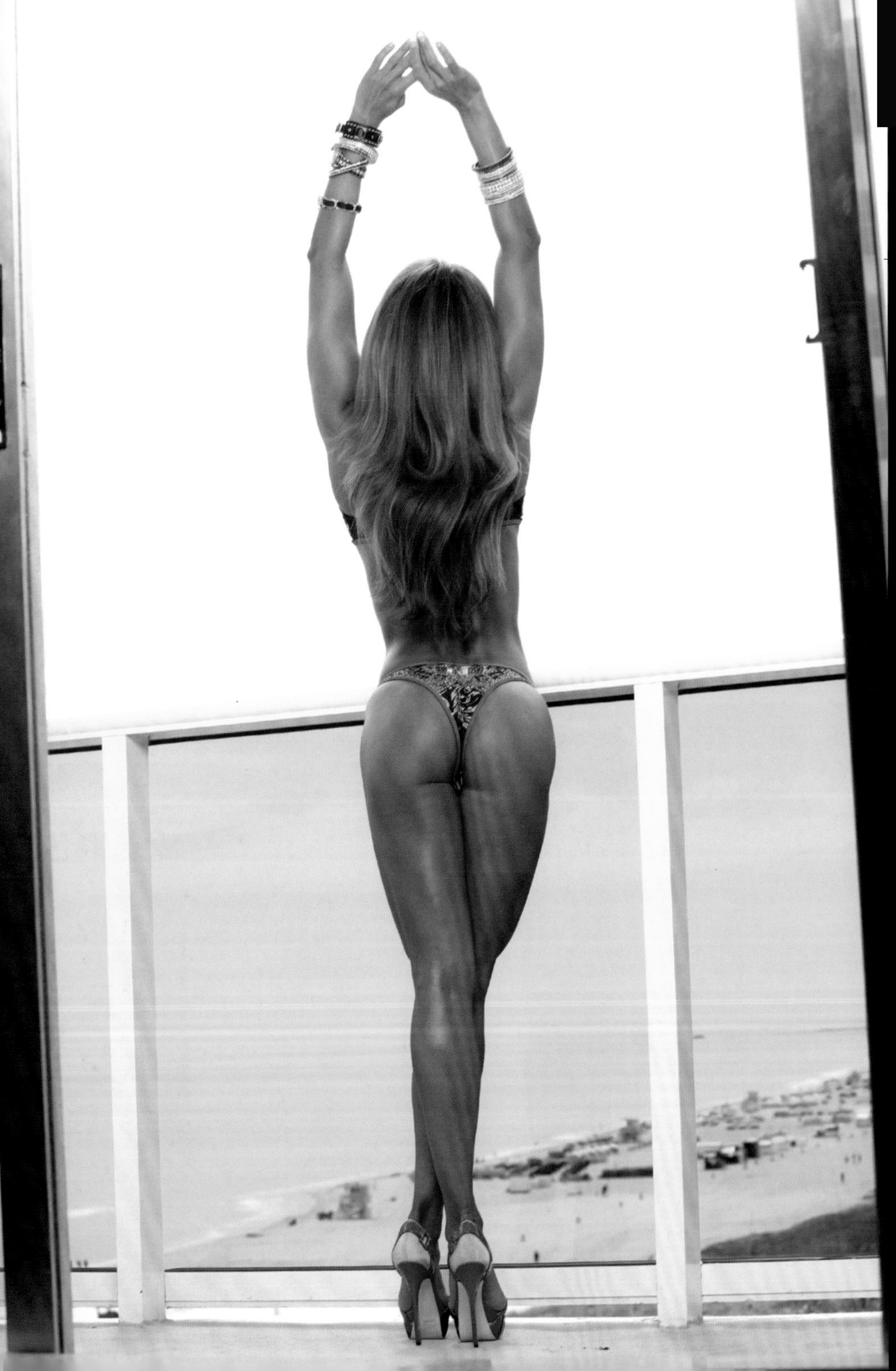

THE FITNESS MODEL PROGRAM CELLULITE/ STRETCH MARKS SOLUTIONS GUIDE

"Outsmarting Mother Nature never felt so good."

—JNL

How do Fitness Models have that cellulite-free skin around their abs, butt, hips and thighs? Well, from my own personal experience and hours of research, I have found a system of getting rid of cellulite that works. I would love to share a personal story with you.

I had been dieting down for a competition, and I was 2 weeks out. I was practicing my posing in my competition suit, and had my friend take some photos of me, so I could see how I looked. To my surprise, I saw that I had extensive cellulite all over the back of my butt, glutes, hamstrings, thighs and the sides of my legs. How could this be? I was dieting down, eating little to no carbs, and working out twice a day – and I still had cellulite. I was infuriated! I felt as if I had been bamboozled and I was desperate to do whatever it would take to banish those ugly little orange-peel dimples from my lower body.

So my search began. I asked all of my fellow fitness experts, beauticians, and even med-spas if they had any advice, tools, techniques, creams or lotions that would smooth out my dimples. And I found the "IT" machine that works! If there is ONE word that you need to know about fighting and winning the war on those darn fat dimples, it's this word right here: ENDERMOLOGIE!

WHAT IS ENDERMOLOGIE?

Endermologie is the painless med-spa procedure that actually breaks down fat cells, allowing fat to be flushed out of your system, thus smoothing out the appearance of cellulite and banishing it for good. In addition, it's been scientifically proven to be as much as 200% more effective than a manual massage for releasing built-up toxins and lactic acid. Many top athletes and sports competitors use endermologie to help "suck out" the built-up lactic acid in their muscles and relieve the soreness in their bodies.

By way of background, the Endermologie machine was created overseas in the early '70s to help "break up" the skin adhesions of severe burn victims. The skin-sucking rollers would roll over the burn scars, helping to smooth them out. By serendipity, the burn patients experienced body contouring as they lost inches, shrunk in size, had less body fat, and shapelier bodies, all due to Endermologie.

I urge all of you to Google med-spas in your area to see which ones offer Endermologie. Be wise and do your homework, because on one side of town you will be charged $90.00-$100.00 per session but in other spas you can get the same procedure done for $40.00-$50.00 per session!

To get more in-depth information on what causes cellulite, along with specific techniques that you can expect in an Endermologie session, please visit www.SHOPJNL.com here to listen to my Instant Audio Download Seminar on "Hollywood's Best Kept Anti-Cellulite Secret: Everyone's Doing it and No One's Talking About It". Log on, listen, learn, and lose that stubborn cellulite!

THE FITNESS MODEL PROGRAM SKIN CARE GUIDE

"Think of your skin as gift-wrapping that covers your true gifts inside. You must protect it, so what's inside is also protected. It's the largest organ of your body so always give it the utmost TLC."

—JNL

Why do Fitness Models have skin that is so healthy and glowing? Because they don't drink, don't smoke, and don't tan in the beds. Just like my mom said: "abstaining" works! Alcohol, cigarettes, and too much sun will make you look old fast. Don't let those aging free radicals run around in your skin.

When I started modeling, I thought that washing my face with a bar of soap and a wash cloth was "skin care"! As I blossomed into a mother, a fitness model, and also entered into my 30's, I learned so much more about real skin care, and just how important it is!

SO, WHAT'S YOUR TYPE? DECIPHERING YOUR SKIN TYPE AND THE BEST WAY TO CARE FOR IT

This list will help you determine your own skin type:

COMBINATION: The most typical skin type: T-Zone is oily with remainder of face dry.

OILY: Oil slick skin, always shiny or you may appear to be sweating oil from your large pores.

DRY: When your skin feels parched, or like a desert. Could be flaky as well with a tight feel to it.

NORMAL: If you have normal skin – CONGRATS! Skin tone is even, and oil production is regular.

SENSITIVE: Very volatile. Anything seems to make you break out. Also blotchy.

JNL's 4-Step Skin Care Routine	COMBINATION ("I have an oily T-Zone and desert-like cheeks—Help!")	OILY ("I'm an oil slick – always shiny")	DRY ("My skin is a desert!")	NORMAL ("Wow, I'm lucky")	SENSITIVE ("Don't touch me, I'm delicate")
CLEAN	Fragrance-free cleanser	Soap-free gel cleanser	Cream cleanser	Anti-blemish foam cleanser	Fragrance-free cleanser
TONE	Balancing toner	Light astringent	Nutrient-rich spray tonic	Blend of rose petal water and witch hazel	Alcohol-free toner
MOISTURIZE	Daily oil-free lotion	Oil-free shine control	Liquid serum	Moisturizing gel	Fragrance-free, paraben-free moisturizer
PROTECT	Moisturizing gel with spf 20+	Oil-free light-weight cream with spf 20+	Time-release hydrating moisturizer with spf 20+	Oil-free, paraben-free cream with spf 20+	Fragrance-free, paraben-free lotion with spf 20+

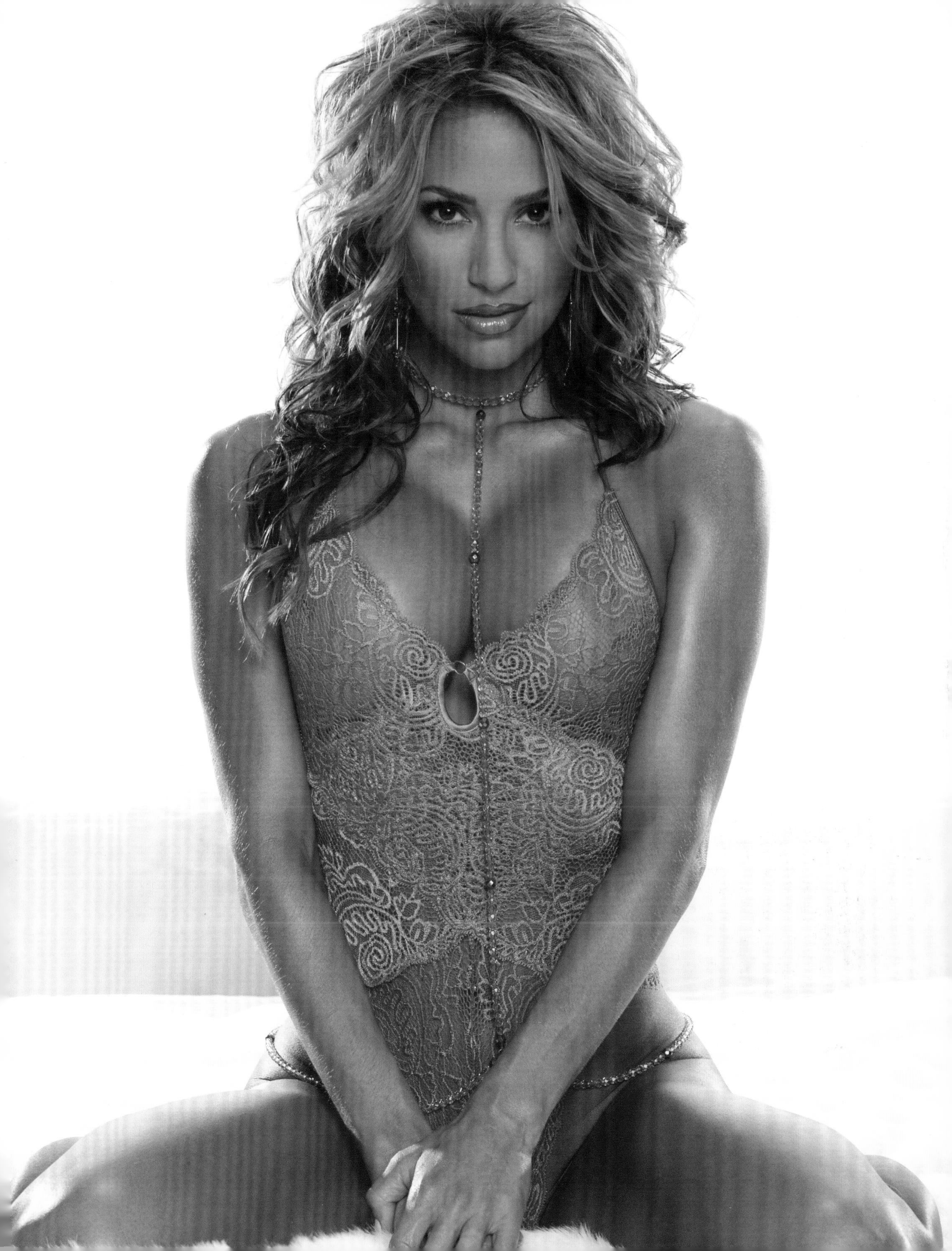

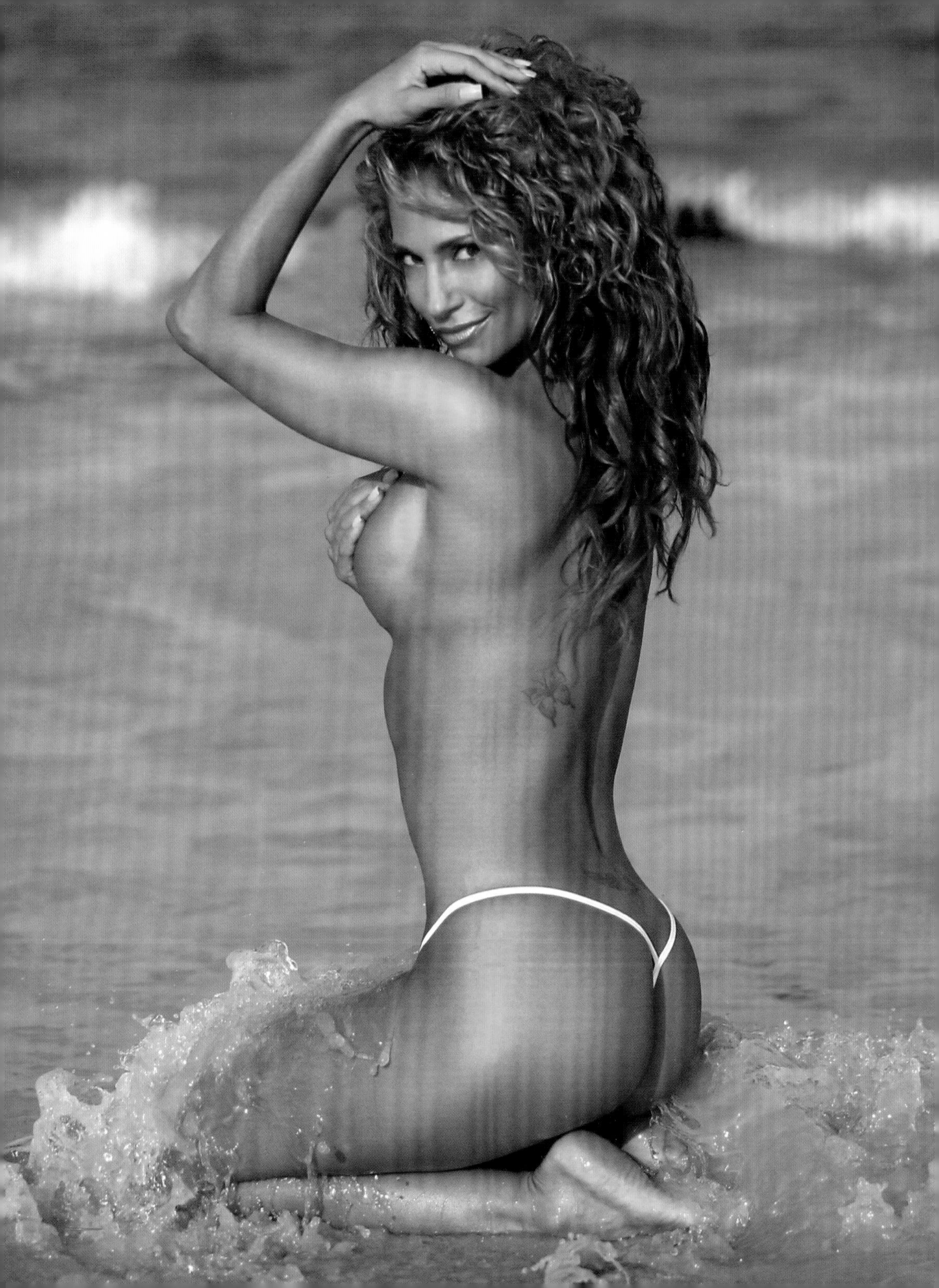

THE FITNESS MODEL FIVE-STEP SKIN CARE SYSTEM

"Beautiful skin doesn't happen by accident. Skin care is a complete science, a step by step process, which one must respect and perform daily to reap the benefits."

—JNL

CLEANSE • EXFOLIATE • TONE • MOISTURIZE • OCCASIONAL FACIALS

1. **CLEANSE:** Cleansing is the foundation of healthy, glowing skin. Make sure that you use an alcohol-free, gentle cleanser that cleanses your skin without stripping it of its natural oils, and is not too harsh.

2. **EXFOLIATE:** This is necessary, but not every day! Aim to use a gentle cleansing paste called gommage, rather than an abrasive cloth, sandy cream, or anything that has those little grains of grit in it. . They do more irritating then exfoliating. My top picks are Yonka's Gommage, and also Chanel's Gommage.

3. **TONE:** Toning is essential! Stay away from strong astringents, but rather select a mild "skin bracer" or "freshener". These are the mildest form of toners; they contain virtually no alcohol, water, and a humectant such as glycerin. Humectants help to keep the moisture in the upper layers of the epidermis by preventing it from evaporating. A popular example of this is rosewater. These toners are the kindest to skin, and are most suitable for use on dry, dehydrated, sensitive and normal skins. My top picks are from the Yonka line.

4. **MOISTURIZE:** This is THE most important part of skin care! Moisturize, moisturize, moisturize! Your aim is to have dewy, "come and touch me" skin that is kissable and irresistible. Forget the days of matte, non-humid looking skin. Your skin needs to look moist and luscious! And use a moisturizer that has an SPF of at least 15.

5. **FACIALS:** This is necessary pampering. The wonders a facial can do for you! Every woman deserves a facial, whether it's once every 6 months or once every 2 weeks. Put yourself back on your to-do list, and your skin will thank you. And don't feel pressured to purchase all the product line your aesthetician will present to you. If you invest in a great cleanser, toner, and a moisturizer with sun block in it, you'll have all you need.

THE FITNESS MODEL PROGRAM HAIR CARE GUIDE

"How can people truly control their entire lives, if they can't even get control over their hair?"

—JNL

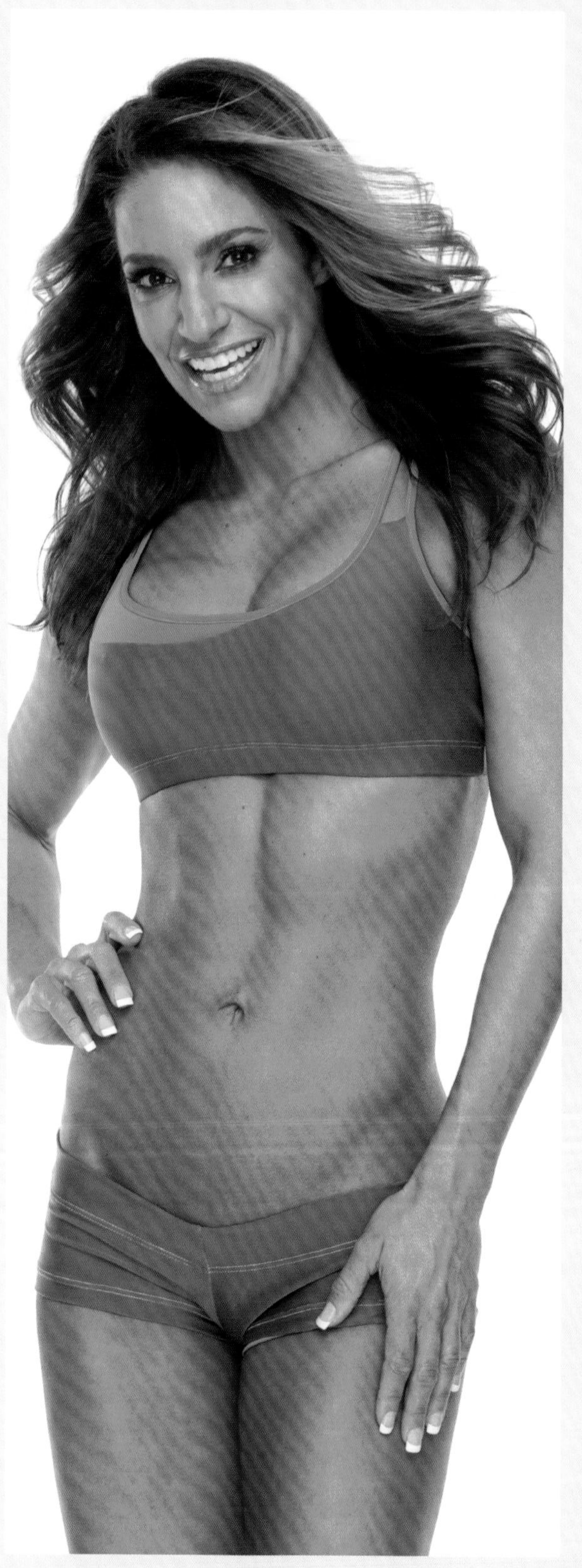

To become a fitness model, or even just look like one, you must radiate the true vision of health, from the top of your head, to the tips of your toes. Therefore, your tresses must be in tip-top shape! Growing long, healthy, lustrous, and brilliantly shining hair requires a combination of proper eating, supplementing your diet with healthy oils, and top-of-the-line hair care products.

What you eat, your supplements, and your deep-conditioning treatments all contribute to how great or not-so-great your hair looks.

PICK THE RIGHT HAIRSTYLE: If your eyes are the window to your soul, your hair is then the frame! So make sure you use your hairstyle to showcase your most stunning features. Find an excellent hair stylist and trust their expert opinion on which cut works best for you.

PICK THE RIGHT PRODUCTS: This is really trial and error! I have used the most expensive products, only to find that sometimes the less-expensive ones at my local drug store work just as well, or better. This is where the fun begins, and I urge you to explore and get creative with products.

ONE RULE: Make sure that you deep-condition, and all other details of your hair will fall into place!

JNL FIT TIP:

Once a week I enjoy an at-home deep conditioning treatment that I actually leave in my hair overnight. First, I wash and gently condition my hair. Then I towel it dry, flip my hair over the bathtub, take a handful of organic, unrefined, virgin coconut oil, and massage it into all of my hair and scalp. I then twist it up into a bun on the top of my head and wrap it with a warm towel, allowing the towel to soak up the excess oil. I either leave the towel on, or wear a small shower cap on my hair all night, so as not to get my pillow oily. When I wake up the next morning, I wash, condition and enjoy super-soft, lustrous hair!

If you want to know other really great fitness model uses for coconut oil, visit www.SHOPJNL.com and download my Audio Seminar on Coconut Oil. In this audio download, you will find out more about this miracle oil that not only makes your hair its healthiest best, but even helps you to lose weight faster.

"Your hair is your 'crowning glory,' and tells the entire world if you truly are healthy."

—JNL

PERKS OF LIVING A FITNESS MODEL™ LIFESTYLE THAT BENEFIT YOUR HAIR

A high-protein and good-for-you-fat food plan is key to the quality and health of your hair.

BASIC FITNESS MODEL™ HAIR DO'S AND DON'TS!

DO: Eat a diet high in good-for-you fats, such as olive oil, coconut oil, flax seed oil, as well as those found in unsalted raw nuts.

DON'T: Diet so stringently that your hair is robbed of essential nutrients. A diet too low in fat can make your hair look dull or lifeless.

DO: Enjoy weekly at-home deep conditioning treatments. Slather on a high-quality deep conditioning treatment, then wrap up your hair with a hot towel, fresh from the dryer.

DO: Rinse your hair with cold water to close the hair shaft, to protect the hair strand and also to make the hair look shinier!

DON'T: Use super hot water to rinse your hair, as it can actually damage your hair's cuticle.

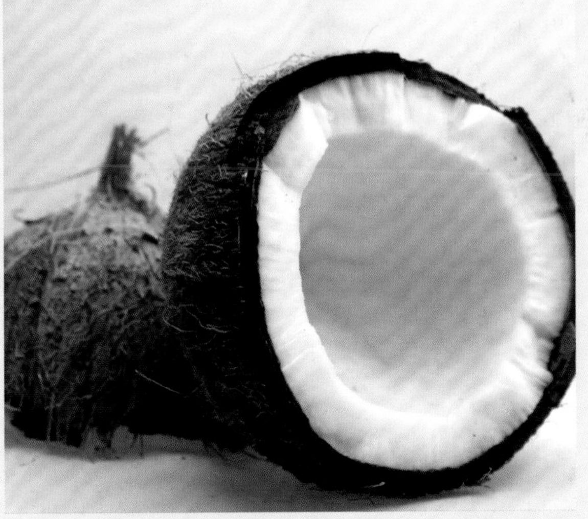

THE JNL FITNESS MODEL™ PROGRAM MAKEUP GUIDE

"Glowing skin, peachy rosy-pink cheeks, flawless complexion, long butterfly lashes, piercing eyes that radiate life, and luscious shiny lips: These are all trademarks of that super-woman, Fitness Model Look!"

—JNL

"I know how to use makeup for a healthy-looking glow, because a real one isn't that healthy."

—CHRISTIE BRINKLEY,
Super Model, International Icon, and past Sports Illustrated Cover Girl

SKIN: Skin is sun-drenched, brushed lightly with bronzers, which give you the look of being radiantly sun-bathed. Choose a foundation as close to your new tan color as possible, blending from the neck up, so as not to allow your neck and face to be two different colors. Use a foundation sponge to gently blend the foundation evenly onto your skin.

CHEEKS: Are neutral toned, and appear dewy if touched. Forgo the matte or heavy color, as your skin needs to breath through the makeup, allowing the shimmery color to enhance, and not detract from, your complexion.

EYES: Some women mistake every day for Halloween. Have you ever seen women who could be mistaken for Cruella DeVille, or Elvira? As the saying goes, your eyes are the windows to your soul — so don't use a heavy hand with the black eyeliner, as it will give you an aged, rather than youthful, look. Raccoon eyes are a big no-no, unless you're a raccoon.

EYEBROWS: Eyebrows are the key to a groomed look. They frame your eyes, and are one feature to which you should always be especially attentive. Make sure not to over-pluck your natural brow shape. Rather, under-tweeze to be on the safe side. If you need to fill in empty spaces, use an eyebrow pencil or shadow with an eyebrow brush.

LIPS: Do not mistake your brown eyeliner for your lip liner! Lips need to be natural, exfoliated, moisturized, and pleasantly plump. There is no real need for injectables, such as Restylane. You can get the same effect with an over-the-counter lip plumper. Two of my favorites are Freeze 24/7 and LipInjection.

NECK: Always use a skin-firming lotion religiously in this area! Prevention of aging of the neck should be an essential part of every woman's beauty program. As the old adage tells us, there are two areas that reveal a woman's age – her neck and her hands. Whether you use a major skin care line's neck-firming cream, or an inexpensive over–the-counter skin-firming cream, it does not matter. Make sure to start application from the back of your neck forward — do not aggressively stroke, but simply pat it on.

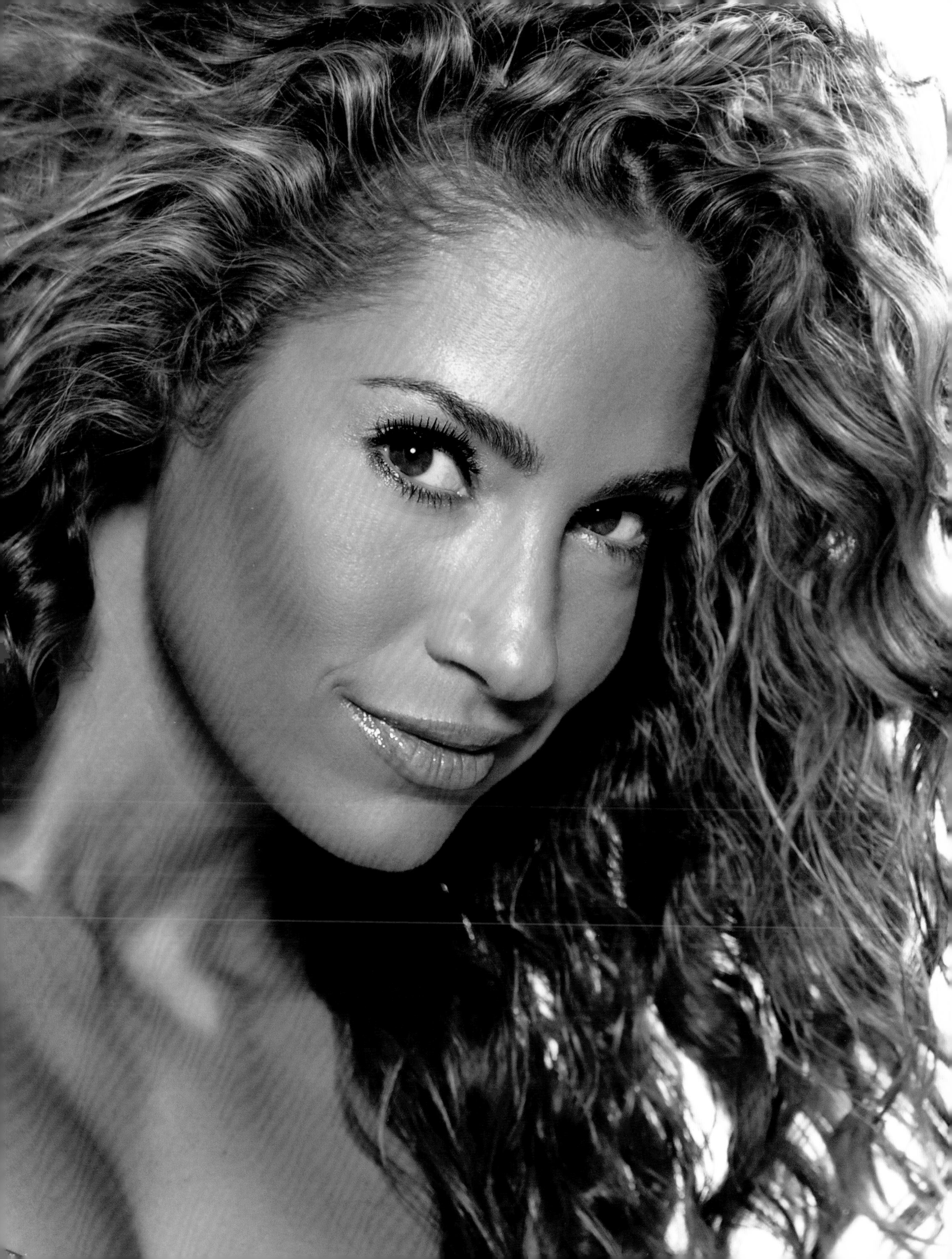

BASIC JNL FITNESS MODEL MAKEUP DO'S AND DON'TS!

DO match your foundation to your neck and to the rest of your body.

DON'T do what many other fitness models do, and walk around with a super-light face and dark body! The camera picks this up mercilessly, so if you are planning a photo shoot, make sure to hire a professional makeup artist to match your skin tones.

DO go light! Remember, less is more! And save heavier makeup for the evening when you're heading out to a big event.

DON'T overdo it or have what I call a "heavy hand" when it comes to applying makeup. You don't want to look like a "drag queen" with heavy black false eyelashes that stick out an inch off your face, "Twisted Sister" blush, or too-big swollen fish lips!

DO learn from classic beauties! For a good example, look at Mariah Carey, who always looks so fresh and put-together.

DON'T follow every trend that you see. Remember ice blue eye shadow? Or the dark lip liner that was filled in with a lighter lipstick shade? No need to say more!

DO take advantage of the free makeup lessons often offered at your local department stores, or even at free-standing MAC stores.

DON'T leave yourself in the dark when it comes to applying makeup! I have been at photo shoots where even the hired, so-called "makeup artist" made me look like Jennifer Lopez from the early 90's! YIKES! I just washed my face (thank goodness I had brought my own makeup case!) and did my own makeup. Me taking action saved the shoot, and also saved me from looking like a bad flashback from the past!

"Never buy your skin care essentials in a hardware store."

—JNL

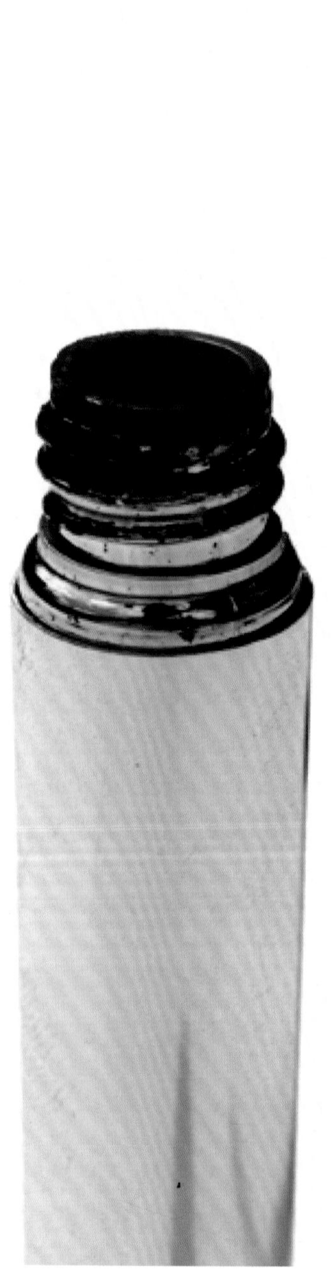

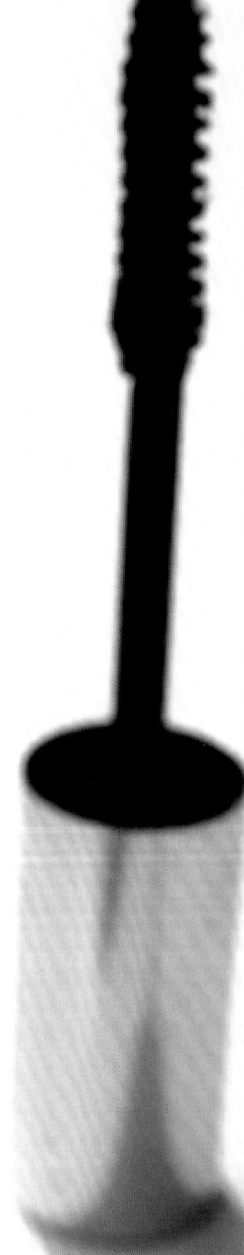

JNL'S ULTIMATE BEAUTY PRODUCT LIST

Many of you email me asking me what my ultimate favorite products for my face, body, and hair are. Here it all is, in one complete, concise list:

FACE:

- Yonka Cleansing Milk Lait Nettoyant — Gentle, everyday cleanser
- Yonka Cleanser Gel Nettoyant All Skin Types — for a more "squeaky" clean!
- Yonka Purifying Antiseptic without Alcohol Juvenile — to clean and disinfect the skin and eliminate bacteria and dirt that could cause blemishes
- Yonka Lotion Toner — alcohol-free toner for normal to oily skin with botanical essential oils
- Elastine Jour — hydrating cream for day
- Elastine Nuit — hydrating cream for night
- Emulsion Pure — Purifying Emulsion with Botanical Essential Oils
- Crème PS — for dry Skin
- Gommage — soft, clarifying gel peel with botanical extracts. Use 303 or 305, depending upon your skin type
- SkinCeuticals Phyto Corrective Gel — complexion-calming gel

BODY:

- Body Excellence Cream by Chanel: Ultra Firming Cream
- Jergen's Skin Firming
- Jergen's Ultra Nourishing Cream
- Nivea Body Good-Bye Cellulite Lotion
- Clarins Total Body Lift for Stubborn Cellulite Control
- Clarins Super Restorative Redefining Body Care
- Palmer's Cocoa Butter
- Nivea Smooth Sensation Daily Lotion for Dry Skin
- Nivea Body Good-Bye Cellulite Patches

HAIR:

For Curly Looks:

- KMS California Line
- KMS Curlup-Bounce Back Spray
- KMS Curlup Curling Balm
- KMS Curlup Control Creme

For Straight Looks:

- Paul Mitchell Skinny Serum
- Deep Conditioning-Organic Virgin Unrefined Coconut Oil
- Kerastase Hair Mask

To Make Curly Hair Straight:

- Paul Mitchell Skinny Serum

JNL FIT SLEEP — THE ULTIMATE GUIDE TO A SUPER FITNESS MODEL'S BEAUTY SLEEP

"What helps me to be better, not bitter; joyful, not jaded; sweet, not sour?

My beauty sleep!"

—JNL

"There is nothing in the world that can replace good old fashioned beauty sleep!"

—JNL

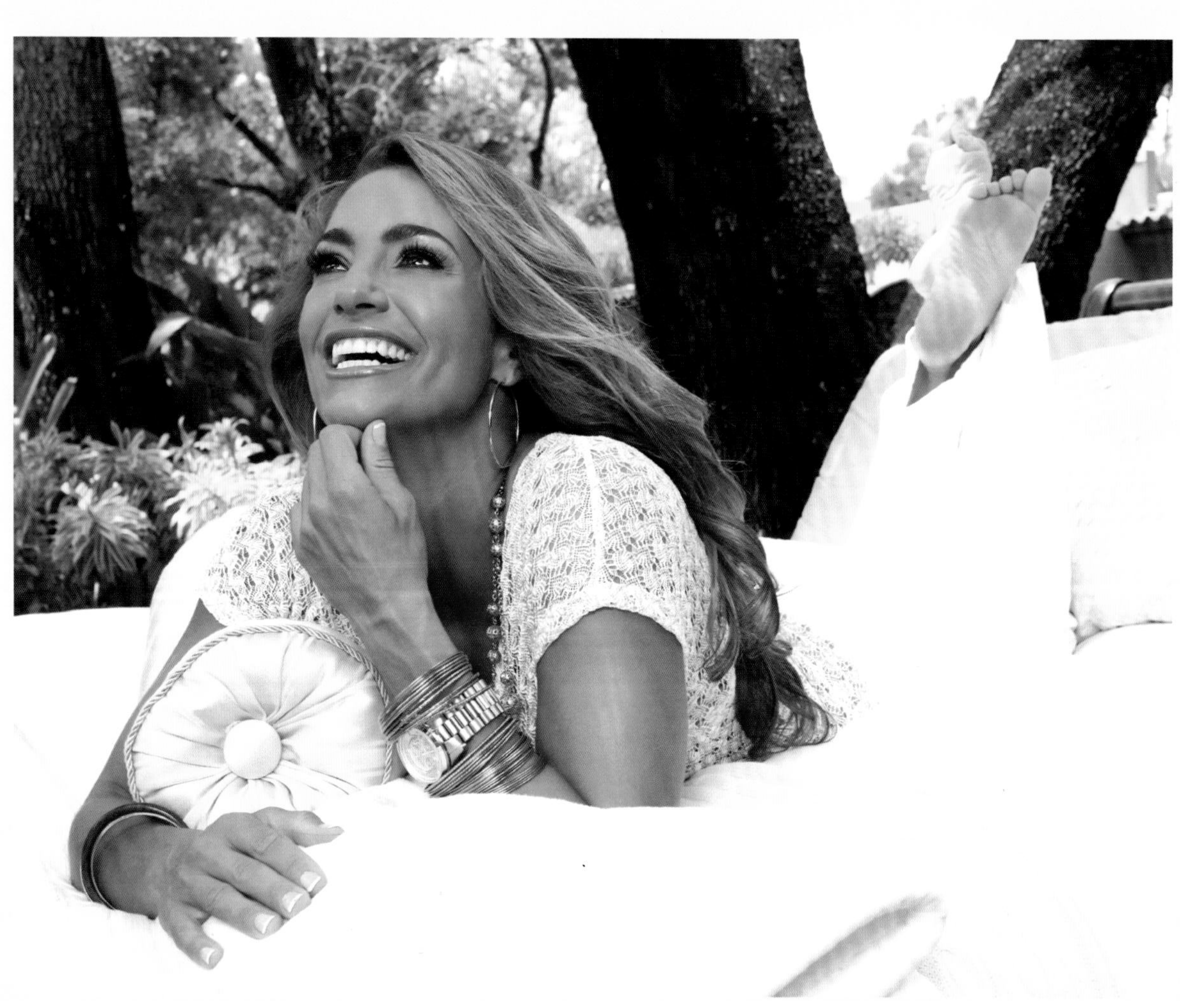

Beauty sleep is an essential part of the Fitness Model lifestyle! You must sleep good to look good and feel good! And you can't skimp out on it for too long, before your body starts to feel it. I make it a point to get a good solid 8 hours of sleep a night. And having the right bedding, sheets, pillows, comforters and mattress covers make ALL the difference!

In my "younger" days, I was able to go out all night, and really sacrifice getting a good night's sleep. But all these late nights ended up showing up in my skin, as it became dull, sallow, and grayish looking. And not getting enough sleep also ate up my energy during the day, and I would drag myself from the morning till the night. That's when I became a mom, and finally realized that I must get on a solid sleep schedule, not only for me, but for my family's sake. I knew that if I got my rest, I would be able to function better, and of course feel and look better too!

This is where I really got interested in the "science" of beauty sleep and making sure that I got the essential rest I needed. And to insure you get your rest, make sure your home is a JNL Fit Home!

WHAT'S A "JNL FIT HOME?"

"My home is a JNL Fit Home, as everywhere you look you will find a tool, accessory, or product which promotes living a healthy lifestyle. Is your home a JNL Fit Home?"

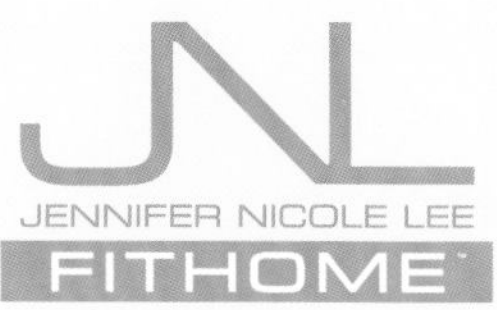

What is a JNL fit home? Well, it's a home that is set up and equipped with the right accessories that promote a healthy lifestyle. This could mean that you have a kitchen appliance that helps you to cook healthier meals, or a bedding line that has built in technology in its designs, to insure that you get a solid night's sleep. In my home, I have found, developed and created products that have helped not only my family, but so many other families around the world live and enjoy a healthier lifestyle, within their budget.

WHAT'S A "JNL FIT SLEEP?"

"'Fit Sleep' is based on using the right kind of bedding to promote, insure, and enjoy the most beneficial sleep to your health, where you will wake up radiating wellness, all from getting a solid, deep, good night's sleep."

—JNL

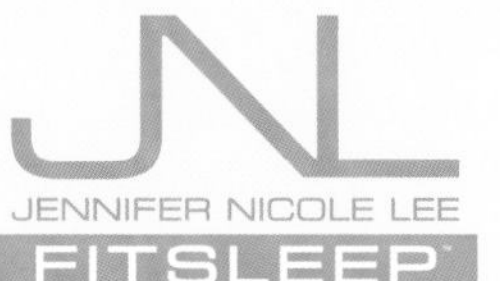

There is the every-night, mundane, run-of-the-mill, 'so -so' sleep, and then there is the JNL Fit Sleep, where you wake up feeling super refreshed and ready to take on the day! What makes the difference? Well, the products you sleep on, of course! I only sleep on the best, and it really makes a difference in how I feel and look the next day.

Bedding is important to making sure you get a fit sleep. We sweat during the night, losing water. We must have bedding that actually keeps us warm, yet allows moisture to be wicked away, so we don't end up in a sauna in between our sheets. I have helped to develop a specific bedding that includes a patented technology that wicks away heat and moisture, giving you a more peaceful, dry – yet warm, way more comfortable sleep.

WHAT'S A "JNL POWER SLEEP?"

"I like to ramp up and get extra sleep before a big week, or when I have an huge workload ahead of me. Sleep is my fuel."

—JNL

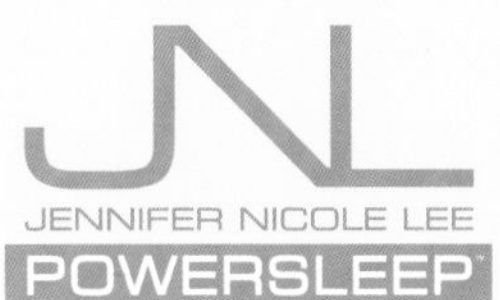

A JNL Power Sleep is getting the additional rest that you know you will need when you have a big work load ahead of you. When I see that I have a huge appearance, or a full 24-hour production schedule, or that I will be in 3 different cities in one week, I make sure that I "pre-rest," or a ramp up on my sleep. I like to go into a "marathon" of a work load extra rested, so I am extra sharp and focused. It's kind of like what my OB-GYN told me before I gave birth, telling me to get my extra rest before my baby was born, so I would be stronger and more prepared. So make sure you take a good look at your schedule and do a pre-rest before that super busy spike in your calendar comes. And yes, bedding is so important! For great JNL Power Sleep bedding ideas and strategies, visit www.JNLFitHome.com

JNL ROBE TIME

"How do I wind down? With my tried and true JNL Robe Time!"

"Every woman needs her JNL robe time!"

My robe time is now one of my beauty and relaxation rituals. At the end of a long work week, or when I have just one of those extra challenging days, I indulge myself with what I call "robe time". I usually start with a long, warm, scented Epson salt bath, with a cup of hot herbal tea. Then I massage my entire body with one of my favorite skin firming and hydrating creams, and then—here comes the best part: I wrap my body in one of my favorite super cozy, super plush, and extremely luxuriously soft JNL Robes. This beauty and relaxation ritual just calms my soul, restores my energy, balances me, and fortifies my spirit. All of my stress just melts away! This ritual helps me to keep my sanity in an insane world, and I always feel at peace and in more control after my robe time. I have designed a line of super plush, cozy robes that are both thick yet light-weight. Every woman needs her robe time!

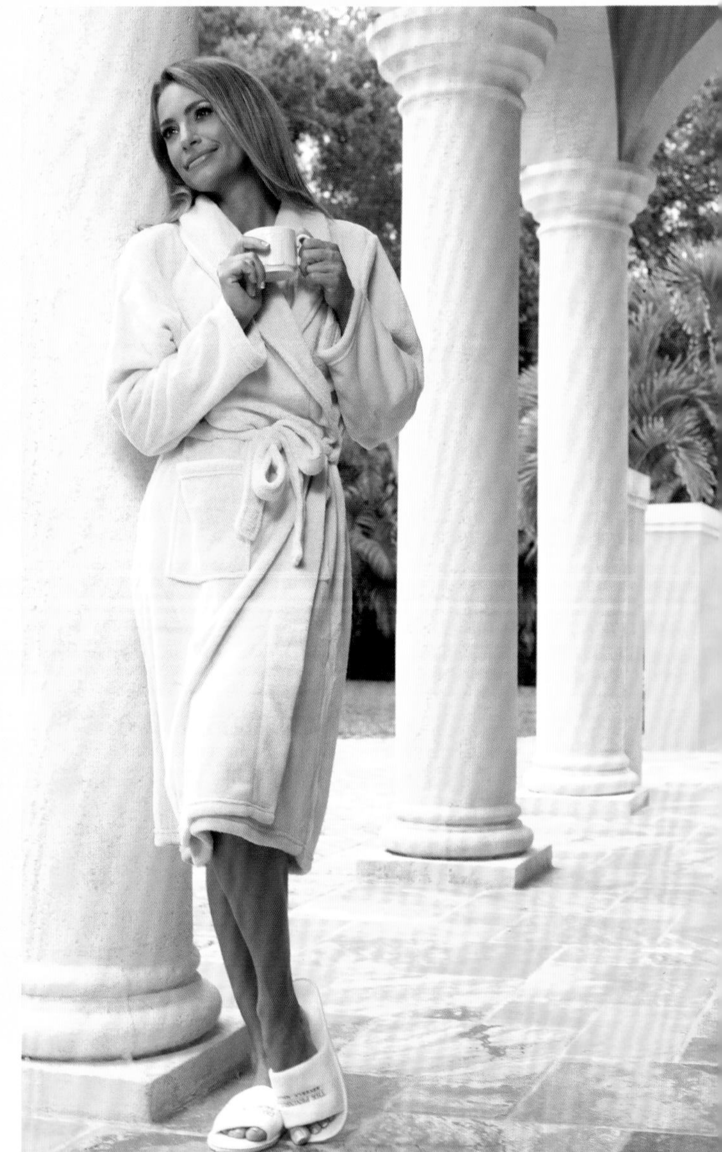

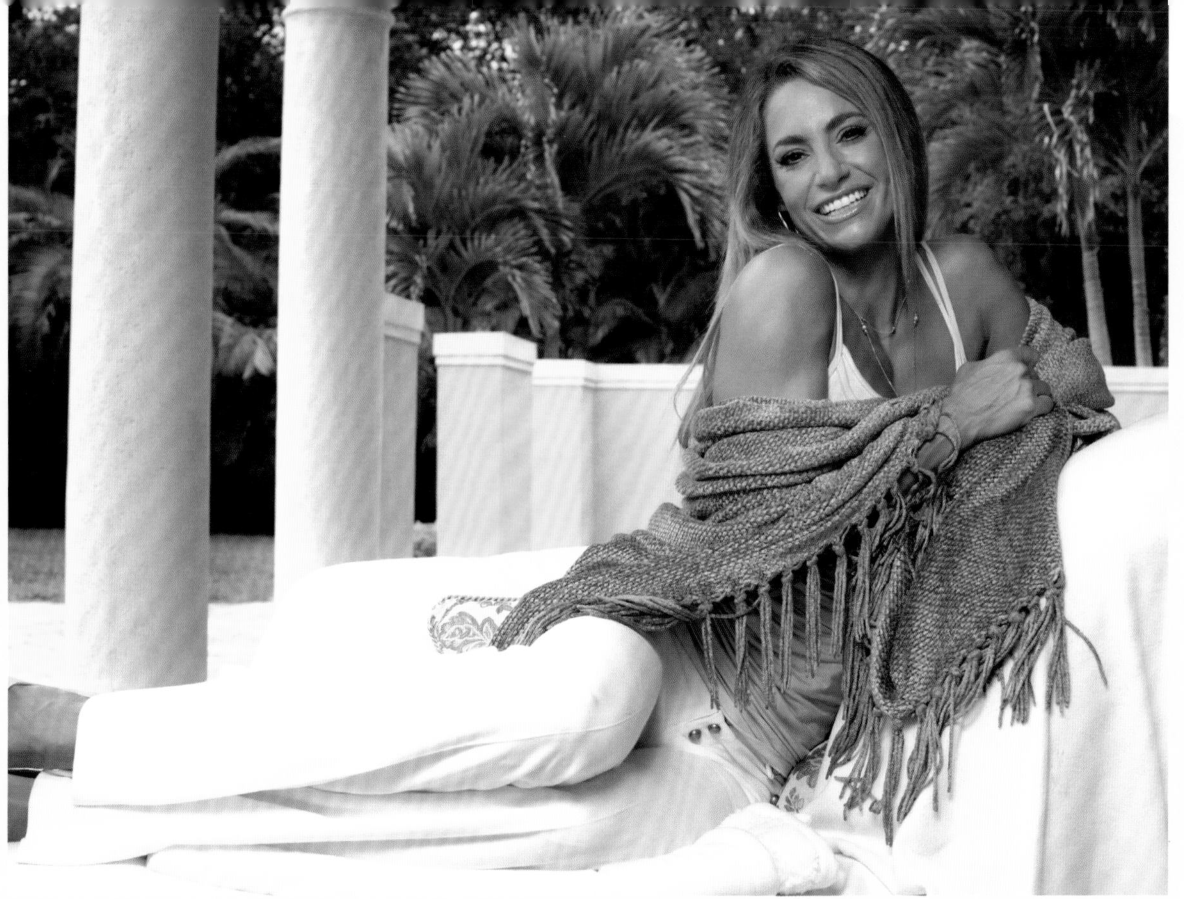

JNL THROW TIME

"I enjoy JNL Throw Time for those power cat naps that will recharge you! All you need is a cozy spot to curl up in, with one of your favorite super soft and plush throws to wrap around your body, sending you out into an instant blissful mental and physical vacation!"

—JNL

JNL
JENNIFER NICOLE LEE
THROWTIME

My JNL Throw Time is something that I created for when I could not afford the time for a full hour nap, and I only had about 10-15 minutes to get a little rest. Taking these "power pauses" throughout the day helps me to stay focused on what is priority, relax my racing mind, and also give my body a much needed break. The power naps from my Throw Time allow me to keep my balance, and remain centered on the most hectic days, allowing me to keep my cool or composure. Also, when I don't want to mess up my bed, I just curl up and get on my chaise lounge with one of my favorite super plush "JNL-Approved" throws that are designed with the ultimate comfort in mind!

For a complete line of all of my JNL-Approved bedding and home products, visit www.**JNLFitHome**.com

CHAPTER FOUR :

FLEX IT, BABY! THE JNL FITNESS MODEL WORKOUTS

How To Exercise Like A Fitness Model

The Fitness Model Exercise Attitude: Change Your Attitude, And You Will See Results

"Fitness and being healthy all starts with your attitude and mindset towards working out, exercising and eating right. It's not torture, it's a gift!"

—JNL

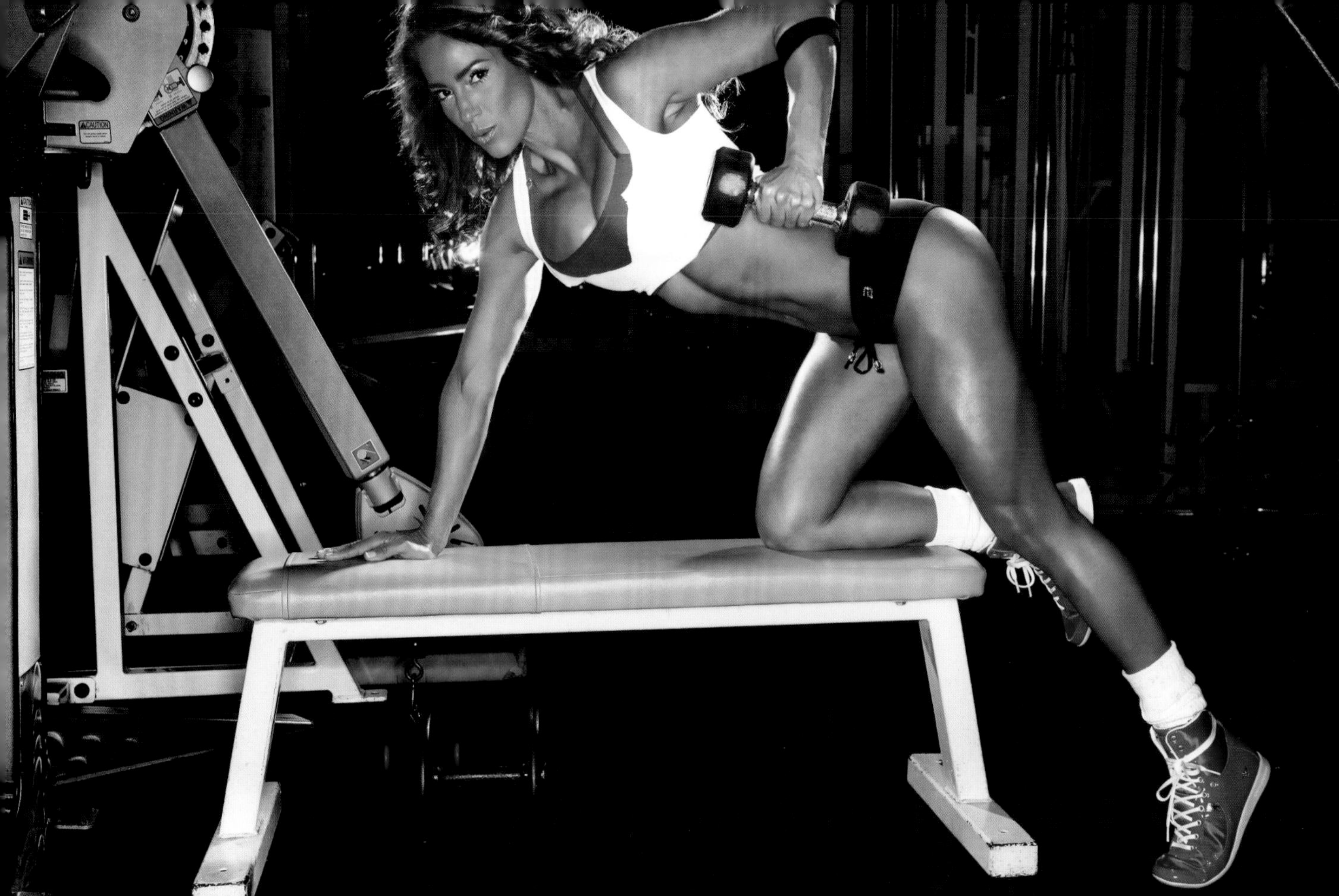

"Welcome to the wonderful world of working out like a Fitness Model!"

—JNL

Improve your 'tude from "I *HAVE* to workout" to "I *GET* to workout!" Just that subtle change in your thinking will help you gain a whole new outlook on working out.

Working out is not a chore to be dreaded. Rather, celebrate the fact that you are getting fresh blood and oxygen to all the cells in your body. And you are giving yourself the best gift ever – the gift of exercise!

THE #1 REASON WHY PEOPLE START & THEN STOP AN EXERCISE PROGRAM REVEALED

"Give yourself the gift of time."

—JNL

I have heard this scenario too many times in my online coaching programs, and in my telephone and in-person live consultations. A client starts a new exercise program, only to quit 2 to 3 weeks later. Why, you ask? It's because they suffer from a pair of dangerous conditions known in scientific terms as of *"Get-there-Itis"* and *"I-Want-My-Results-Now-Itis".*

They want to "get there," and they "want results now"! With this self-sabotaging mindset, they are setting themselves up for failure.

PERFECTION VS. PERSISTENCE

Once you understand that it's not about "being perfect" but, rather, about being persistent, you will be successful and see the results are you longing for! Remember to never stop, never give up and never quit. Only losers quit. Winners carry on, always taking their program one day at a time.

JNL PERSONAL MOTIVATIONAL STORY: NEVER GIVE UP!

"Winners never give up or quit. Only losers do. And sometimes you have to fail your way to being successful. That's part of the journey."

—JNL

When I had given birth to my second son and, months later, took my infamous "before" photo, I went on a mission to become my healthiest. I started this Fitness Model™ Program, but I did not see results. Even when I was two and a half months into it, I still saw no real results. I almost gave up, gave in, and threw in my towel. But a little, positive, self-loving voice inside my head told me not to quit, and to carry on. That even if I didn't see results I wanted, I would still be benefiting from a super healthy lifestyle.

Then it happened!

A week later, it was as if my body finally started to respond drastically to my new healthy lifestyle. The fat floodgates finally opened, allowing my body to release the fat that it had been storing for years. Muscle mass started to show.

To hear my personal story with all the details, and to really get to know me, please visit my instant downloadable audio seminars at www.SHOPJNL.com and click on "My Story." It will inspire you to never give up, and to keep your momentum in life.

And if you ever need that personal, non-judgmental fitness coach and friend to talk to, you can consult with me one-on-one on a confidential basis by applying at www.clubjnl.com

JNL'S FITNESS MODEL PROGRAM WEEKLY WORKOUT EXERCISE PLAN

"Plan your workouts like important business meetings that you can't be late to, cancel, or not show up to, with the most important person in the world: YOU!"

—JNL

I have come a long way from my early "cardio queen" days, and have mastered crafting the basic fitness model workout formula. I learned the hard way, training like a gerbil on a wheel, getting nowhere fast by doing endless, mindless cardio. I have learned the big "do's" and "don'ts" of exercising to get that coveted super-fit, healthy look that goes with being a top fitness model. Yes, it's true! Doing endless hours of cardio doesn't get you the rock-hard, round, shapely body of a fitness model. But my program will!

You see, many of us women have been conditioned to be afraid of the "guys' side of the gym," so we cling onto the cardio machines as if they are our safe havens. I have to admit, when I started working out, it was easier just to get on and push the "start" button. But when I saw that all of this cardio wasn't getting me the sexy athletic build that I desired, I started my quest for the right way to train like a top fitness model.

Through long hours of research, reading, and discovery, I have compiled all that I have found into my JNL Fitness Model Exercise Program. I've got it boiled down to a science, an easy step-by-step guide that will get you amazing, major results in minimum time.

The JNL Fitness Model Exercise Program is as simple as this:

Work out with weights 4 days a week, and if you have some fat you need to blast, add 2 days of Fitness Model™ Cardio, no less than 25 minutes and no more than 45 minutes.

Below, you see a sample week. This is an outline that I strongly suggest you follow and stick to. It's a solid plan, you won't be lost, and you'll know what you're doing and what to do next, taking out all the guess work.

JNL'S FUSION METHOD

WWW.JNLFUSION.COM

- **MONDAY** is always going to be **SHOULDERS & TRICEPS.**
- **TUESDAY** is always going to be **LEGS.**
- **WEDNESDAY** is **CARDIO AND ABS.**
- **THURSDAY** is **CHEST AND BICEPS.**
- **FRIDAY** is **BACK.**
- **SATURDAY** is **CARDIO AND ABS.**
- **SUNDAY IS YOUR OFF/ACTIVE REST DAY,** and also Food Prep Day (grocery shopping and meal planning).

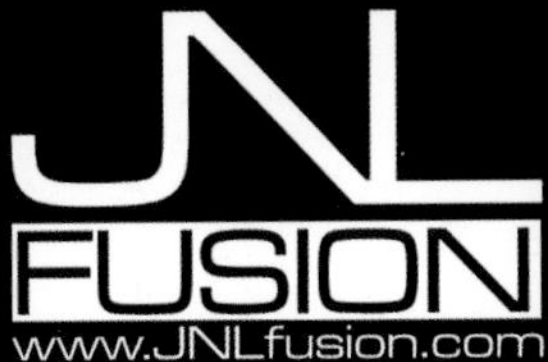

THE JNL FITNESS MODEL WORKOUT GUIDE

SUN	MON	TUES	WED	THURS	FRI	SAT
Off-Grocery Shopping, Food Planning, And Prep Day	Shoulders & Triceps	Legs & Butt	Abs & Fitness Model Cardio	Chest & Biceps	Back	Abs & Fitness Model Cardio

BASIC NOTES: Start every workout with a warm up. Warm up simply by walking in place, then moving side to side, then picking up the intensity to jumping-jacks, then running in place. Aim for a warm up of at least 5 minutes. One of my all-time favorite ways to warm up is with my speed rope. I jump for about one minute, take a rest for 30 seconds, and then jump again for about 1 minute, followed by another 30 second rest. After about 5 minutes of speed rope jumping, my entire body is warmed up, and my heart rate is in the fat-burning zone.

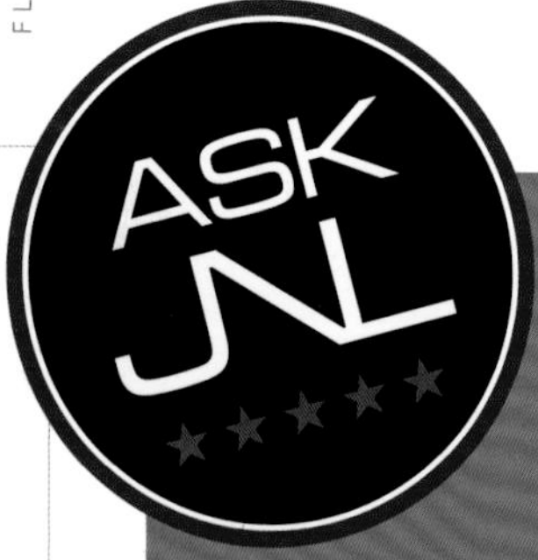

"But JNL-I'm confused! How Many Sets and How Many Reps? Help!"

—ELIZABETH,
Full-time college student and part-time waitress, LA, California

ELIZABETH, THAT'S A GREAT QUESTION. And here is my answer: IT DEPENDS!

IF YOU DON'T HAVE MATURE MUSCLE MASS, AND WANT TO INCREASE YOUR MUSCLE MASS:
Perform 8-12 reps for 3 sets, at a challenging weight at which the last 8-12 reps are hard to Finish.

IF YOU HAVE MATURE MUSCLE MASS, AND WANT TO SIMPLY MAINTAIN IT, WITHOUT ADDING SIZE:
Perform 18-21 reps for 3 sets, at a challenging weight at which the last 18-21 are hard to finish.

I fall into this category, since I am not out to gain any more girth or size in my body. Also, for those of you who gain muscle easily, or bulk up easily, or who have gotten too big from exercise weight training, or feel too muscular, you can bring down your size by performing the 18-21 reps.

THE ESSENTIAL PIECES OF FITNESS MODEL WORKOUT EQUIPMENT

"You don't need an entire gym to get outstanding weight loss, muscle toning, and fat blasting results."

—JNL

Contrary to popular belief, you only really need some core, fundamental pieces of exercise tools and equipment to achieve the "Fitness Model" look. You don't need an expensive gym membership, or a "glorified counter" who calls himself a trainer, or tons of useless gadgets and equipment to achieve Fitness Model, magazine-cover-worthy results!

All you need are the following:

- A Workout Mat
- Three Sets of Dumbbells — one heavy, one medium, and one light (I suggest one pair of 15 or 12 lbs for heavy, one set of 10 lbs for medium, and one set of 5 lbs for light).
- A Inclining/Reclining Bench
- Straight Bench
- A Straight Bar
- An EZ-Curl Bar
- Exercise Tubing with Handle
- A Stability Ball
- Ab Circle Pro or a Complete at home workout gym (visit www.JenniferNicoleLee.com for ideas & suggestions)
- A Piece of Cardio Equipment (Jump Rope, Elliptical Machine, Stair Master, or an Air Stepper)

And I LOVE to hit my entire core while burning calories with cardio with my Ab Circle Pro! Visit www.JNLAb-CirclePro.com and find out where you can order yours right now, to whittle your waist, dial in your mid-section, and carve out your core.

JNL FIT TIP: Designate an area of your home to be your "Fitness Model" Program Workout zone. I suggest you create an area with a TV nearby, so you can watch your favorite program while you work out, or even by a window to enjoy the scenery. I have coached too many people from too many different countries who try to "hide" their equipment or not allow it to be in the way, so they end up placing it in the garage or basement. Don't be embarrassed by your at-home gym! Leave it out in your living room in a corner, so "in sight, in mind". When you see it, you will exercise! If you leave it in the smelly, dark basement or garage, you may not want to go to there, and you'll only end up not doing your workout.

THE JNL FITNESS MODEL 25-MINUTE CARDIO WORKOUT

"Like a gerbil on a wheel, you are going nowhere fast when you perform endless amounts of cardio. Your body will not get the same amazing fat-blasting and muscle toning results that it does with weights. However, cardio, if performed correctly, is an essential component to the Fitness Model Exercise program."

—JNL

When I started my own weight loss transformation from flabby to super-fit, I studied intensely what the hottest and hardest bodies did for their workouts. I was surprised to discover that the female athletes who were fitness models did not focus their energy on high-tempo, fast paced monotonous cardio for hours on end. Rather, the foundation of their training was weight training, with some cardio added to their workouts when needed.

I knew I was on to something BIG here! I was my own "guinea pig" and I practiced what I had discovered. Now, coming from someone like me, who had done the endless amounts of cardio, only to become a "skinny fat person" and gain all the weight back – I WAS READY FOR THE CHALLENGE!

So I switched my program from cardio-heavy, to weight-focused with some cardio. And let me tell you – IT WORKS! My body started to trade the flabby fat for rock-hard, sexy lean muscle. And the greatest part is that, when you have sleek, sexy muscle tone, your body "keeps" its desired healthy lean weight easier and longer.

But that doesn't mean that cardio is not important. It is. But there is an exact science to achieving the super-healthy, athletic build of a super fitness model. There is a delicate balance to cardio, and the great news is that, when you perform it right, your body will respond by keeping your hard earned muscle tone, while melting off the fat. So, let me explain how you should perform cardio, if you want to get the look of a fitness model.

FITNESS MODEL CARDIO

"Getting fresh blood and oxygen to all of the cells of your body leaves you feeling recharged, more mentally and emotionally stable and strong. So give yourself the gift of exercise daily-and your body will thank you!"

—JNL

The secret to performing "Fitness Model" cardio is to not exceed your target heart rate of 75%. If you get your heart rate up too high, you start burning muscle mass, and not fat. So aim to stay in your fat-burning zone, which is 65%-75%.

Below is the formula for calculating your Target Heart Rate— Here's how:

1. First thing in the morning, while still in bed, calculate your heart rate (HR).
2. Subtract your age in years from 220 to get you standard maximal HR.
3. Subtract your morning HR from your standard maximal HR.
4. Multiply the result of step 3 by 0.60.
5. Multiply the result of step 3 by 0.70.
6. Add your morning HR to the result of step 4.
7. Add your morning HR to the result of step 5.
8. Your target HR training zone is between the two results of steps 6 and 7.

JNL FIT TIPS:

▸You should be warmed up and breathing more heavily, but still able to talk without pauses while working out within your target zone.

▸If your fitness level is good or excellent, include exercising at 80 percent of your maximal HR for at least 20 minutes, at least 3 times a week.

▸To ensure the sufficient level of your resting metabolism, include strength-training exercises for at least 20 minutes, at least 3 times a week.

▸You can also wear a heart rate monitor while you are working out, which will tell you instantly when you are in your fat burning zone.

FITNESS MODEL BULLET POINTS TO REMEMBER:

- Fitness Models focus on keeping their heart rates down, so as not to burn off their hard-earned muscle mass.
- Fitness Models rarely run, because this too "eats at their muscle mass," and makes them flabby. I'm not saying not to run, but make sure you don't make it the majority of your training regiment.
- Fitness Models perform no more than 25 to 45 minutes of cardio, unless it's time to compete, when they bump it up.

When we begin to see the effects of Sarcopenia (the term for muscle loss as we age), we should kick up the weight training and back off of the cardio, to prevent any further unnecessary muscle loss.

FITNESS MODEL EXERCISE DO'S AND DON'TS!

DON'T run! I'm not telling you never to run, but don't ever make it the foundation of your cardio. Try to embrace another form of low-impact cardio. Believe me, your muscle mass and your joints will thank me! Fitness models and other fitness professionals lean towards the "no running" principle because running is known to "eat away" at the muscle you work so hard to gain.

DON'T work against yourself and defeat your progress by running. It takes a lot of energy with no real gains, except for cardiovascular. You can receive cardiovascular benefits from other low impact exercise, such as using the Elliptical, Nordic Track, AirStepper, and the Stair Master.

DON'T do less than 25 minutes, or more than 45 minutes. This "magic zone," between 25 and 45, burns fat. If you do more than that, your body "hits a wall," and you slow/stop your progress.

DON'T focus on cardio! In order to have that strong, sleek and sexy muscle tone, you need to focus more on weight training to build it up. Remember, excessive cardio will "eat away" at your muscle mass.

DON'T over-train! If you over-train, your appetite will increase and you will start eating like a 250-pound football player, not a fitness model. Rather, do just enough to blast fat, not to hit a plateau. When you over-train, your body will "lock up" and not allow you to burn off the fat that you need to.

DO understand that fitness is a journey to be enjoyed, not a one-time event. Like the old adage says, "Rome wasn't built in a day." Your body, too, is a masterpiece in progress. Take it one day at a time, and enjoy the process.

"Give yourself the greatest gift ever – the gift of exercising!"

— JNL

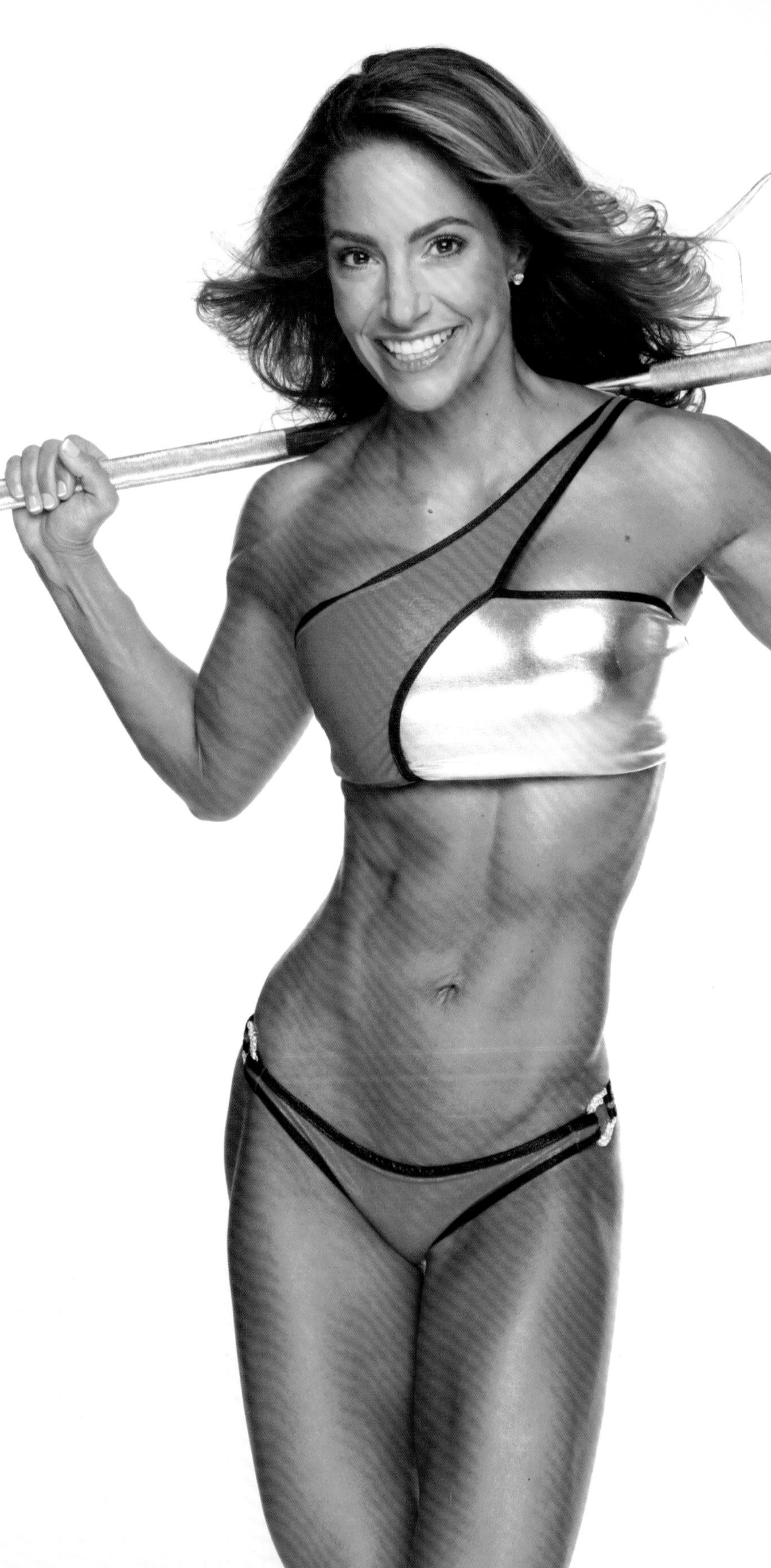

PHOTOS AND EXPLANATIONS OF FITNESS MODEL EXERCISES

Congrats on making it this far in my Fitness Model Program — a round of applause for you! Now comes the real fun part: proving to yourself that you can do it!

The upside to my Fitness Model workout is that you do not need an expensive gym membership, fancy equipment, or a costly trainer to achieve the Fitness Model body! As you will see from my photos, I am simply working out, and these movements can be done anywhere! Try them in your living room, family room, that extra room that no one really uses, or even outside! And the great thing is that you can take this book with you to the gym, and use it as a guide there to work out.

The key here is to just do this program. It's as simple as that! And whether it's at your home, or at the gym, it doesn't really matter where you are. The piece of equipment that I prefer to perform my cardio on is the Stairmaster, but you can use a Nordic track, elliptical machine, a steady walk on an inclined treadmill, or jumping rope, for your cardio.

FITNESS MODEL EXERCISE PROGRAM FORMULA

"To get the body of a super fitness model, you must follow my tried and true formula. You don't just throw stuff against a wall, and hope it sticks. With my JNL Fitness Model Diet, you will get results!"

—JNL

Refer to the seven-day calendar that was outlined previously in this chapter. Focus on the part of your body that is assigned each day, and choose 3 exercises from the exercises listed and illustrated below.

Depending upon your current fitness level and goals, perform 3 sets of 8-12 reps (for beginners) per exercise, or 3 sets of 18-21 (for intermediate to advance) reps. Make sure you choose a weight that is challenging enough so that you have to really focus to finish the last 8-12/18-21 reps!

Don't cheat yourself! Make sure you follow through and complete your entire weight-training session.

MAJOR MUSCLE GROUPS

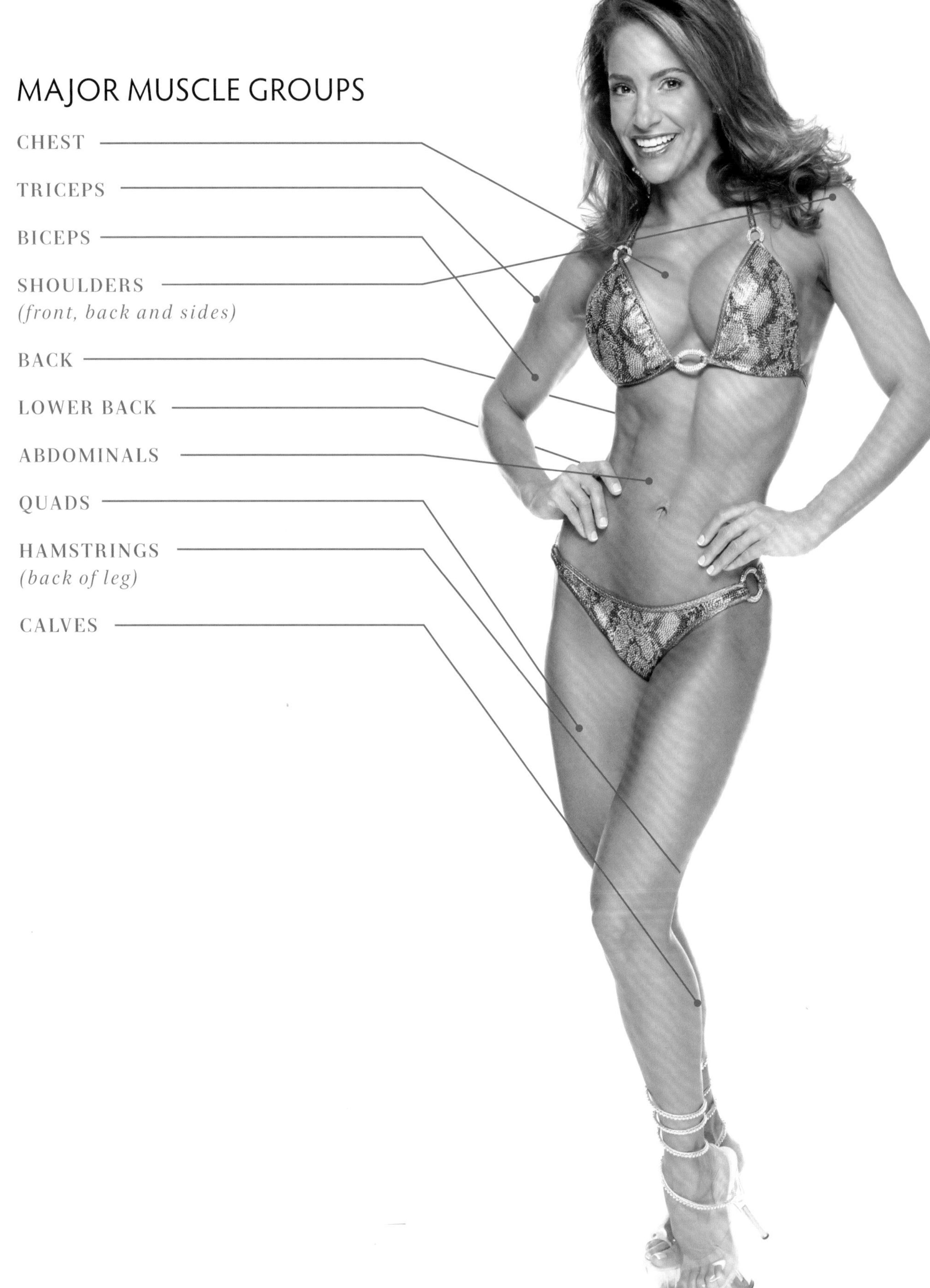

UPPER BODY

List of Exercises for Shoulders

- Seated Dumbbell Press
- Shoulder Press on Stability Ball
- Standing Dumbbell Press
- Side Raises
- Bent Over Raises
- Front Raises
- Bent Over Side Lateral Raises with Bands
- Upright Row with Barbell
- Front Raises with Tubing
- Upright Rows with Tubing

SEATED DUMBBELL PRESS START

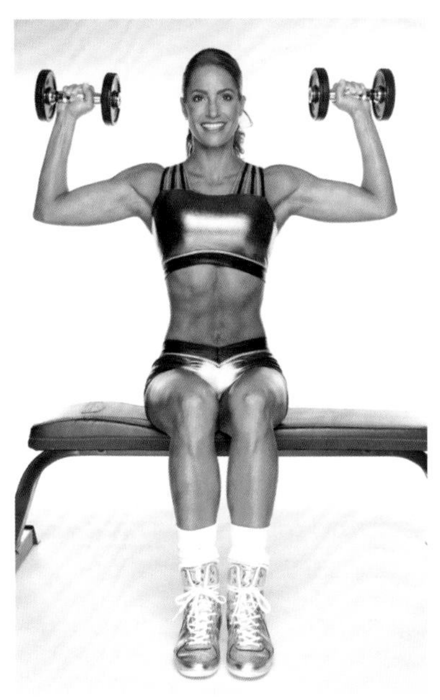

SEATED DUMBBELL PRESS

Start out by inclining your bench. Sit on the edge of it with your feet flat on the floor. Hold a dumbbell in each hand at shoulder height, elbows out and palms facing forward. Press the dumbbells up and in so that they almost touch above your head. Press them up until your arms are almost straight and slowly lower them back to starting position.

SEATED DUMBBELL PRESS FINISH

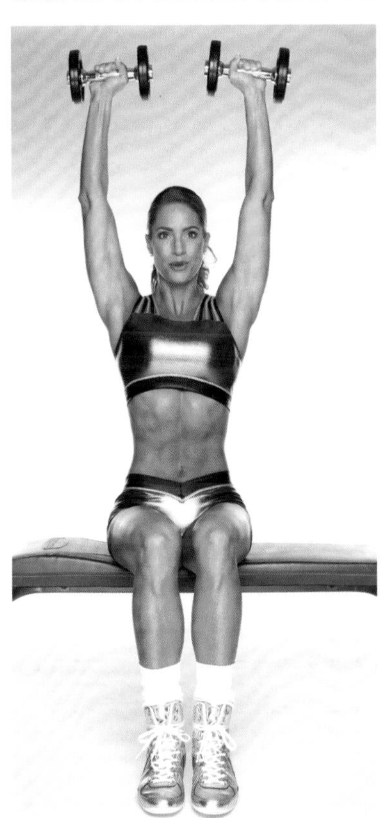

JNL FIT TIP: don't lean your head too far back; always look straight forward with your chin up and chest high.

SHOULDER PRESS ON STABILITY BALL

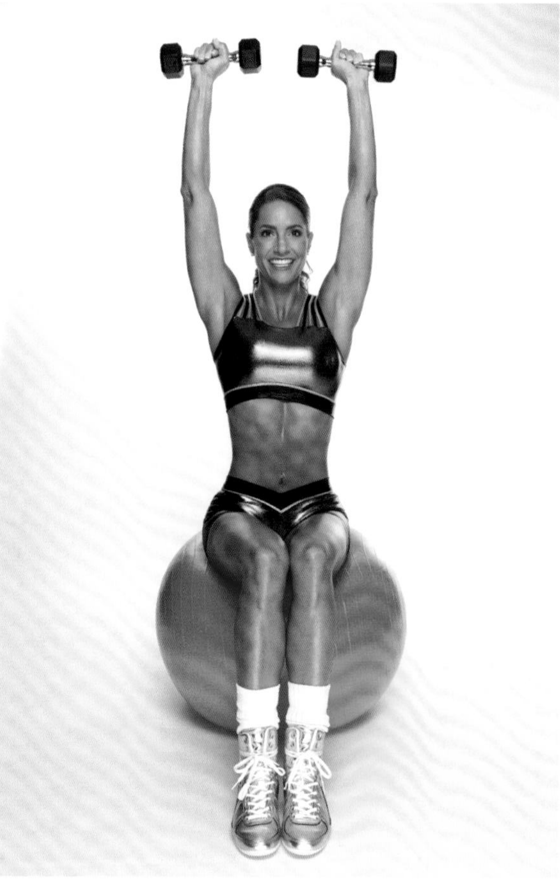

STANDING DUMBBELL PRESS

Stand with your feet shoulder width apart; knees slightly bent. Hold your dumbbells with your palms facing you and press the weight up until your arms are fully extended over your head. Pause for a count of one before slowly lowering your weight to the starting position.

JNL FIT TIP: do not arch your back as you press the dumbbells upward as it may cause back injury.

SIDE RAISES

Stand upright with your feet shoulder-width apart and your arms at your sides. Holding a dumbbell in each hand (palms facing your body) lift the weights out and up to the sides until they are right about level with your chin and hold them for a count of one. Lower them slowly back down to your sides.

JNL FIT TIP: Do not lean and swing the weights up or lean your torso forward and bring the dumbbells down in front of your body – let the weights down to your sides instead.

SIDE RAISES START

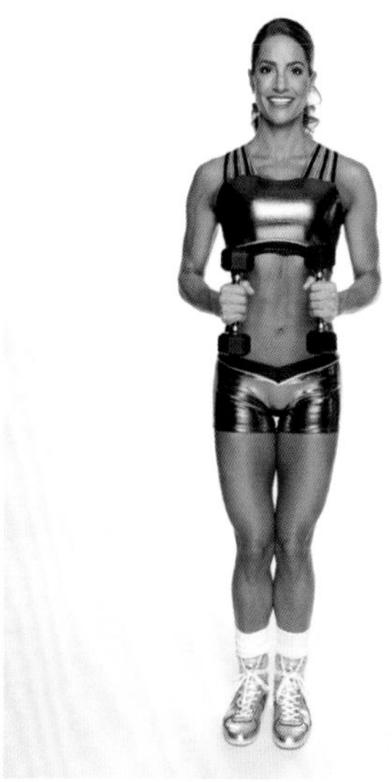

SIDE RAISES FINISH

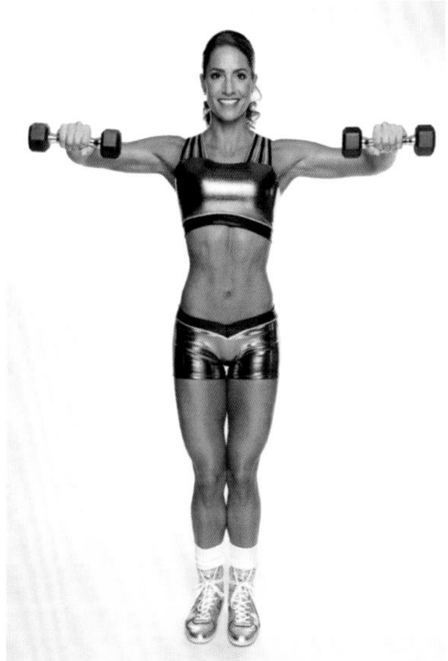

JNL FIT TIP: Don't hunch your back by leaning over too much. Your back should be straight and your torso should be almost parallel to the ground.

BENT OVER RAISES

Holding a dumbbell in each hand, keeping your feet shoulder width apart, bend forward at the waist so that your upper body is parallel with the floor. Let your arms hang straight down, palms facing each other. Raise the dumbbells, pulling your arms apart and moving your elbows up.

BENT OVER RAISES START

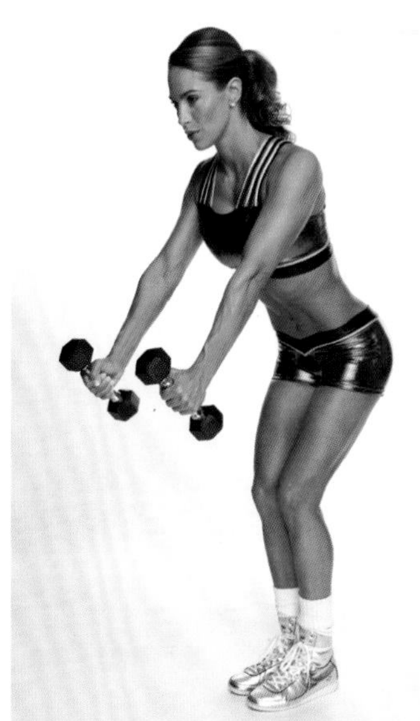

BENT OVER RAISES FINISH

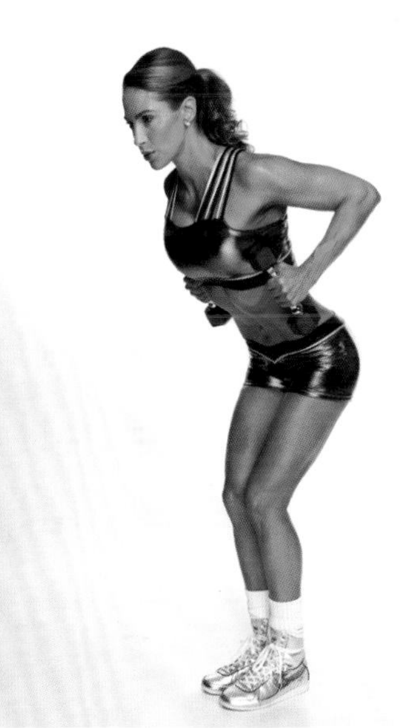

FRONT RAISES

This is an essential move to create sexy and shapely upper body muscles! Hold your dumbbells in your hands to your sides, palms facing inward. Raise the dumbbell up, hold at the top, and gently lower down.

FRONT RAISES START

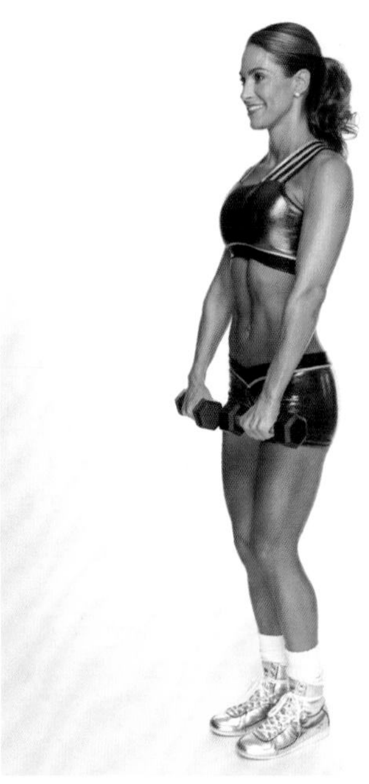

FRONT RAISES FINISH

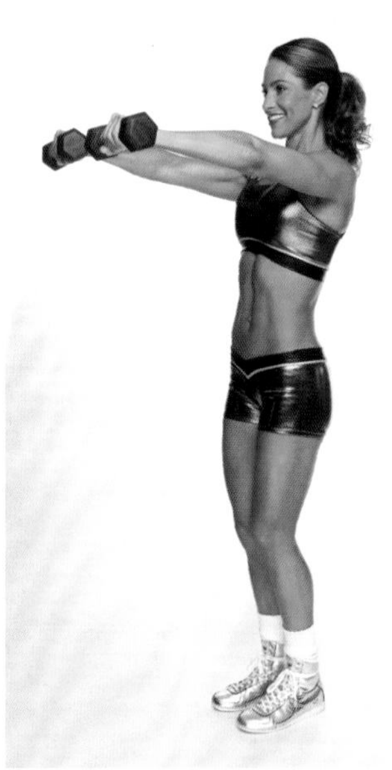

BENT OVER SIDE LATERAL RAISES WITH BANDS

Its always great to get in some upper body band work. By bending over a touch, you are engaging your core and activating more back muscles.

BENT OVER SIDE LATERAL RAISES WITH BANDS START

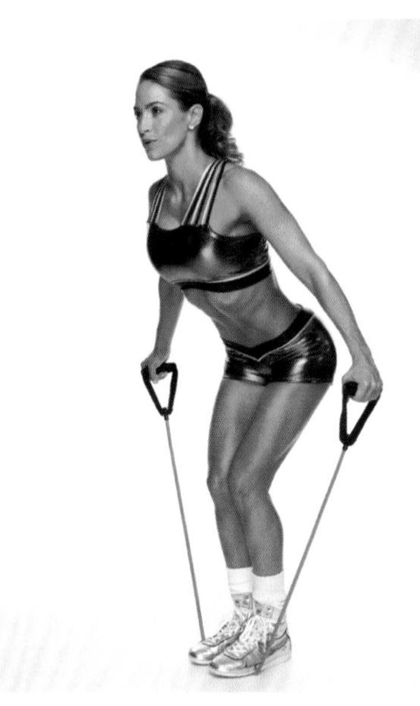

BENT OVER SIDE LATERAL RAISES WITH BANDS FINISH

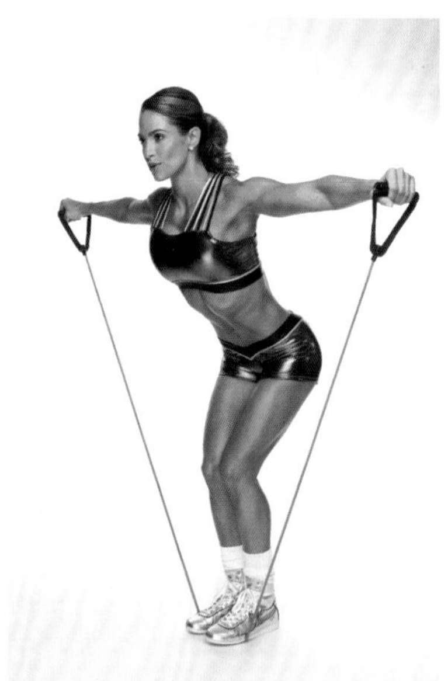

UPRIGHT ROW WITH BARBELL

UPRIGHT ROW WITH BARBELL START

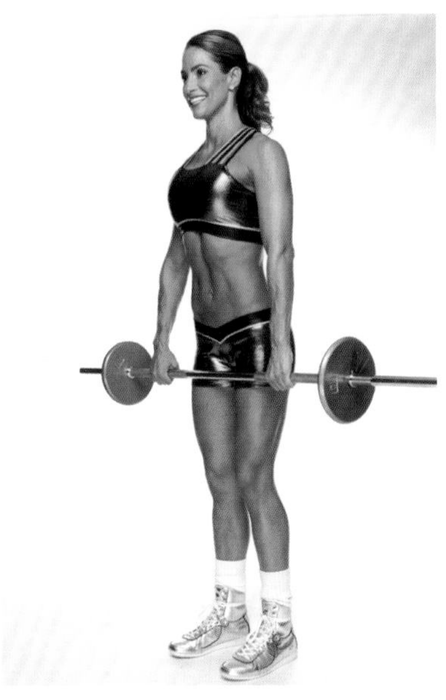

UPRIGHT ROW WITH BARBELL FINISH

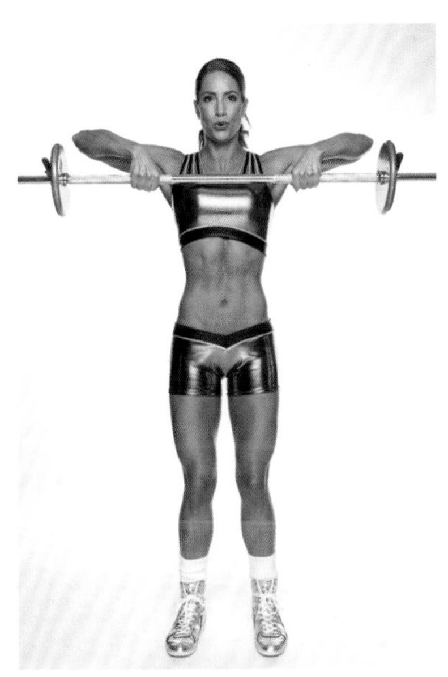

FRONT RAISES WITH TUBING

FRONT RAISES WITH TUBING START

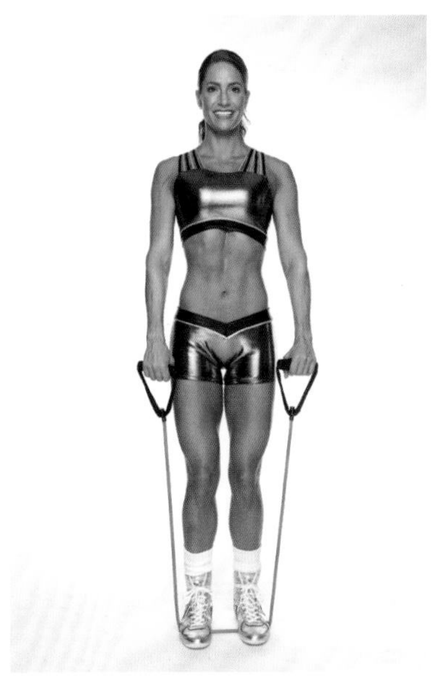

FRONT RAISES WITH TUBING FINISH

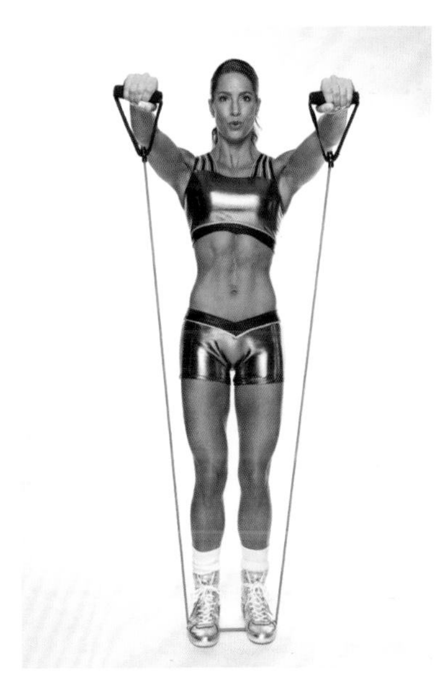

UPRIGHT ROWS WITH TUBING

UPRIGHT ROWS WITH TUBING START

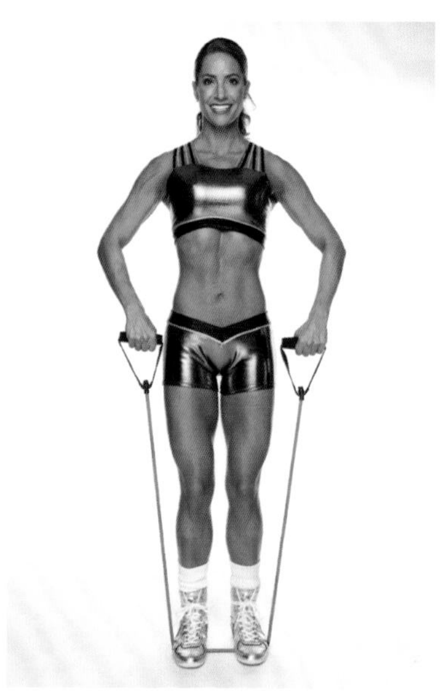

UPRIGHT ROWS WITH TUBING FINISH

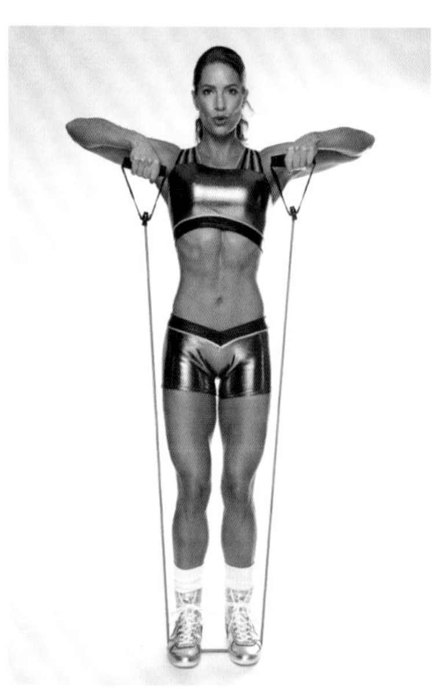

BICEPS

List of Exercises for Biceps

- Seated Dumbbell Curls
- Hammer Curls
- Barbell Curl
- Bicep Curl on Stability Ball

SEATED DUMBBELL CURLS

Sit on the edge of your flat bench with your arms at your sides and a dumbbell in each hand. With your palms facing forward, curl both arms lifting the dumbbells towards your shoulders.

JNL FIT TIP: Avoid swinging the weight up and do not lean back or forward as you lower the weights.

JNL FIT TIP: don't lift with your palms facing down; the proper way is for your palms to face each other.

SEATED DUMBBELL CURLS START

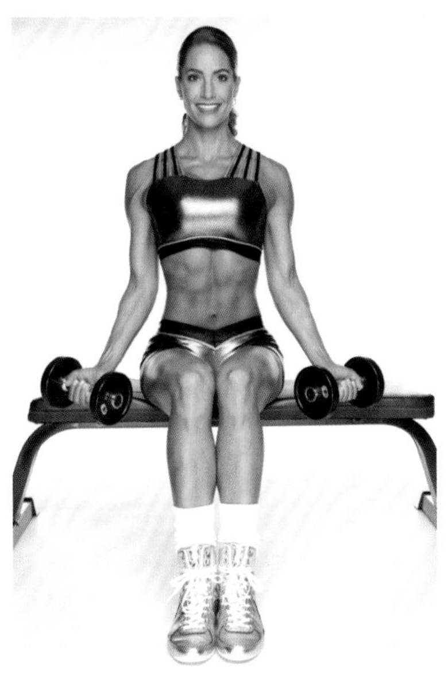

SEATED DUMBBELL CURLS FINISH

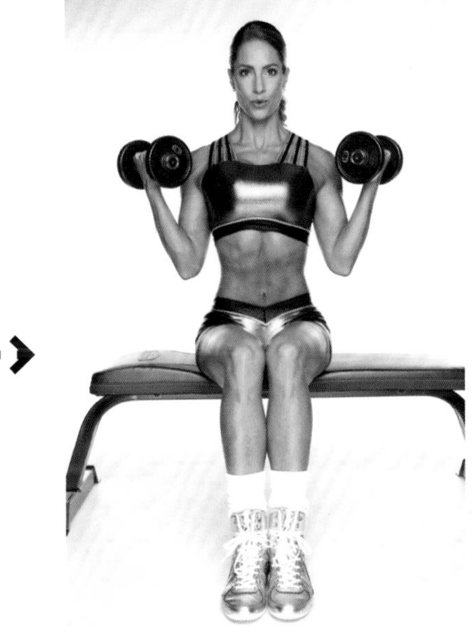

HAMMER CURLS

Stand with your feet shoulder-width apart with a dumbbell in each hand. Your arms should be extended down at your sides and palms facing each other. Curl both arms up and lift the dumbbells toward your shoulders. Remember to keep your upper arms and torso still as you curl.

HAMMER CURLS START

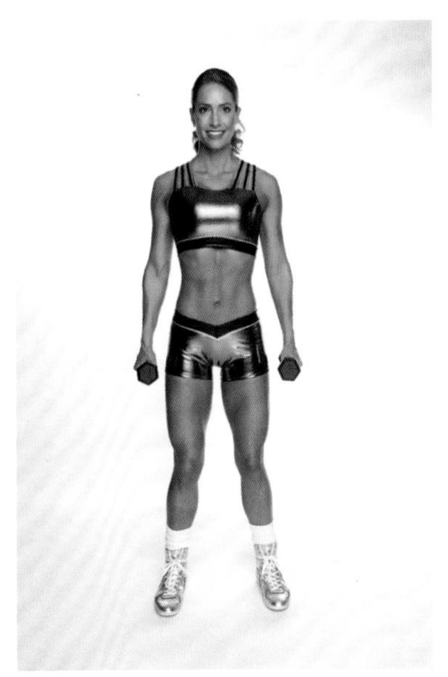

HAMMER CURLS FINISH

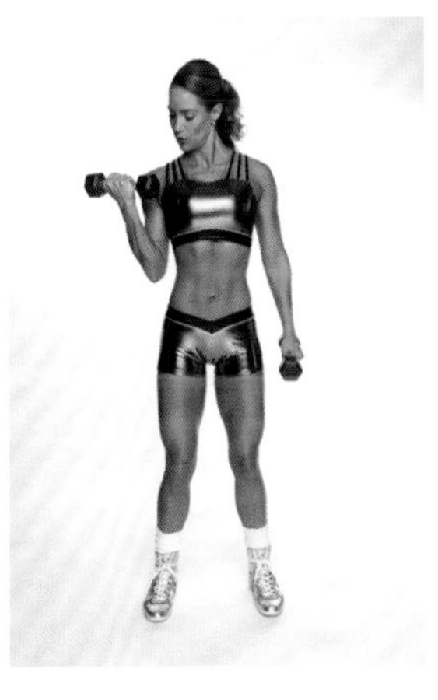

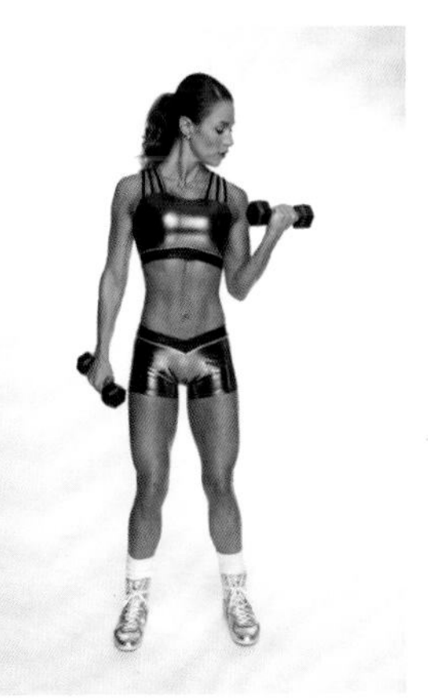

BARBELL CURL

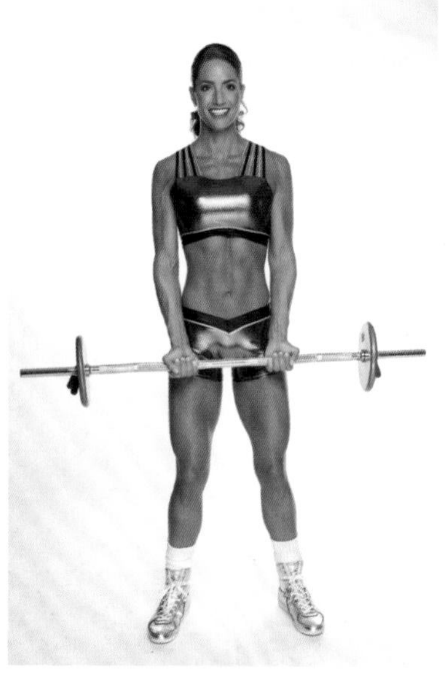

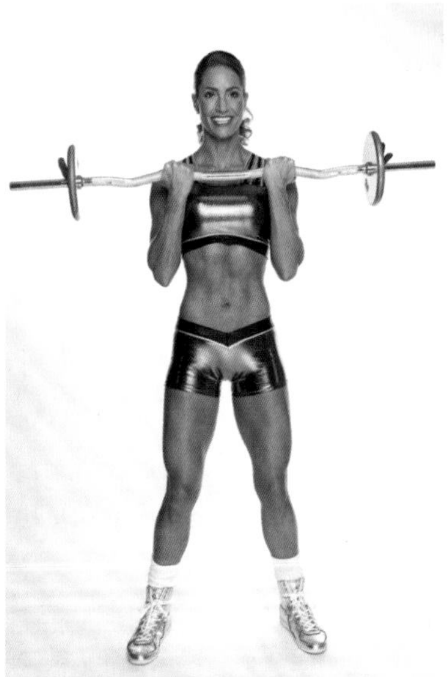

BICEP CURL ON STABILITY BALL

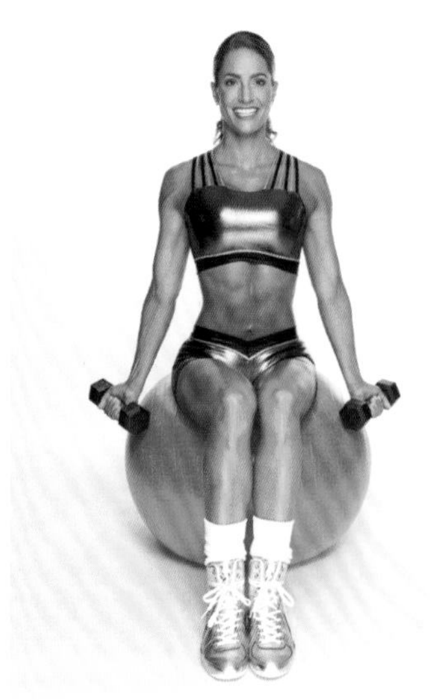

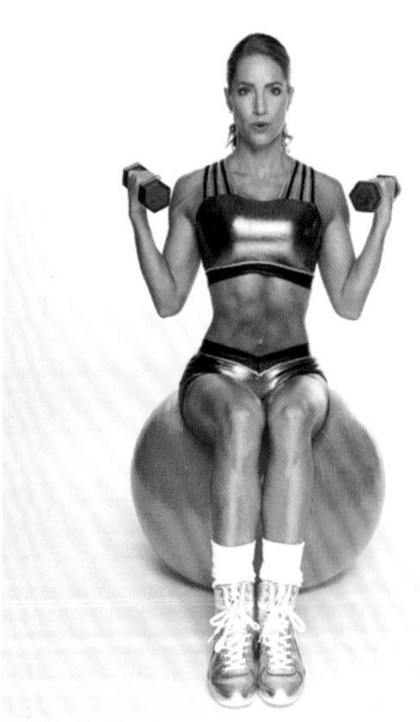

JNL FIT TIP: don't let the dumbbells sway back toward your head and over your face and do not lift your head off the bench as you do this exercise.

CHEST

- Dumbbell Bench Press
- Inclined Dumbbell Bench Press
- Push Ups
- Push Ups on Stability Ball

BARBELL BENCH PRESS

Lie on your back on your bench with a barbell or a dumbbell in each hand. Bring your weights to a point just above your shoulders. Your palms should face towards your feet and elbows out. Press your weights straight up until they are locked out right over your collarbone and slowly lower them to starting position.

BARBELL BENCH PRESS START

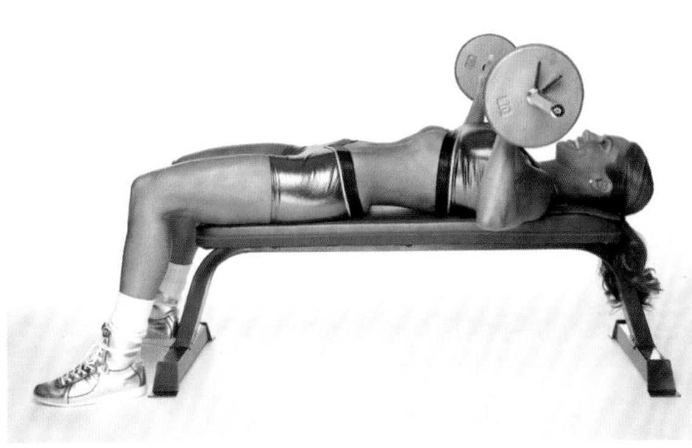

BARBELL BENCH PRESS FINISH

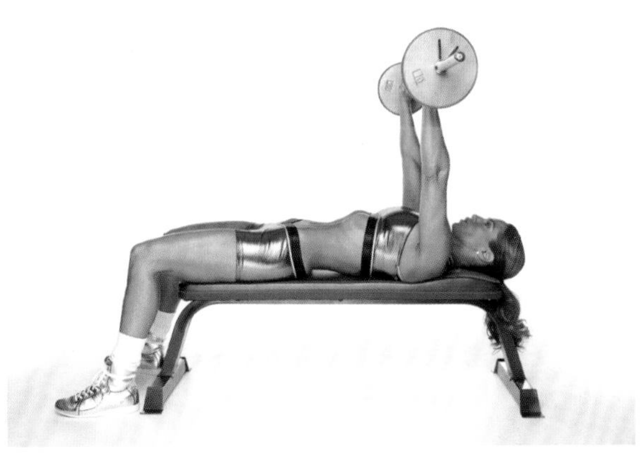

INCLINE DUMBBELL CHEST PRESS

INCLINE DUMBBELL CHEST PRESS START

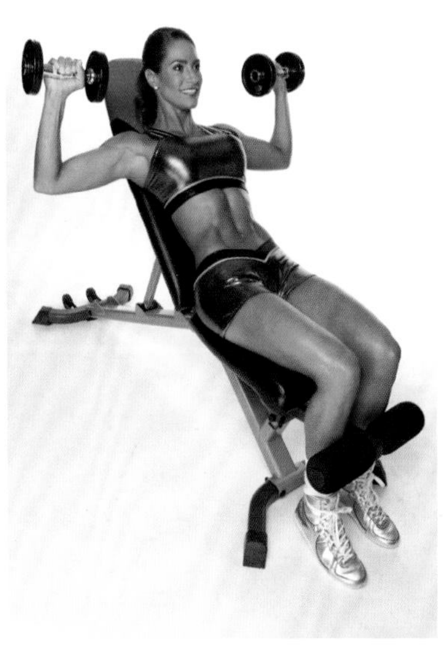

INCLINE DUMBBELL CHEST PRESS FINISH

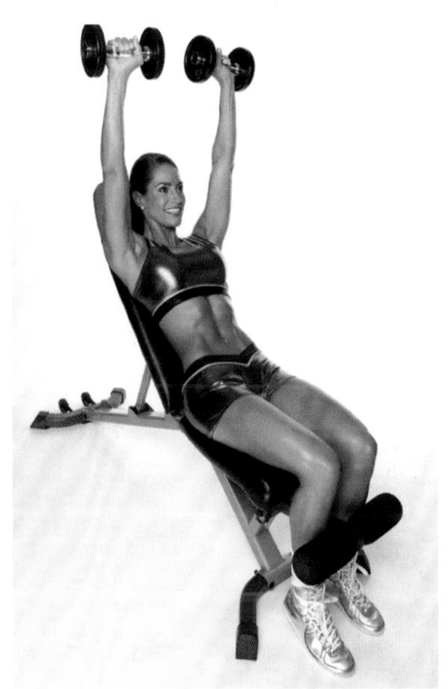

PUSH UPS

PUSH UPS START

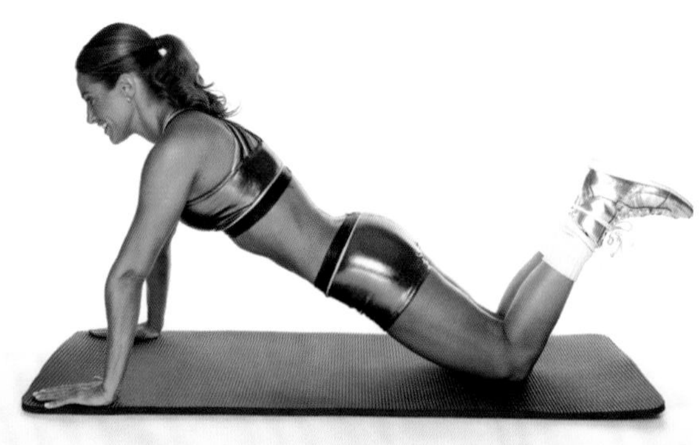

PUSH UPS FINISH

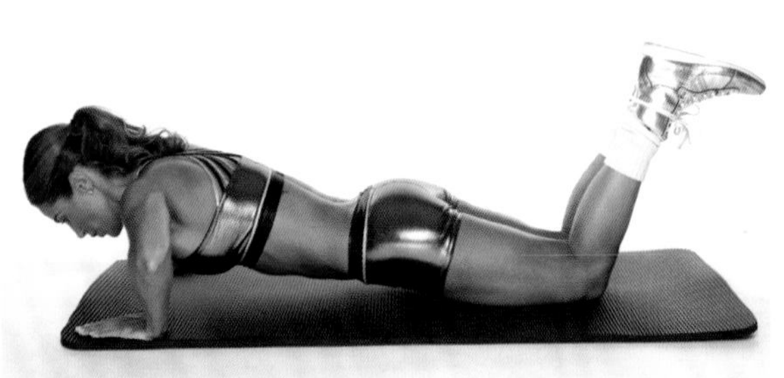

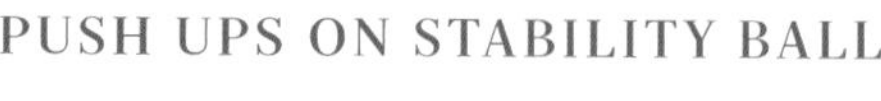

PUSH UPS ON STABILITY BALL

PUSH UPS ON STABILITY BALL START

PUSH UPS ON STABILITY BALL FINISH

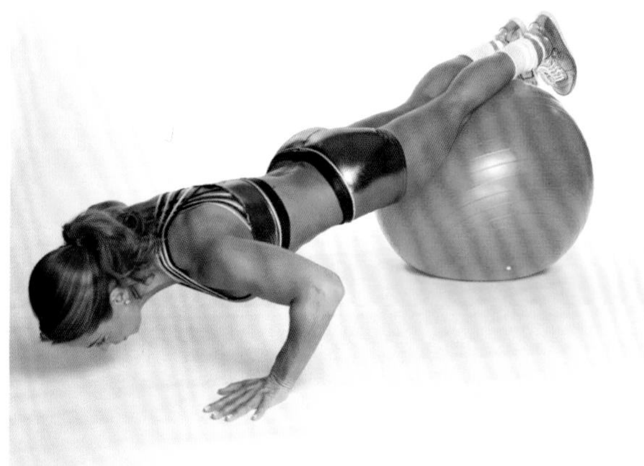

BACK

List of Exercises for Back

- Bent Over Row
- "Superwoman"
- Standing Dumbbell Row
- Dumbbell Pullover
- Super Woman on Stability Ball with Dumbbells
- Back Flies on Stability Ball
- One Arm Rows with Tubing

BENT OVER ROW

Start with your right foot flat on the floor and your left knee resting on a flat bench. Lean forward so that you're supporting the weight of your upper body with your left arm on the bench. Your back should be almost parallel to the floor. Concentrate on pulling the elbow as far back as it can go. After you have rowed the dumbbell as far up as you can, slowly lower it to the starting position.

JNL FIT TIP: Don't hunch your back as you do this exercise – keep it flat.

BENT OVER ROW START

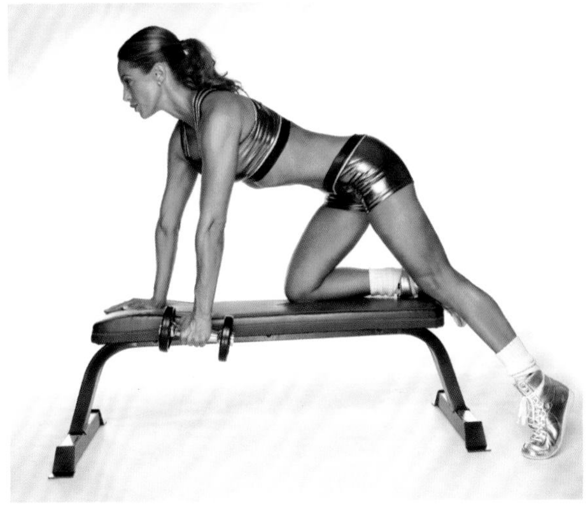

BENT OVER ROW FINISH

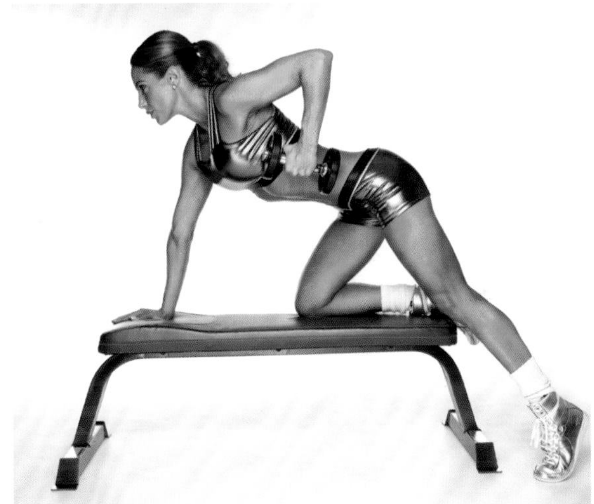

"SUPERWOMAN"

Lie on your stomach, either on floor, or on the stability ball bench as shown here. Start in a neutral position then bring up your upper body keeping your legs planted down squeezing your back area.

SUPERWOMAN START

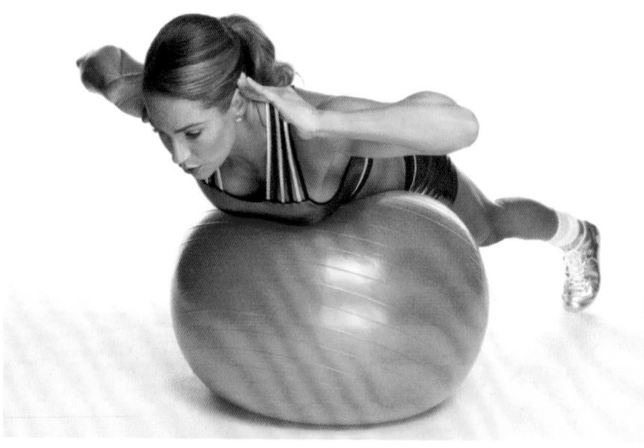

SUPERWOMAN FINISH

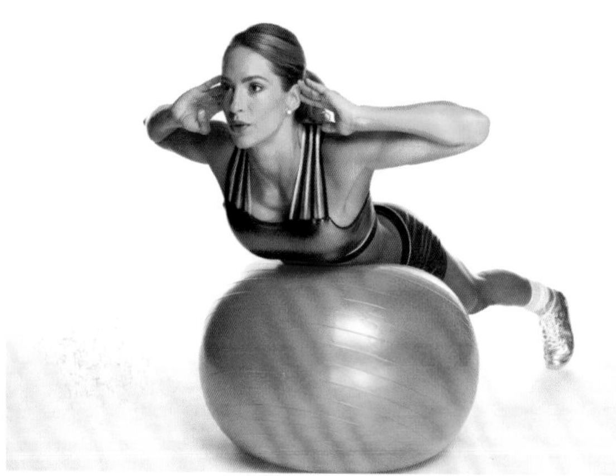

STANDING DUMBBELL ROW

This move is essential to the covergirl's program because it helps her to achieve a strong sexy back! Bend knees slightly and grasp your dumbbells. Keep your abs locked in tight, chest is up and put, and bend over. Make sure you have an arch in your back. Pull weights in, hold for a small pause and gently lower down in a controlled negative motion.

STANDING DUMBBELL ROW START

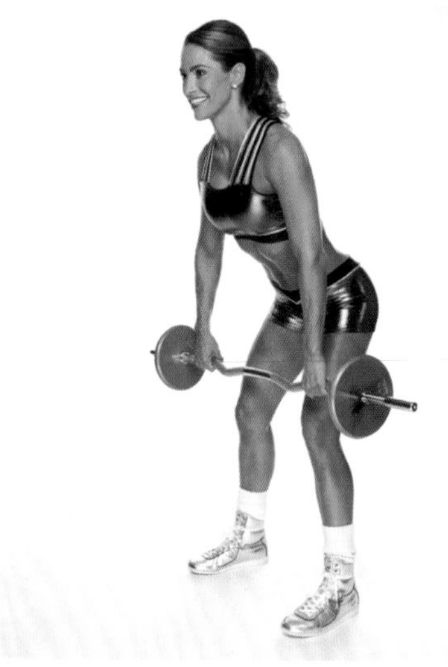

STANDING DUMBBELL ROW FINISH

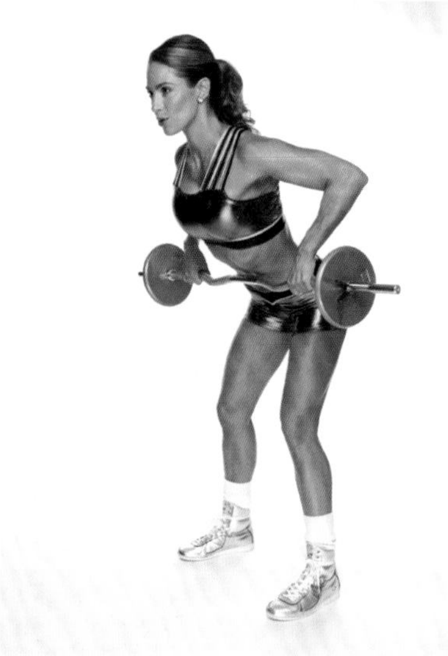

DUMBBELL PULLOVER

Start by lying across a flat bench with only your upper back making contact with the bench. Lift a dumbbell overhead and hold it at arm's length over your face. Without raising your hips, lower the dumbbell in an arc as you slowly breathe. Once you have reached a fully stretched position, hold it for a quick count of one and then raise it back up as you exhale.

JNL FIT TIP: Keep your hips in the same spot and don't let your hips rise.

DUMBBELL PULLOVER START

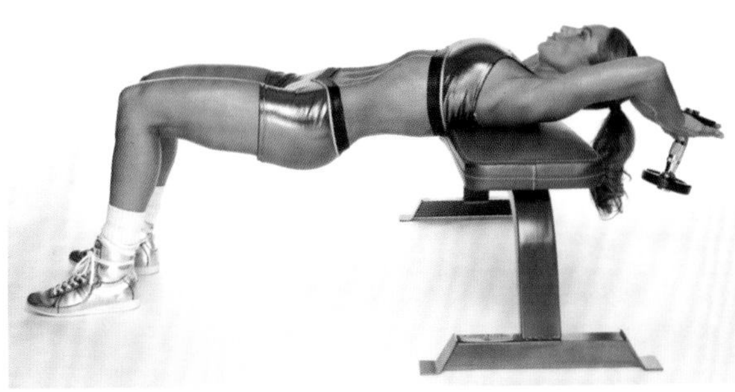

DUMBBELL PULLOVER FINISH

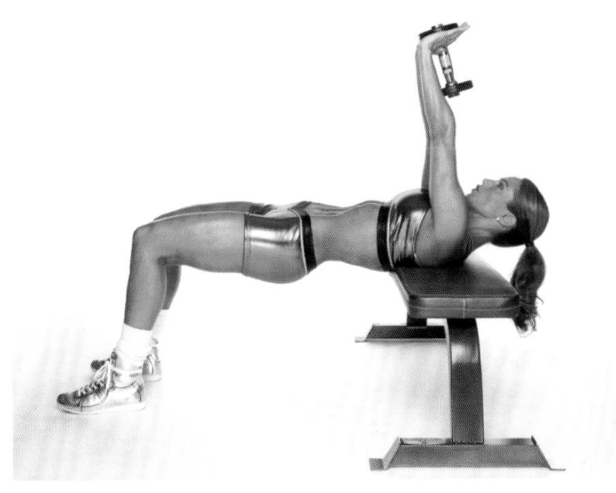

SUPER WOMAN ON STABILITY BALL WITH DUMBBELLS

SUPER WOMAN ON STABILITY BALL WITH DUMBBELLS START

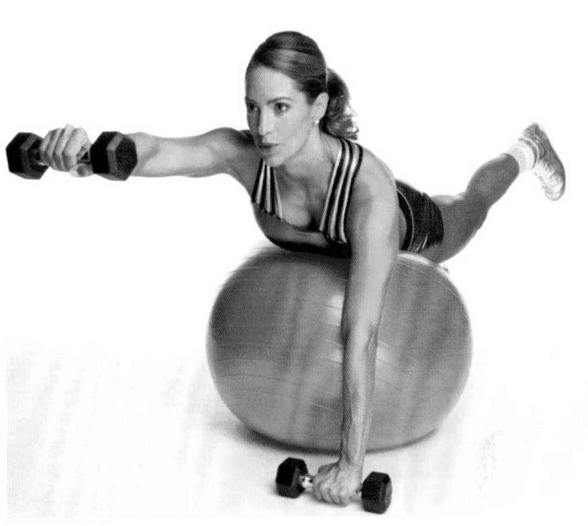

SUPER WOMAN ON STABILITY BALL WITH DUMBBELLS FINISH

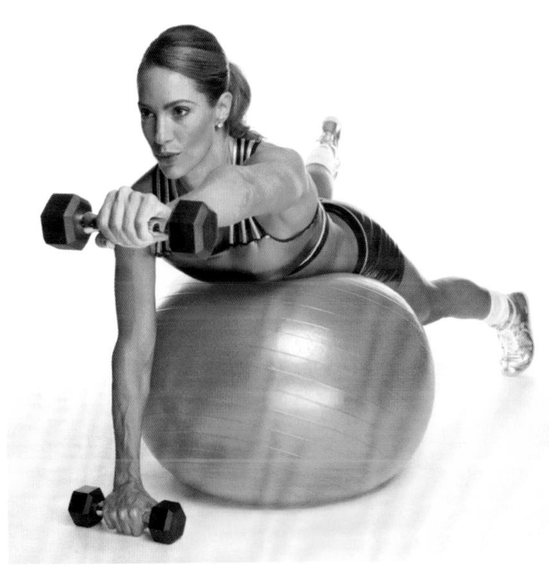

BACK FLIES ON STABILITY BALL

BACK FLIES ON STABILITY BALL START

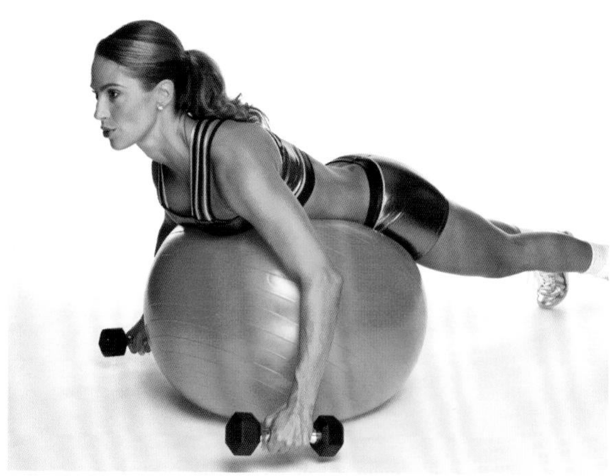

BACK FLIES ON STABILITY BALL FINISH

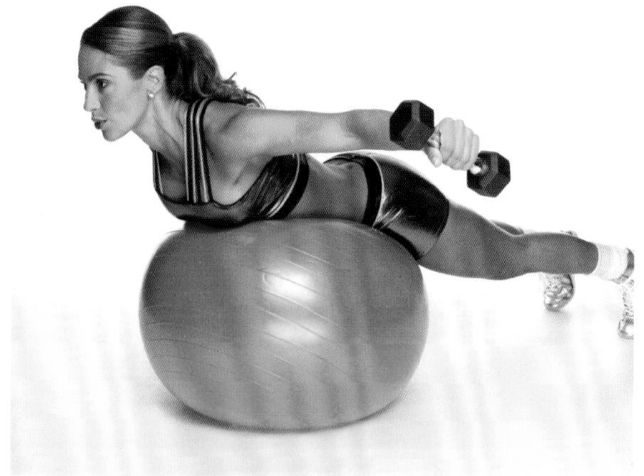

ONE ARM ROWS WITH TUBING

ONE ARM ROWS WITH TUBING START

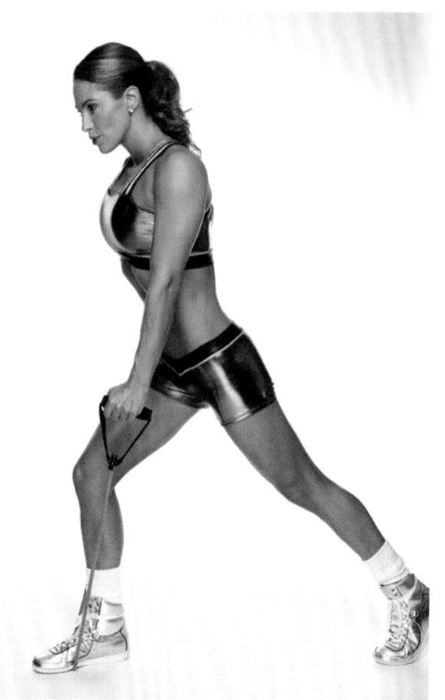

ONE ARM ROWS WITH TUBING FINISH

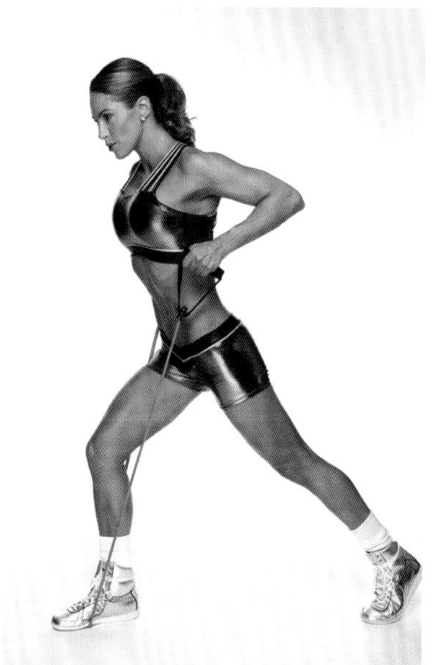

TRICEPS

List of Exercises for Triceps

- Seated Dumbbell Extension
- Close Hand Pushups
- Dumbbell Kickbacks
- Lying Dumbbell Extension
- Dips
- Tricep Kickbacks With Tubing
- Skull Crushers with Bar

SEATED DUMBBELL EXTENSION START

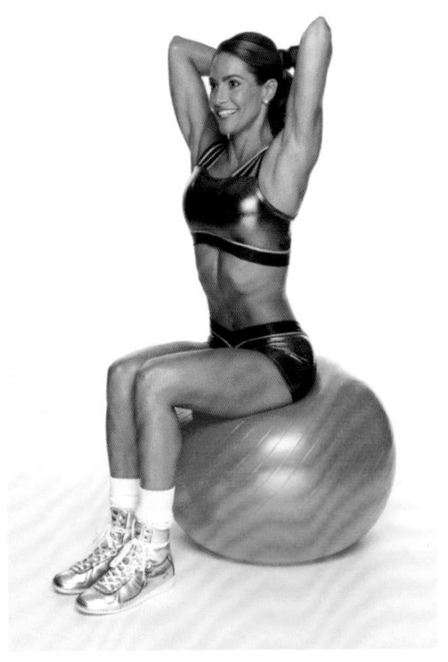

SEATED DUMBBELL EXTENSION

Sit on the bench and grasp one end of the dumbbell with two hands and raise it above your head. Start slowly lowering the dumbbell behind your head, keeping your elbows close to your head and pointed straight up throughout the exercise to keep the focus on your triceps. Lower the weight until you feel the stretch and hold it for one count, then press the weight back up.

SEATED DUMBBELL EXTENSION FINISH

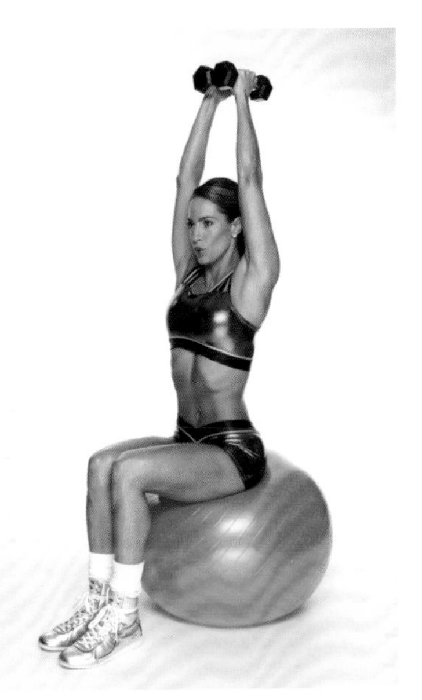

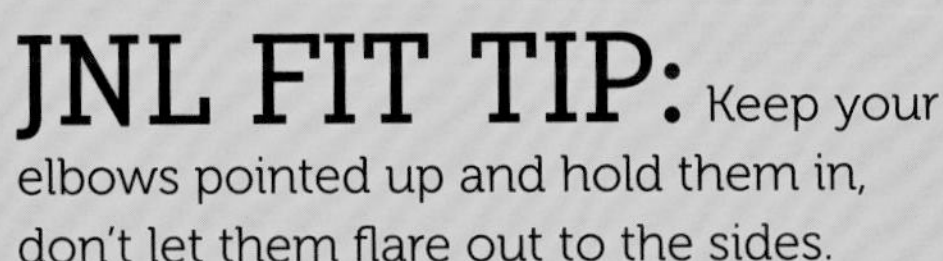
JNL FIT TIP: Keep your elbows pointed up and hold them in, don't let them flare out to the sides.

CLOSE HAND PUSHUPS

This is an excellent move for the entire upper body, but especially the triceps! If you can't perform them on your toes, then do them on your knees and work your way to your toes. Place your hands close together. Perform pushups, squeezing at the top of the movement. If it's hard for you to execute this move with your hands really super-close, keep them further apart and build up to closer.

DUMBBELL KICKBACKS

Gently bend your knees, keeping your abs tight; shoulders are up and back, chest is out, and neck and spine is in neutral alignment. Bend over from the waist and bring your arms up and back, bending at the elbows. With your wrists in neutral alignment, focus on your triceps, pushing the weight back, holding at the top of the movement. Gently release and lower down.

DUMBBELL KICKBACKS START

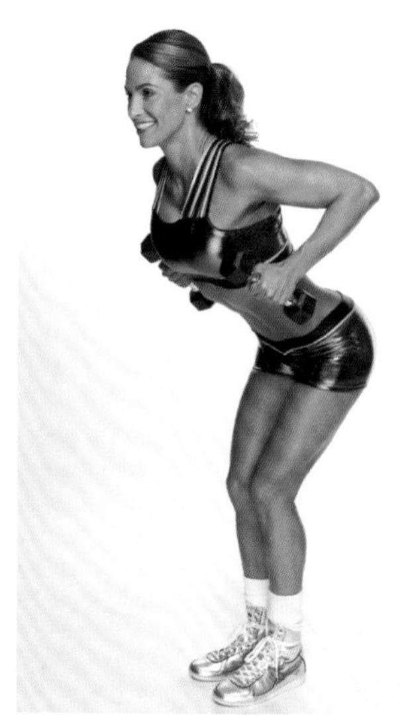

DUMBBELL KICKBACKS FINISH

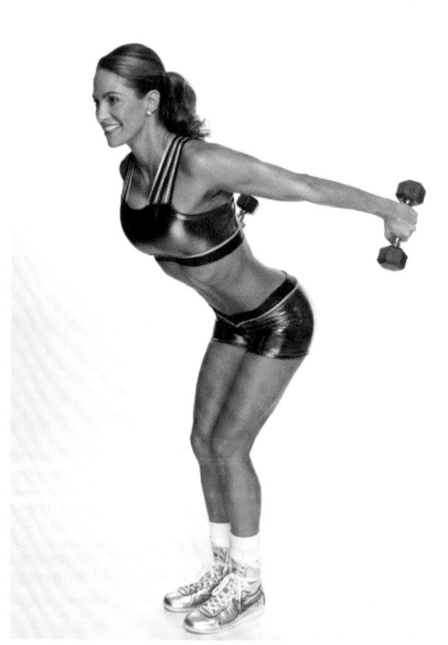

LYING BARBELL EXTENSION

Lie on a flat bench with a barbell, arms extended over your head so you are looking straight up at them. Bend the elbows and slowly lower the barbell toward your shoulders, not your head.

JNL FIT TIP: Don't let your elbows flare out and keep them in and pointed straight up.

LYING BARBELL EXTENSION START

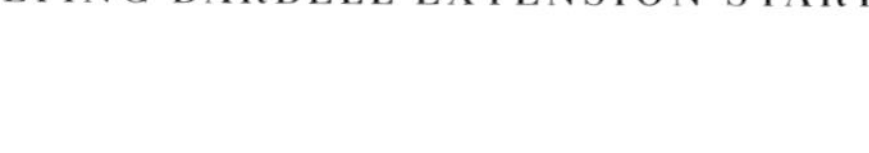

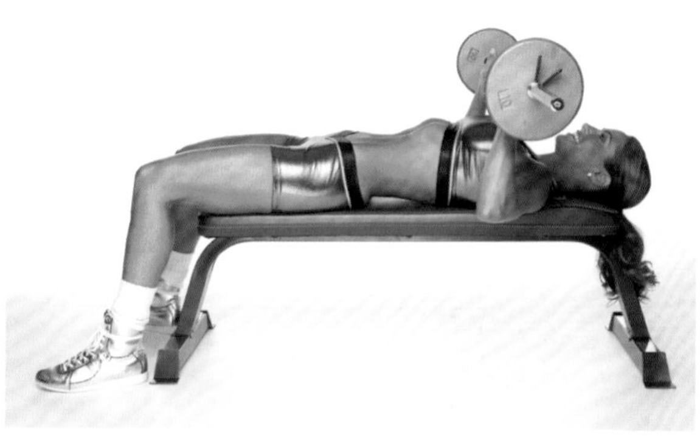

LYING BARBELL EXTENSION FINISH

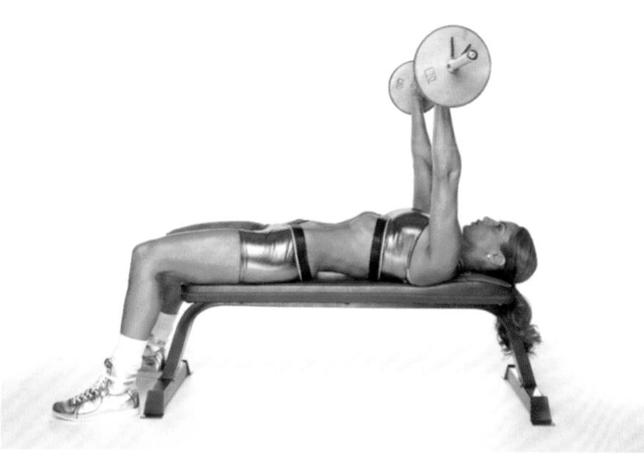

DIPS

Come to the edge of the bench. Firmly grasp onto the edge and bring your elbows back. Make sure your shoulders are back and down withyour chest out, allowing proper alignment of your spine. Gently bring your feet out in front of you. Lower down, focusing on contracting your triceps, and the entire back of your upper arms. Hold at the bottom for a small pause, and then bring it back up, squeezing your triceps as you bring yourself back to the starting position. Repeat.

DIPS START

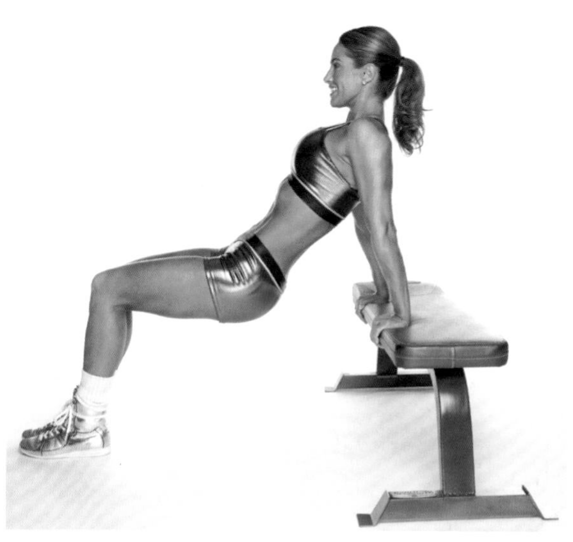

DIPS FINISH

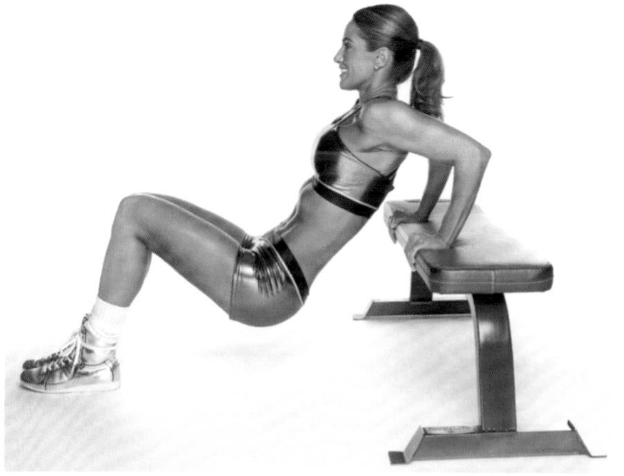

TRICEP KICK BACKS WITH TUBING

TRICEP KICK BACKS WITH TUBING START

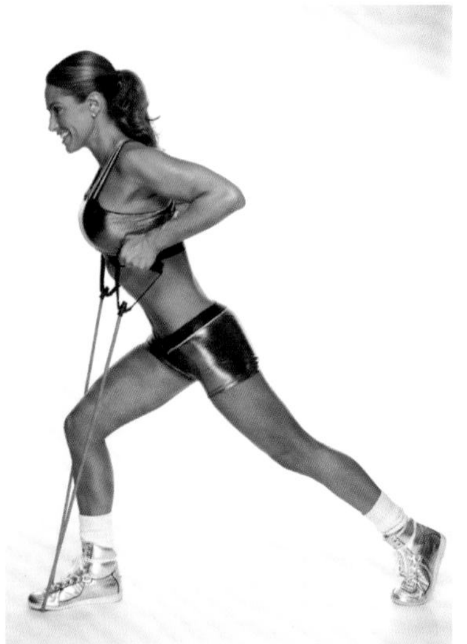

TRICEP KICK BACKS WITH TUBING FINISH

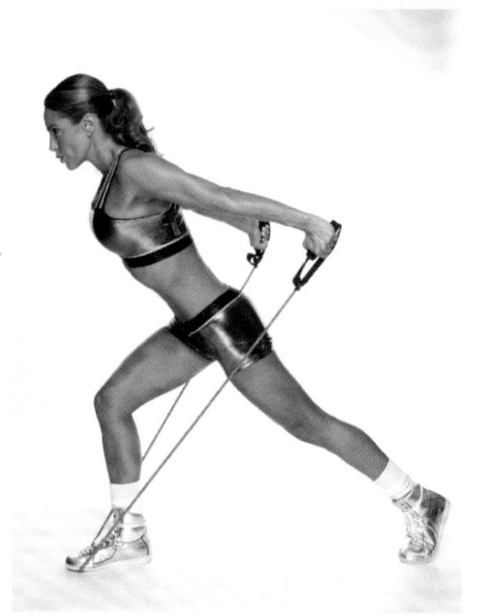

SKULL CRUSHERS WITH BAR

SKULL CRUSHERS WITH BAR START

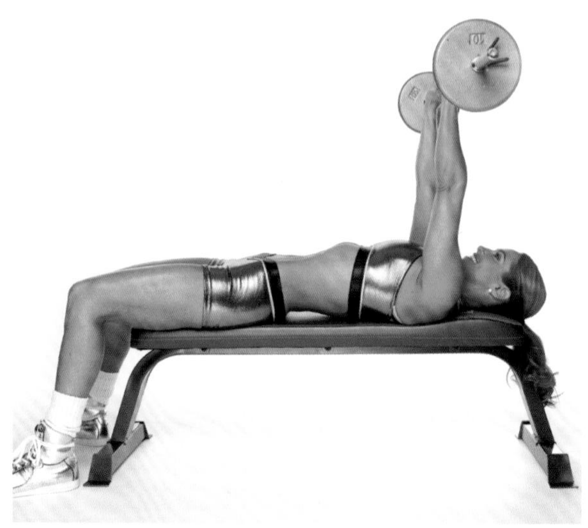

SKULL CRUSHERS WITH BAR FINISH

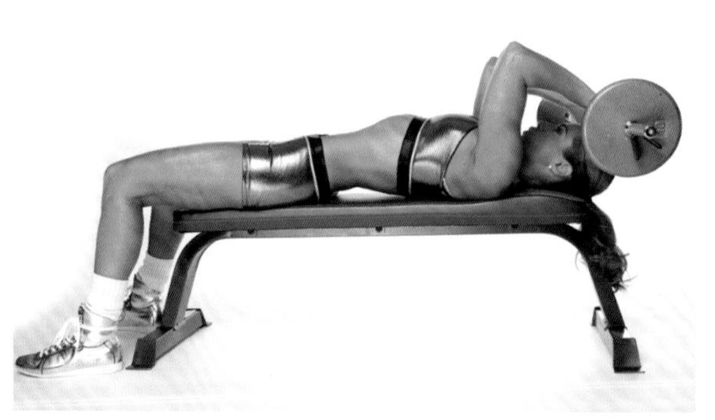

LOWER BODY

List of Exercises for Quads

- Dumbbell Squats
- Dumbbell Lunges
- Barbell Squats
- Dumbbell Side Plié Zipups

DUMBBELL SQUATS

Holding dumbbells in both hands and to your sides, stand with your feet a little wider than shoulder width apart. Hold your abs in tight, shoulders are up and back and your chest is out. Slightly arch your lower back, sticking your glutes out in a natural manner. Keep your knees slightly bent. Gently lower down into a squatting position keeping your spine in neutral alignment and your chest up.

DUMBBELL SQUATS START

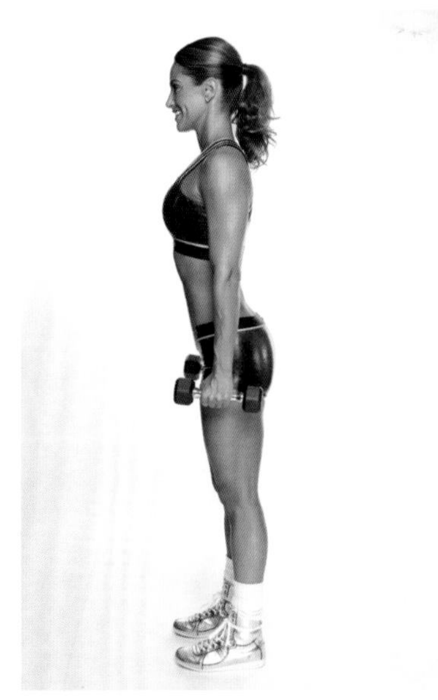

DUMBBELL SQUATS FINISH

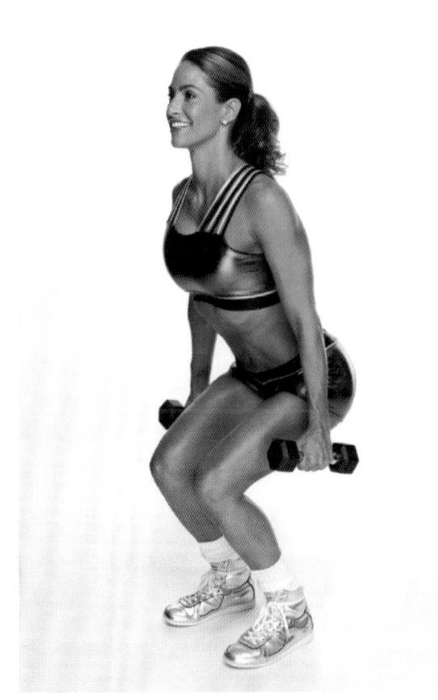

DUMBBELL LUNGES

Stand with your feet together, toes pointed straight forward and a dumbbell in each hand. Step forward with your right foot, then bend at the knees as you lower your hips until your left knee is just a few inches off the floor. Push with your right leg as you raise yourself back up to your starting point. Repeat until you have completed the amount of reps you planned on and then do the same with your left leg.

DUMBBELL LUNGES START

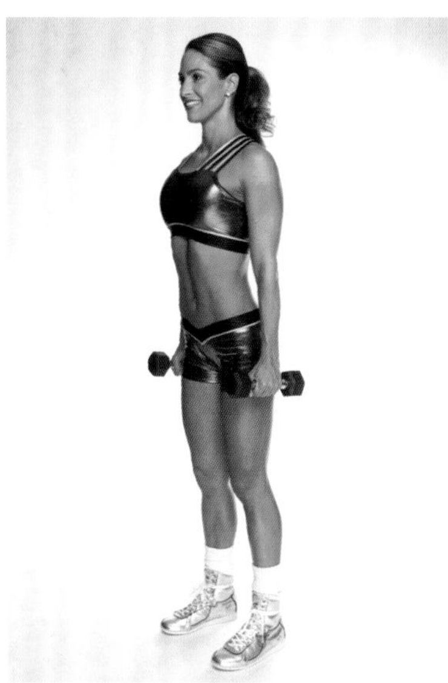

DUMBBELL LUNGES FINISH

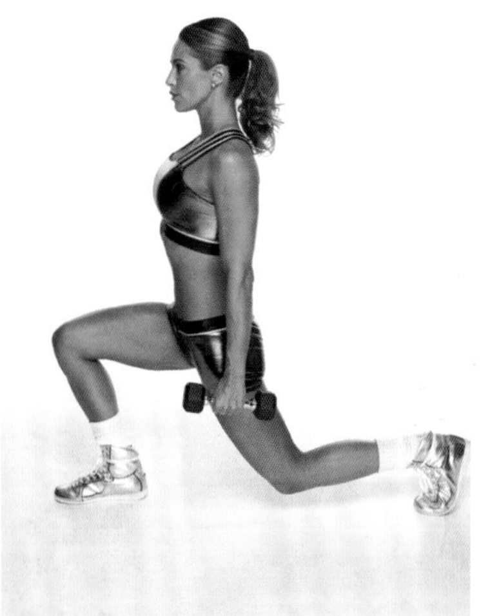

BARBELL SQUATS

BARBELL SQUATS

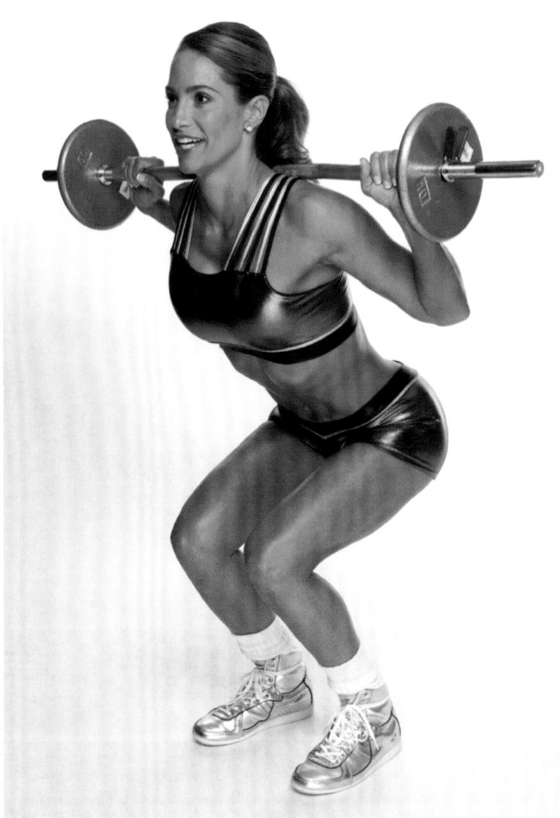

JNL FIT TIP:

Don't lift your foot up or point your toes in/out — keep your feet firmly planted on the floor, pointing straight forward.

DUMBBELL SIDE PLIÉ ZIPUPS

I love this move! It blasts the entire leg, especially the inner thigh! Start with your feet together, holding your dumbbells. Then lunge out gently to the side, keeping your knee bent and aiming to land softly. Then drag your foot up to the starting position.

PLIÉ ZIPUPS START

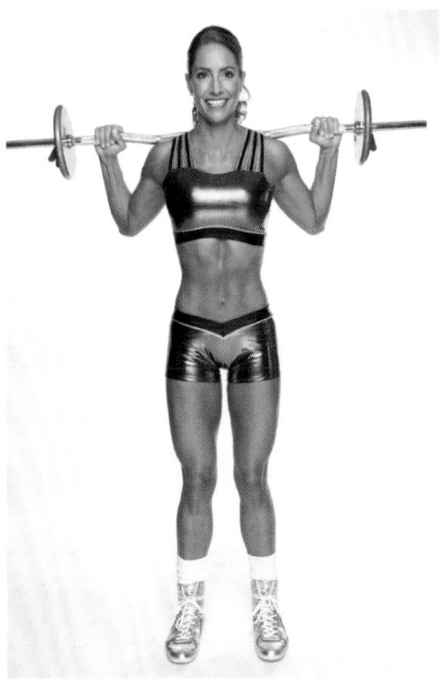

PLIÉ ZIPUPS FINISH

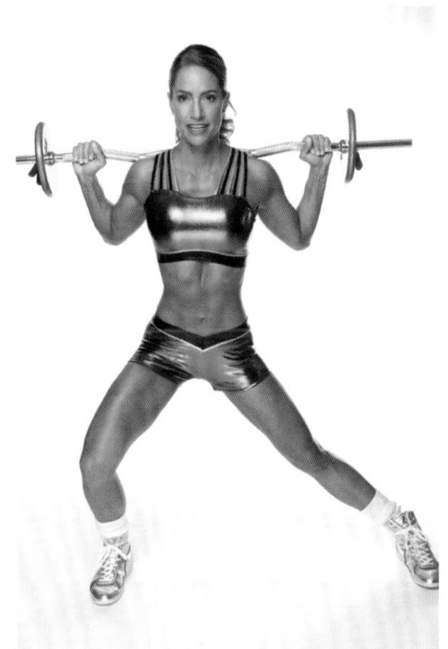

HAMSTRING

- Dead lifts

DEAD LIFTS

Stand up straight, with your feet shoulder width apart and a dumbbell in each hand, palms facing toward your legs. Bend forward at your hips and slowly lower the dumbbells in front of you until the weights touch the floor. Keep your back straight and raise your upper body and weights to the starting position.

> **JNL FIT TIP:**
> Don't hunch over. Keep your back fairly rigid throughout this exercise.

DEAD LIFTS

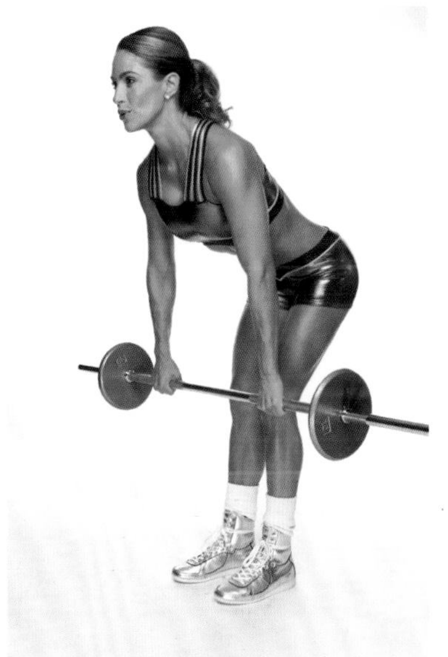

HIPS, BUNS AND THIGHS—THE BUTT AREA

- Fitness Model Dumbbell Step Ups
- JNL's Butt Blasters
- JNL's Bench Squats
- JNL One Leg Squeeze Up
- Pelvic Thrusts

FITNESS MODEL™ DUMBBELL STEP UPS

Clasp dumbbells in both hands. Place your foot firmly onto the bench. Step up, engaging all of your lower body muscles, squeezing throughout the glute area. At the top of the movement make sure you tighten your butt. Lower down in a controlled manner, working this negative motion of the movement. Repeat for 12 reps on the same leg, and then switch legs.

STEP UP START & FINISH

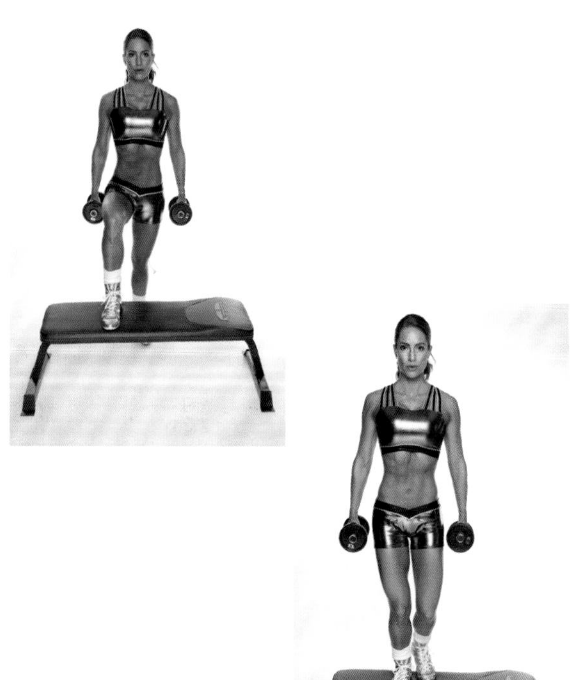

JNL'S BUTT BLASTERS

START

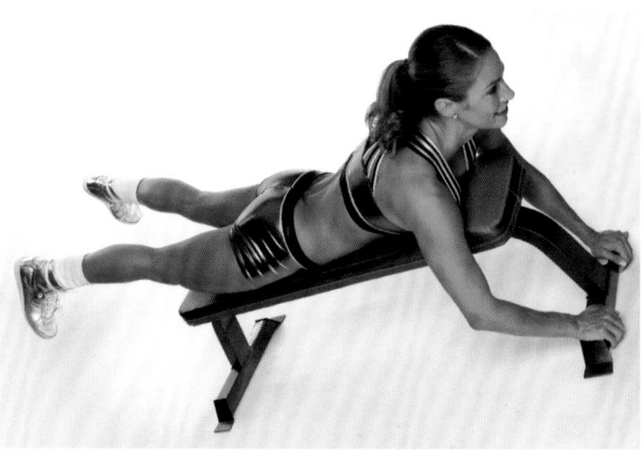

FINISH

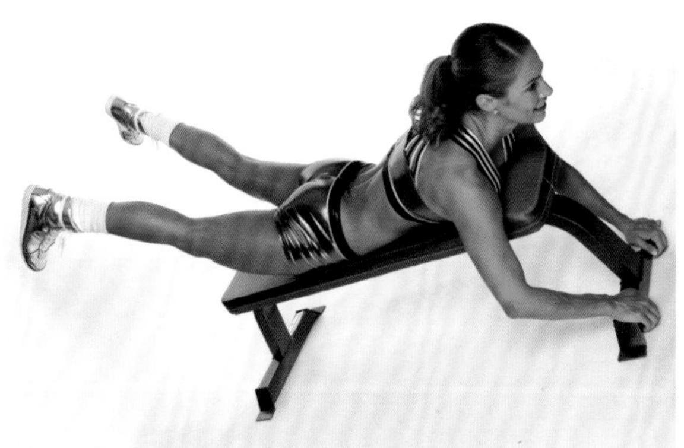

JNL'S BENCH SQUATS

START

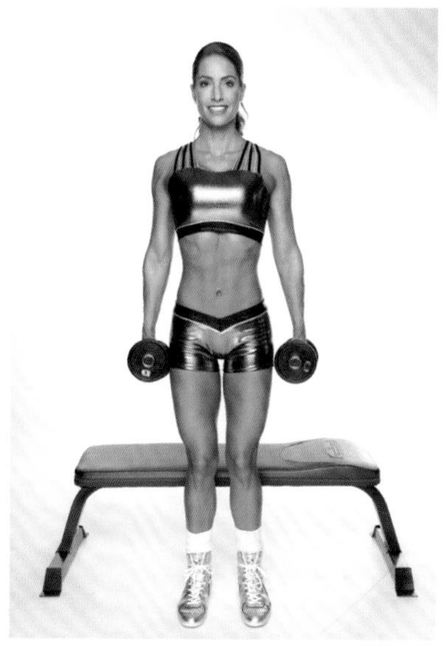

FINISH

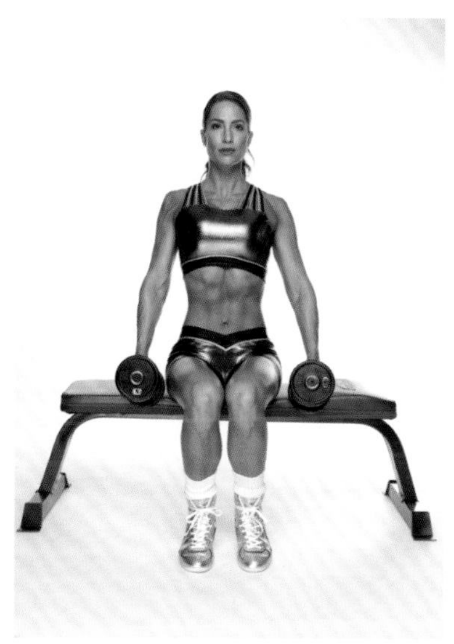

JNL ONE LEG SQUEEZE UP

START

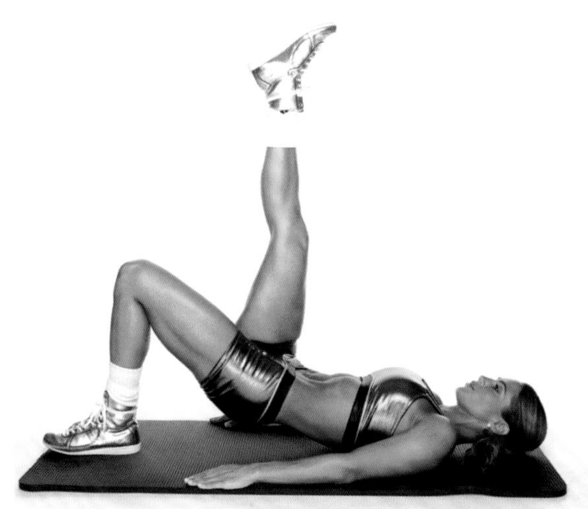

FINISH

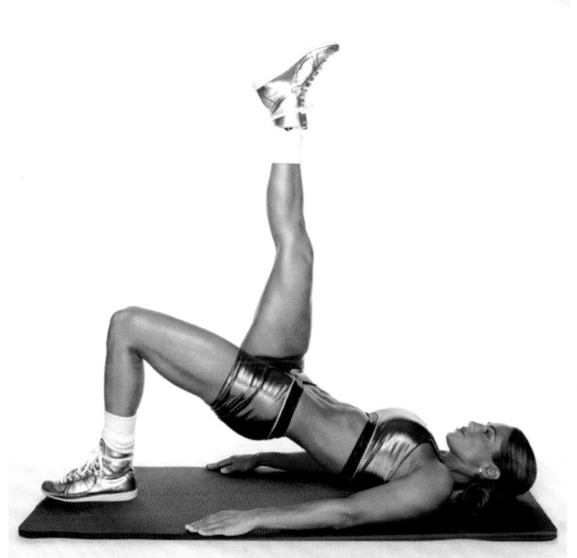

PELVIC THRUSTS

START

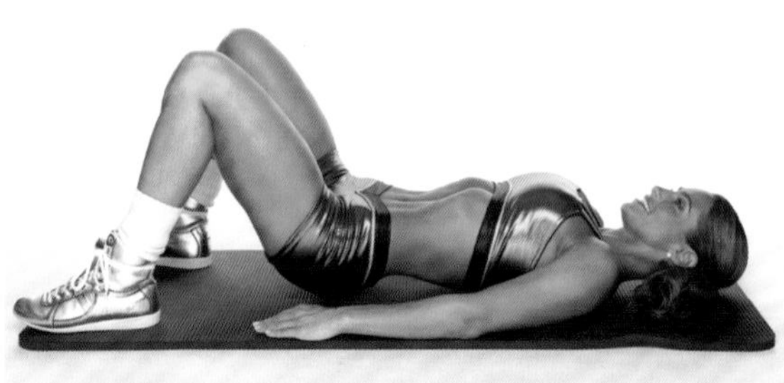

FINISH

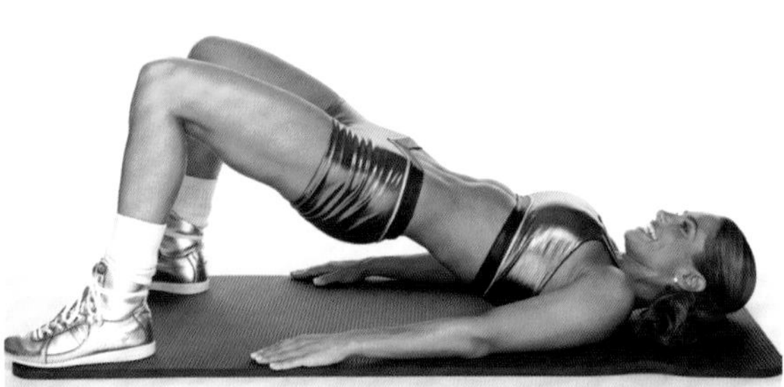

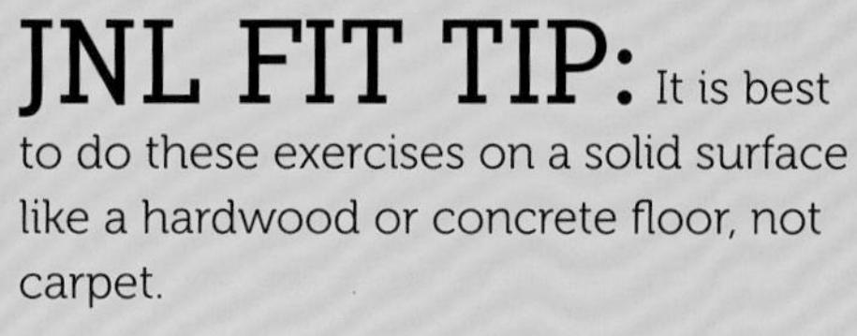

JNL FIT TIP: It is best to do these exercises on a solid surface like a hardwood or concrete floor, not carpet.

CALVES

- Standing Calf Raises
- One Leg Calf Raises
- Angled Calf Raises

STANDING CALF RAISES

Simply stand in place with a dumbbell in each hand and put your weight on the ball of your foot as if you were standing on your tip-toes. Repeat for 3 sets of 15.

START

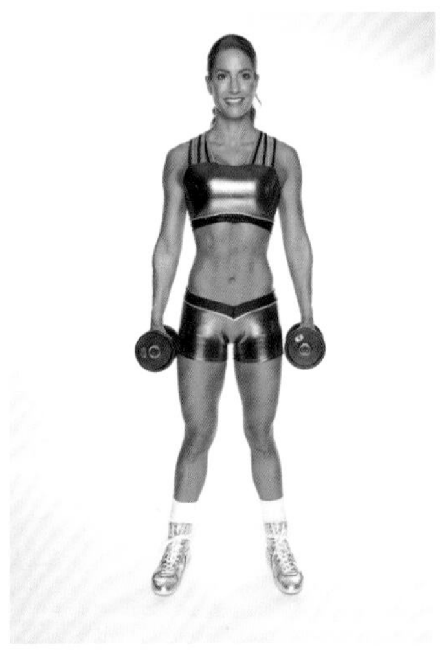

FINISH

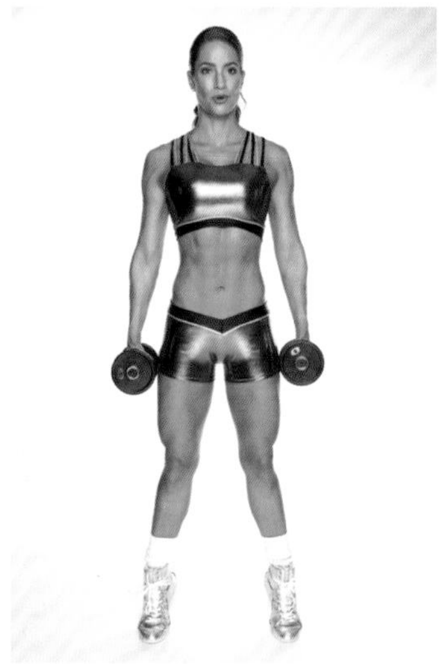

ONE LEG CALF RAISES

Implement the same movement as the Fitness Model Standing Calf Raises but do it one leg at a time. Repeat for 3 sets of 15.

START

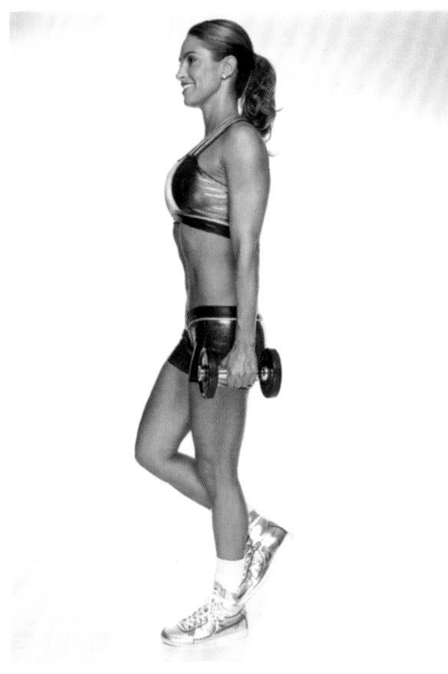

FINISH

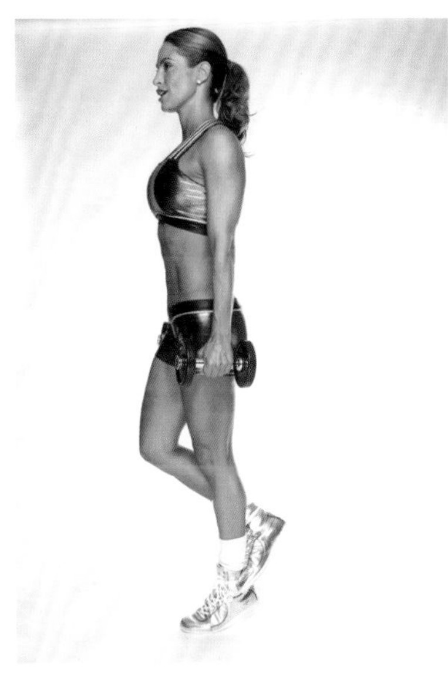

ANGLED CALF RAISES

Start by holding a dumbbell in each hand and stand with feet shoulder-width apart. Turn your toes out so that your feet form a 45-degree angle. Keeping your legs straight, raise up on your toes as high as possible, pause for a count of one and slowly lower to the starting position.

START

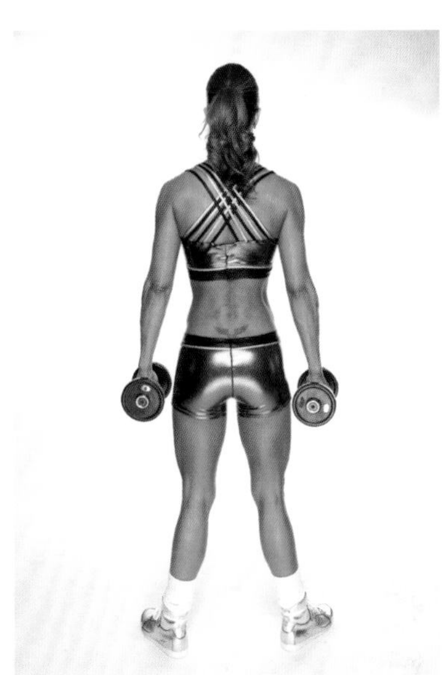

FINISH

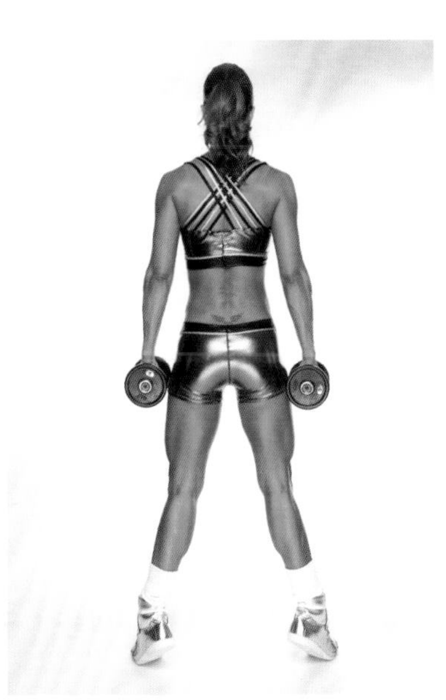

ABDOMINALS

List of Exercises for Abdominals

- Floor Crunches
- Twist Crunches
- Ball Crunches
- Bent Knee Leg raises
- Firecracker Abs
- Standing Twists
- Knee Roll Ins on Stability Ball
- Ab Circle Pro Exercises!
- Ab Roll Up with Medicine Ball

FLOOR CRUNCHES

Lie on your mat and put your hands beside your head. Bring your knees together and place them flat on the floor about a foot from your hips. Start by pushing your lower back down and begin to roll your shoulders up, keeping your knees and hips stationary. Continue to push down as hard as you can with your lower back. The range of motion of this exercise is very limited and your shoulders should only come off the ground a few inches. Hold this position and flex your abs as hard as you can for a count of one and then slowly lower your shoulders to the ground; never stop pushing down with your lower back.

JNL FIT TIP: Don't lock your hands behind your head — they should be cupped at the sides of your head and not used for leverage)

FLOOR CRUNCHES START

FLOOR CRUNCHES FINISH

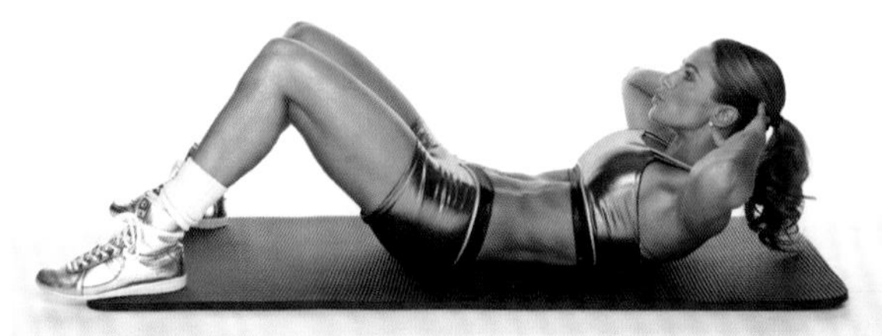

JNL FIT TIP: Don't lock your hands behind your head

TWIST CRUNCHES

Lie flat on your back with your knees bent and your hands beside your head. Let your legs fall as far as they can to your left side so that your upper body is flat on the floor and your lower body is on its side. Press your lower back down into the floor while you roll your upper body slightly up until your shoulder blades reach the ground. Concentrate on your obliques and contract and hold the crunch for a count of one. Hold the contraction and slowly lower to the starting position, count one and perform the next rep. Switch to the other side after you completed your planned number of reps.

TWIST CRUNCHES START

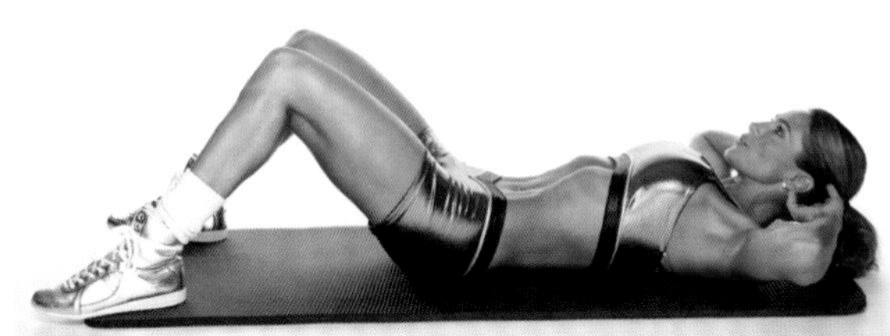

TWIST CRUNCHES FINISH

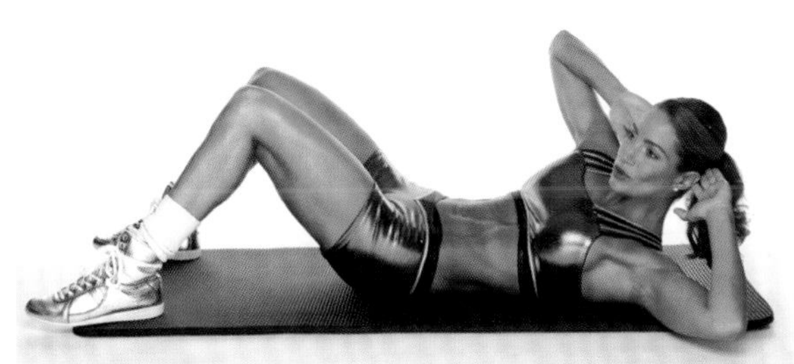

BALL CRUNCHES

Gently sit on your exercise ball and walk your legs forward to roll back onto the ball. Once you stabilize yourself, put your hands behind your head, keeping your spine in neutral alignment with your chin towards the sky. Exhale as you crunch up and inhale as you release back down. This is great for targeting your entire ab area.

BALL CRUNCHES START

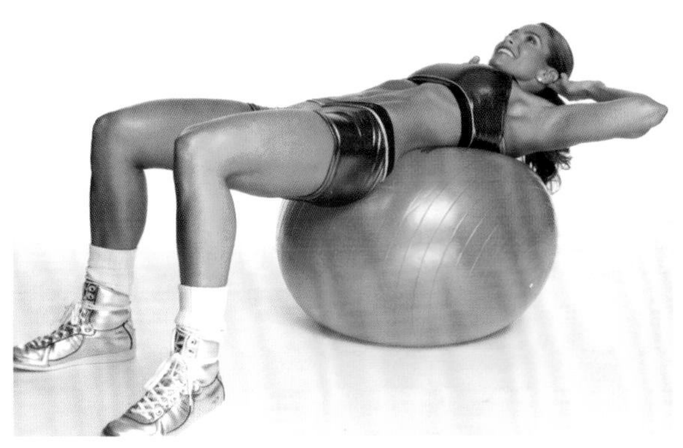

BALL CRUNCHES FINISH

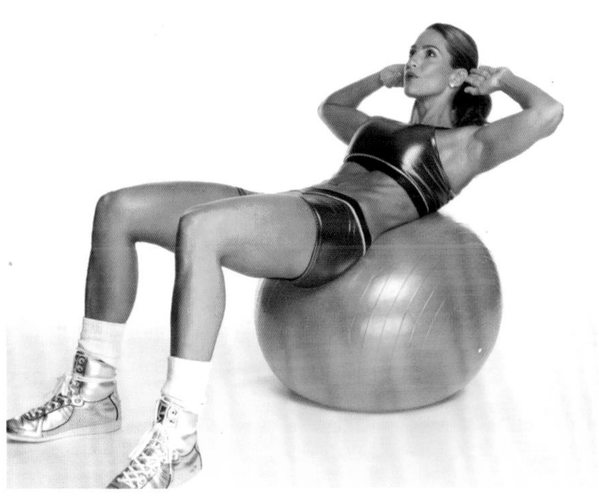

JNL FIT TIP: Don't lift your head up too far or let your lower back arch.

BENT KNEE LEG RAISES

Lie flat on your back on your mat with your hands under your hips, palms down for support. Lift your head up slightly off the floor and lift your legs off the floor while you bend them at your knees, pulling your thighs up towards your chest slowly. With your knees approaching your chest, contract your abs and slightly lift your pelvis off the floor. Slowly straighten your legs and bring them back down towards the floor but don't let them rest on the floor. Hold them in that extended position for a count of one and then bring them back up.

BENT KNEE LEG RAISES START

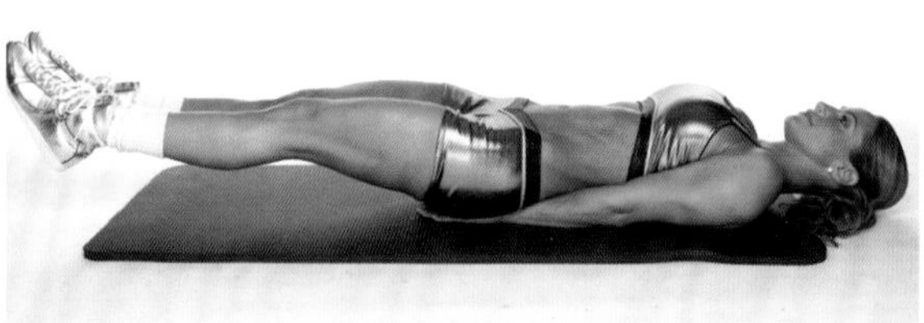

BENT KNEE LEG RAISES FINISH

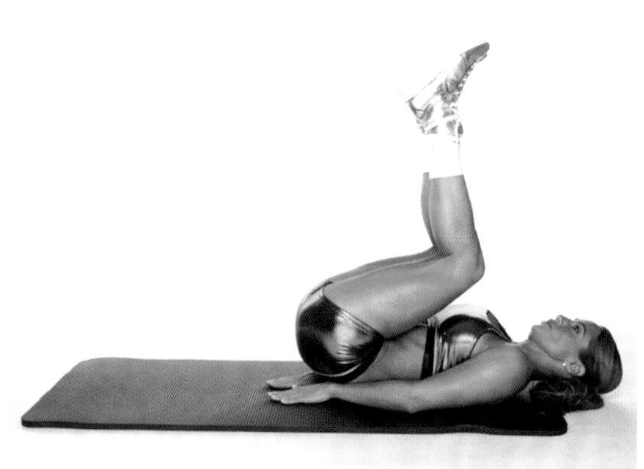

FIRECRACKER ABS

Lie down on the ground with your hands underneath your bottom and lift both your legs up to about 90 degrees and lift your legs upwards.

FIRECRACKER ABS START

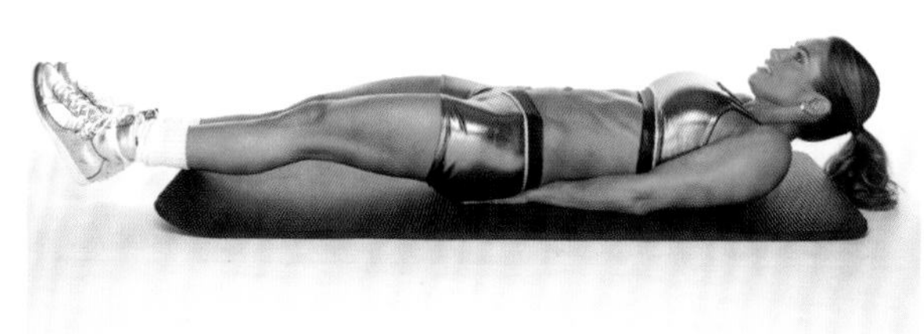

FIRECRACKER ABS FINISH

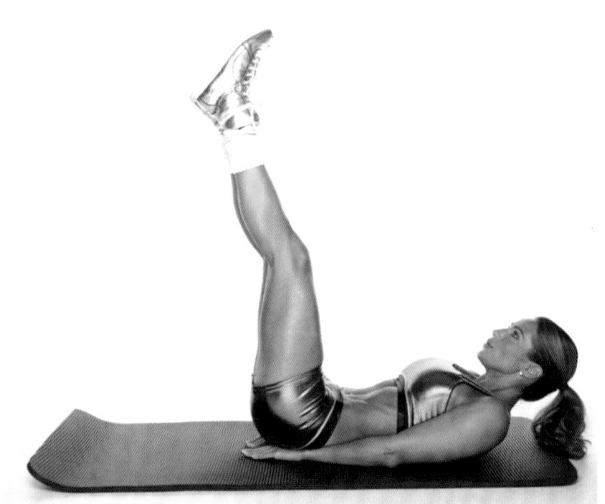

STANDING TWISTS

STANDING TWISTS START

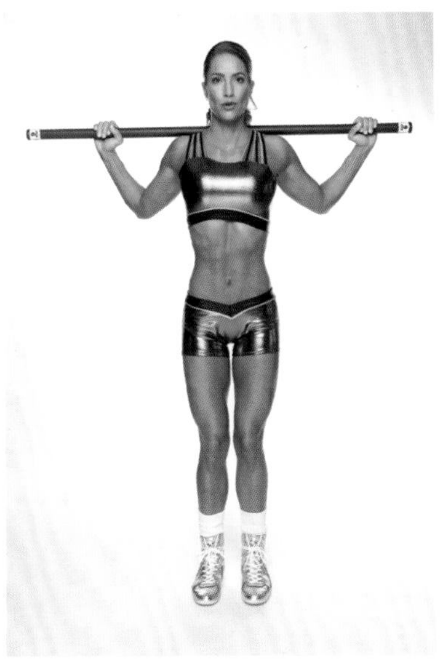

STANDING TWISTS FINISH

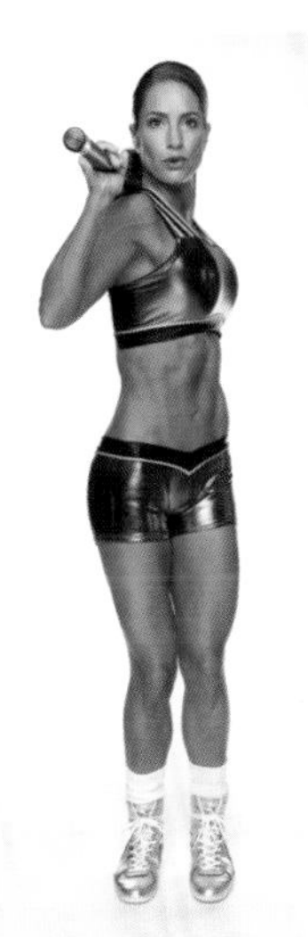

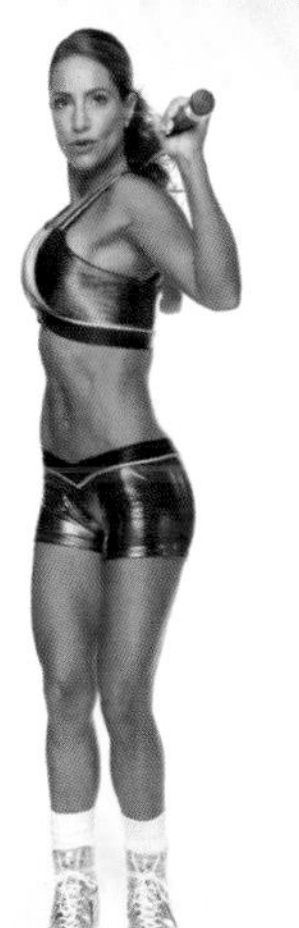

KNEE ROLL INS ON STABILITY BALL

KNEE ROLL INS ON STABILITY BALL START

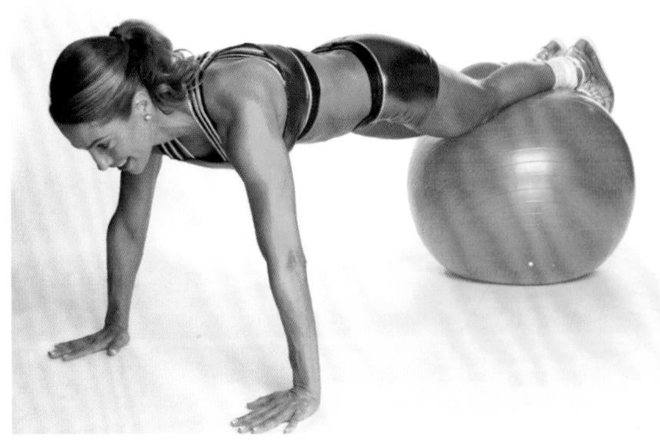

KNEE ROLL INS ON STABILITY BALL FINISH

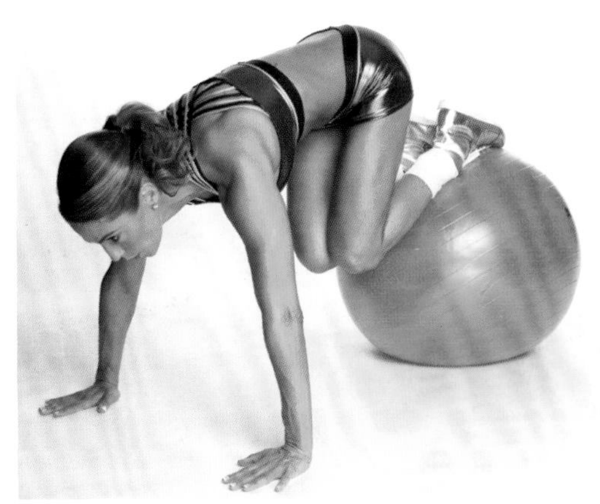

AB CIRCLE PRO EXERCISES!

You must get an Ab Circle Pro! Its absolutely indespensible because of its circular technology, that no other machine has. Plus they are very inexpensive and way worth the results! Visit www.JNLAbCirclePro.com to get yours today!

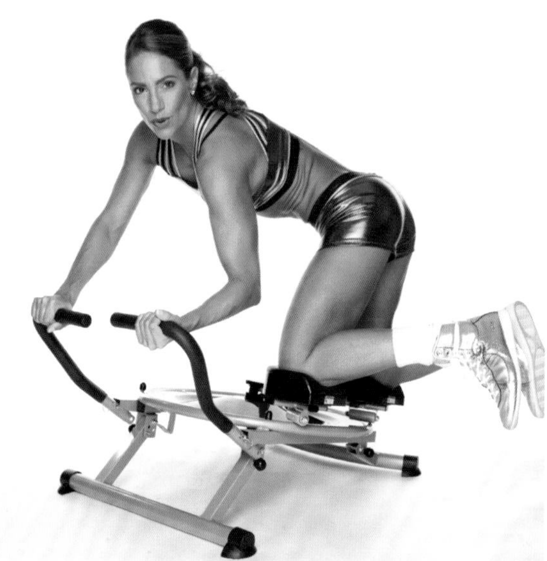

AB ROLL UP WITH MEDICINE BALL

START

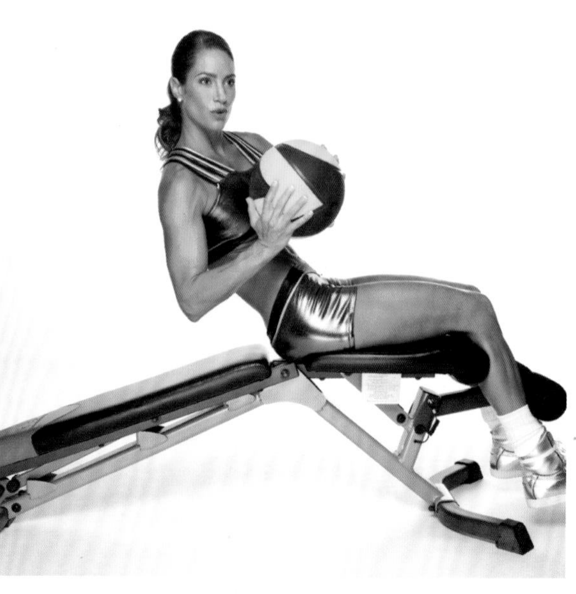

FINISH

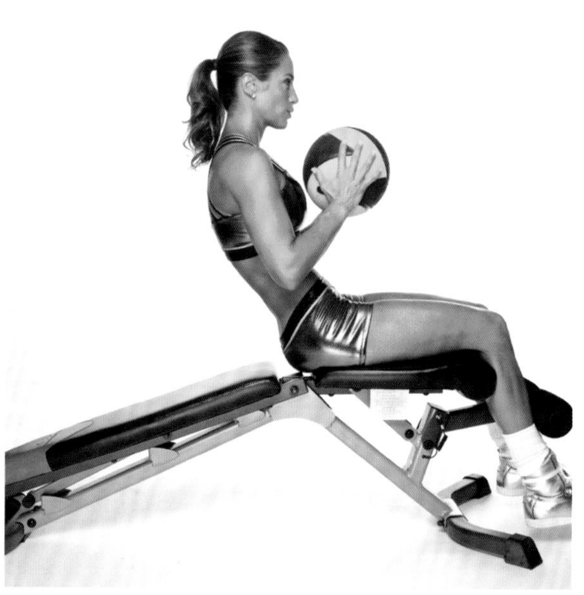

"R&R" FORMULA

You may know that the abbreviation 'R&R' means rest and relaxation. But in my Fitness Model diet, 'R&R' stands for recovery and recuperation. Again, I would like to emphasize that, in order to see results, do not over-train! You must allow your body time to heal and rebuild itself back up from the weight-training sessions.

"JNL-APPROVED" METAPHORS THAT MAKE FITNESS SIMPLE AND EASY TO UNDERSTAND

SANDPAPER METAPHOR

There are two sides of the coin when it comes to resistance training. When you work out, you must also allow your body time to recover and recoup. For your muscles to heal and rebuild, rest and recuperation is essential. Think of this metaphor: When you lift weights and engage your muscles into resistance training, it's as if you are taking sandpaper and scraping it on your skin, irritating it so much that you get an abrasion. Therefore, you must allow your muscles to "heal," allowing time for a "scab" to form on top of the muscles. In other words, you must allow time to form a "callous" from the sandpaper. If you don't allow yourself time to heal in between weight training sets, you are "irritating" your muscles too soon, not allowing the "callous" to form and heal, just opening the wound again and again.

If you over-train, you are cheating yourself and not letting the "wounds" heal. I cannot stress this enough; please don't over train and rush the process. Instead, give yourself the gift of time and follow this program.

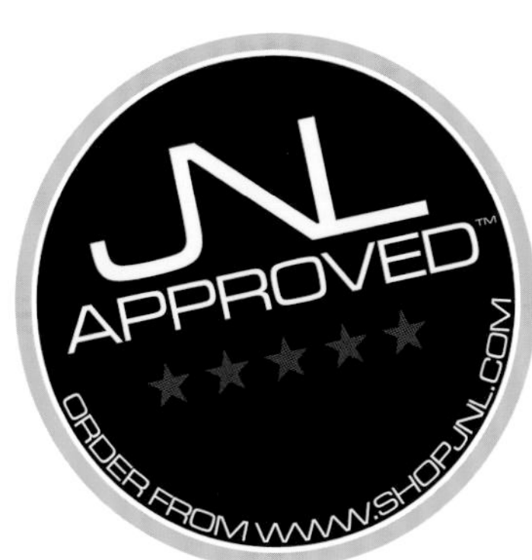

THE FIRE HYDRANT PRINCIPLE

Your body is like a fire hydrant; it only takes one tool to unlock it. Once it's unlocked, it shows its ultimate potential with an at-times uncontrollable, extremely forceful release. The Fitness Model Diet is that one wrench that can unlock your body's full potential. It took me 2 months of working with the Fitness Model Diet to begin seeing results. My body lay dormant for that 2 months, then it happened! The floodgates opened and my body started releasing the fat. I urge you not to give up and know that it's not about being perfect, but being persistent.

THE DYNAMITE PRINCIPLE

Don't cheat yourself by using weights that are easy for you to finish the last 8-12 reps. Make sure you are challenging yourself, in that by the 8-12th rep, it is very difficult for you to finish. Let me illustrate with the stick of dynamite analogy: You can have a stick of dynamite and tap it with a pencil and nothing happens, you can tap it with a pencil 10 times and still nothing happens, or you can take sledgehammer and hit it once, and the stick of dynamite will explode. In the same way, it is imperative to use a weight that is heavy enough to hit your muscles, not with a pencil tap but with the power of a sledgehammer!

CARDIO

CARDIO CORE PRINCIPLES

Fitness models never run; they do cardio at 65-75% of their target heart rate. When you over-train cardio, you start eating your muscle and your appetite goes out of control. I have been there. I would get out of the gym with such a big appetite that I would eat spaghetti, chocolate donuts, or anything in sight that was high-carb to refuel my body.

You need to train like a Fitness Model, and Fitness Models don't over-train, or overdo cardio. That way, we don't overeat or "burn off "our muscle mass.

Another great fitness model technique is to weave cardio into your weight-training workout, in between sets. Many of you have seen me perform about 45 seconds to one minute of speed rope in between my weight sets, to help keep my heart rate up in the fat burning zone. This allows me to get the best of both worlds: to burn off fat with the bursts of cardio, and also to build muscle while weight training.

SPEED ROPE

Jumping rope with a speed rope is a great toning and cardiovascular workout. Start slow, take your time, and get enough rest between exercises to re-energize your body.

The following is a suggested routine that will help you get the most from your jump rope workout, and have fun doing it:

- Perform one jump rope exercise for 45 seconds to a minute.
- Rest for a few seconds, or until your body feels re-energized.
- Perform the next jump rope exercise for 45 seconds to a minute.
- Rest for a few seconds, or until your body feels re-energized.
- Perform the next jump rope exercise, and so on.

For beginners, follow the above pattern for 10 minutes. As you progress, work your way up to 10 to 15 minutes for an intense workout.

For the first couple of exercises, turn the rope slowly to warm up. Then, gradually speed up the pace, until you are performing faster moves about halfway through your workout. Then, gradually slow your pace down, until you are turning the rope very slowly on the last two to three exercises to cool down. Below are some fun, basic exercises to get you started and to add variety to your jump rope routine.

- The baseline (also simply called "line") refers to a starting line to be used as a point of reference on feet placement and jumps. Unless otherwise specified, the baseline should be horizontal to your body. Only certain exercises will specifically call for a vertical baseline, which will be vertical to your body and between your feet.
- A balancing bounce is the bounce used between rope turn jumps. The balancing bounce can be a simple jump, or a more complicated movement. Some exercises call for balancing bounces, others don't.

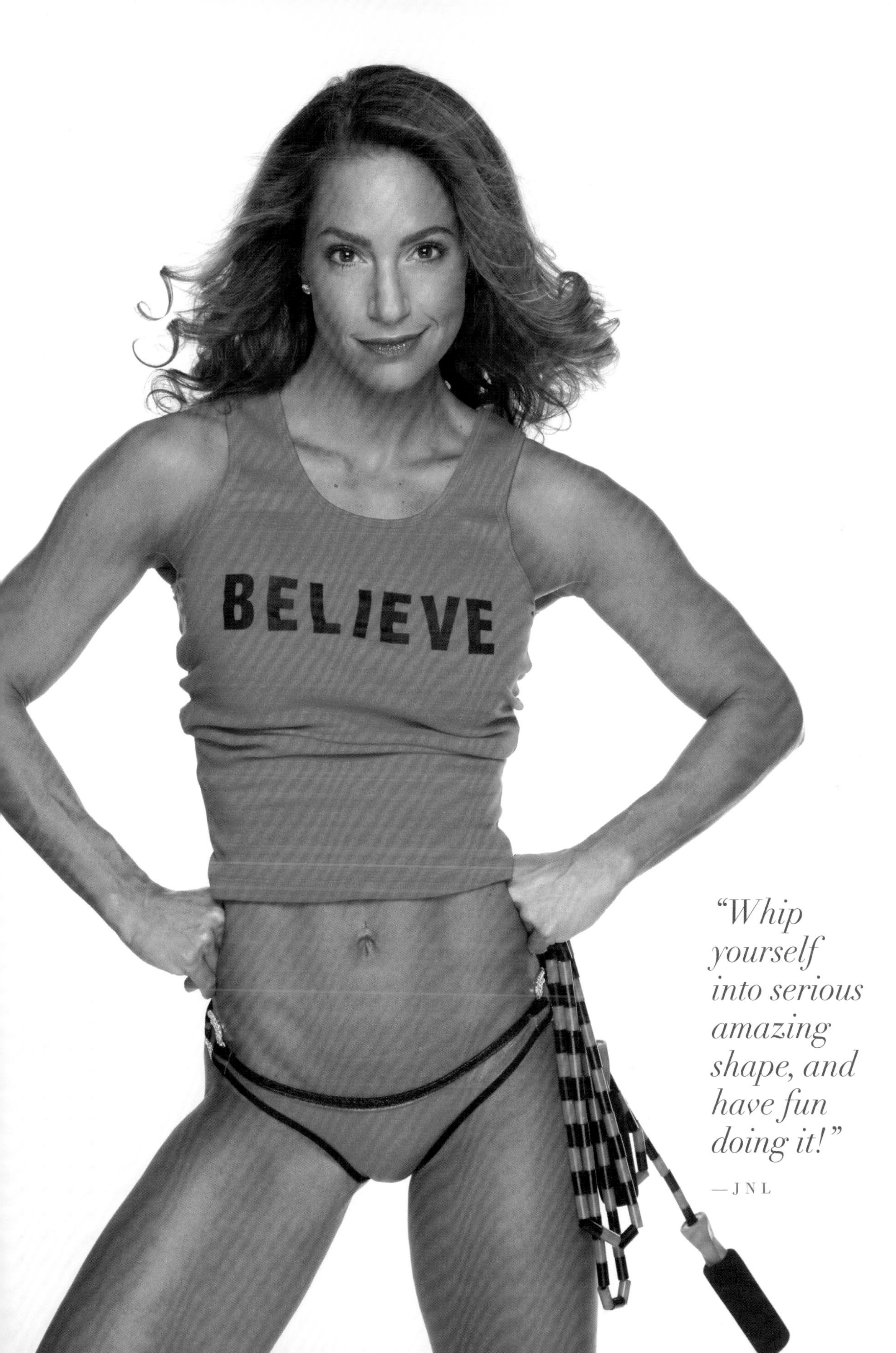

"Whip yourself into serious amazing shape, and have fun doing it!"

—JNL

CHAPTER 5:

Short on Time and Long on Needing a Workout?

JNL'S ALL-TIME FAVORITE WORKOUT ROUTINES

"It's about working out smarter, not harder to get maximum results in minimum time."

—JNL

"The method to my madness is called JNL Fusion"

—JNL

WWW.JNLFUSION.COM

THE JNL TOTAL BODY WORKOUT

"I call my training methodology JNL Fusion. I have blended the best fields of fitness into one, and infused it with intensity and power yet also focus and grace. And your body will prove its powerfulness in the results that it gets."

—JNL

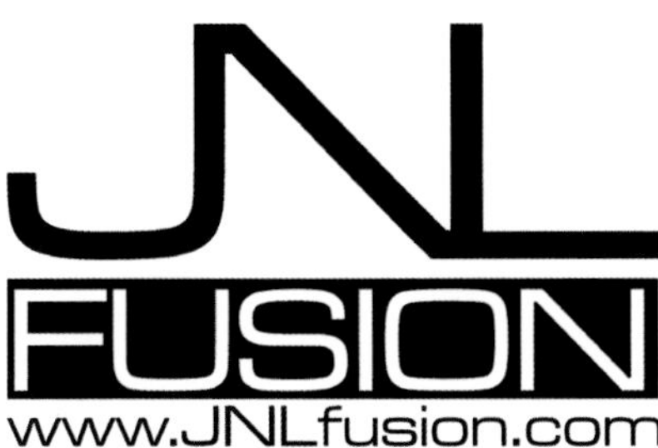

Here's my favorite fast-paced circuit, for when I'm short on time and long on needing a workout! This is the exact workout that I do, to hit all of the major muscle groups of my body from top to bottom. It involves three circuits, performed one right after another.

JNL'S FAST-PACED CIRCUIT

Warm up for 5 minutes, walking in place, pumping arms.

CIRCUIT #1:

3 sets each of 18-21 reps of:

- Lunges with either straight bar behind the head, or dumbbells Squats
- Standing Shoulder Presses with Dumbbells
- Bicep Curls with dumbbells
- Triceps Kick-Backs with dumbbells

REPEAT THIS CIRCUIT 3 TIMES, FROM START TO FINISH THEN MOVE ONTO CIRCUIT #2

CIRCUIT #2:

- Standing Shoulder Press Bar
- Standing Triceps Extension with Bar
- Side Lateral Raises with Dumbbells

CIRCUIT #3

- Ab Crunches on Ball
- Knee Roll Ins on Ball
- Ab Circle Pro for 3 min. (www.JNLAbCirclePro.com)

THE JNL QUADRUPLE THREAT BUTT-BLASTING CIRCUIT

(When you Need an Instant Booty Lift & Want to Tighten and Tone Your Entire Tush!"

Repeat this Circuit 3 Times with little rest in between. Perform 8-12 reps if you want to build muscle, 18-21 reps if you need to want to maintain your muscle tone and build endurance

- Dead lifts with dumbbells
- Step-Ups with Dumbbells
- Bench Squats with Dumbbell
- JNL's Butt Blasters; Perform 30 reps per set.

THE JNL "NO MORE WIGGLE WHEN YOU WALK & WAVE" WORKOUT

JNL Tackles Those Hard-to-Hit Target Areas; Arm Flab, Back Fat & Inner Thigh Wiggle, Be Gone!

The areas of a woman's body most prone to being jiggly and wiggly are the back of her arms, or the triceps area, and her inner and outer thighs. This workout will target these trouble zones, tightening and toning them up to blast off the jelly!

- Lying Dumbbell Extension, aka Skull Crushers
- Close Hand Pushups
- Dumbbell Kickbacks
- Dips
- Overhead Triceps Kickbacks. on Stability Ball
- Triceps Kickbacks. with Tubing
- Pelvic thrusts
- Ab Circle Pro for 3 minutes; remove interlocking pin and perform Inner & Outer Thigh Movement (www.JNLAbCirclePro.com

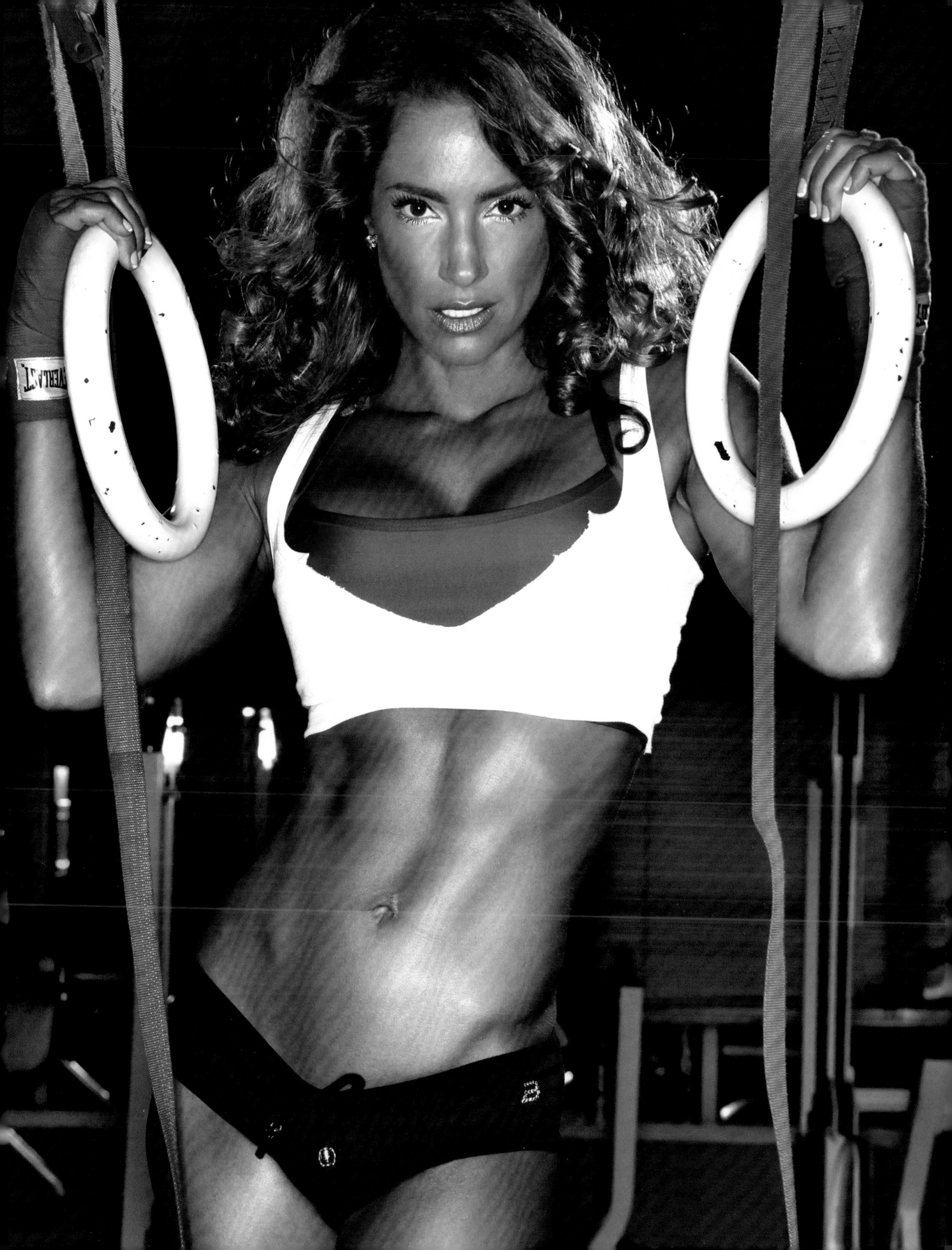

CHAPTER 6:

THE FITNESS MODEL FOOD PLAN & GUIDE TO SUPPLEMENTS

"I've got a big bag of super fitness model tricks, that will help you get maximum results in minimum time!"

—JNL

"Fitness Models EAT! They don't starve themselves, and they don't eat accidentally!"

–JNL

THE FITNESS MODEL FOOD PLAN FORMULA

There is a certain formula to eating like a Fitness Model. Fitness models eat breakfast like a queen, lunch like a princess, and dinner like a peasant! This cute adage will keep you focused on how important it is to trickledown your calories through out the day.

Follow this formula, except at dinner, where you take out the whole grain carb. Fitness models take out the whole grain carb at dinner, because they are working with their bodies to burn off fat and build muscle in their workouts the morning after. If you were to eat that complex carb at night, you would wake up with more carbs to burn off. Make sense?

BREAKFAST

This is the most important meal of the day! Don't do what I used to, long ago, and NOT eat breakfast thinking it was going to help me save calories. If you skip breakfast, you will only become super-ravenous by midday and end up eating more than you should. Skipping breakfast will also slow down your metabolism, which you don't want.

LEAN SOURCE OF PROTEIN +

CUP TO 1 CUP OF FIBROUS CARB
(1/2 if fruit, 1 cup if vegetable) +

WHOLE GRAIN CARB (1/2 CUP) =

FITNESS MODEL FOOD PLAN FORMULA

LUNCH

Lunch is very important. Don't forgo lunch to help you save time at the office, or because you are running errands. If you do, you are setting yourself up for failure at dinner. You will end up eating the paint off the walls or whatever is in sight by the time dinner rolls around, if you forgot to eat lunch.

LATE AFTERNOON SNACK

This meal is crucial! From my countless consultations, I have learned that this late afternoon time period is so tricky! I call it our "Withcy-ithcy" hour, when we are prone to slipping. Don't do it! We have had a long day, our patience is running out, and we are feeling the effects of all of the day's duties. Our office friend shows up with a box of cookies from the bakery down the street, and we end up giving in! But I promise you, if you ate a great big breakfast, had your mid morning protein shake, and your satisfying lunch, you won't give in.

Please make it a point to enjoy another protein shake, small protein bar, or a Mini-meal to keep your hunger at bay and under control until dinner.

DINNER

Finally we are home, with our family and loved ones. Sigh of relief as we all gather together for a meal at home. Dinner is a meal to be enjoyed with our friends and family, but don't overdo it! Remember this very important key; focus on your lean source of protein and also your fibrous carb. Aim to focus on a steamed vegetable, such as broccoli, asparagus, spinach, or a large green salad to keep the complex carbs at bay.

POST-DINNER SNACK

In order to work with my body, and not against it, I always aim to have a protein shake made with water before I go to bed. Why? Well, number one, I'm hungry! My metabolism has gotten to be so efficient that I am always burning off my calories effectively. Secondly, I want to have adequate amounts of "bio-available" protein in my system, so that I may repair and recover my muscle mass during my rest. I wake up with tons of energy, knowing that I "fed" my muscles.

JNL FIT TIP: An excellent way for you to ensure that you are getting adequate amounts of high quality protein in your body is to supplement your food plan with protein shakes. I rely on BSN's Lean Dessert Protein and also Syntha-6 powder. But make sure you always make your shakes with water, not soymilk or regular milk, as they will bloat you.

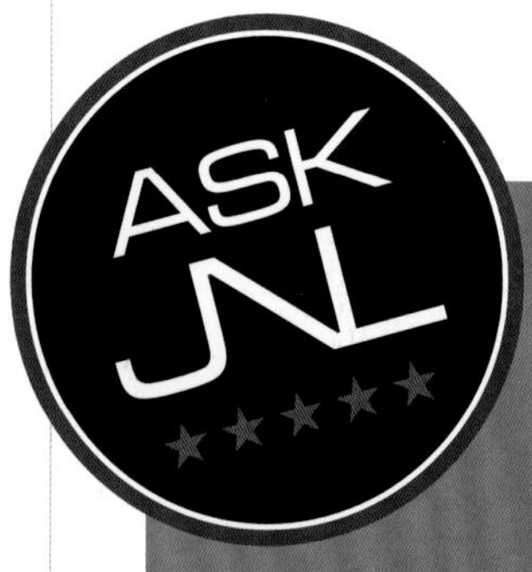

"But, JNL, how much protein should I be consuming daily?"

THIS IS AN EXCELLENT QUESTION! The U.S.R.D.A rate for protein for adult women is 1 gram per kilogram or about .4 grams per pound of body weight. (A kilogram is 2.2 pounds.) If you're exercising, though, you need more—usually between .5 to .6 grams per kilogram, or up to .7 to 1.6 grams per pound or more if you're trying to gain muscle. In general, .5 to .6 grams per pound is a good range for an active woman, but many women simplify the math even more by trying to consume about 1 gram of protein per pound. This is what I follow, multiplying by my weight of 130 lbs. Thus I consume around 130 grams of protein per day.

THE FITNESS MODEL ULTIMATE GROCERY LIST

Fitness Model Foods You Must Eat to Lose Weight & Build Sexy, Strong & Sleek Muscles

"The great news about my diet is that you must EAT to LOSE weight and build sexy feminine muscle!"

—JNL

PROTEINS

- Boneless, Skinless Chicken Breast
- Tuna (water-packed)
- Fish (salmon, sea bass, halibut)
- Shrimp
- Extra-Lean Ground Beef or Ground Round (look for 4% fat, antibiotic-free)
- BSN Lean Dessert Protein Powder
- Egg Whites or Eggs
- Rib eye Steaks or Roast
- Top Round Steaks or Roast (AKA Stew Meat, London Broil, Stir Fry)
- Top Sirloin (AKA Sirloin Top Butt)
- Beef Tenderloin (AKA Filet, Filet Mignon)
- Top Loin (NY Strip Steak)
- Flank Steak (Stir Fry, Fajita)
- Eye of Round (Cube Meat, Stew Meat, Bottom Round, 96% Lean Ground Round)
- Ground turkey, Turkey Breast Slices or cutlets (fresh meat, not deli cuts)

COMPLEX CARBS

- Oatmeal (Old-Fashioned or Quick Oats)
- Sweet Potatoes (Yams)
- Beans (pinto, black, kidney)
- Oat Bran Cereal
- Brown Rice
- Farina (Cream of Wheat)
- Multigrain Hot Cereal
- Pasta
- Rice (white, jasmine, basmati, Arborio, wild)
- Potatoes (red, baking, new)

"Being fit and sexy never tasted so good!"

—JNL

FIBROUS CARBS

- Leaf Lettuce (Green Leaf, Red, Leaf, Romaine)
- Broccoli
- Asparagus
- String Beans
- Spinach
- Bell Peppers
- Brussels Sprouts
- Cauliflower
- Celery
- Cucumber
- Green or Red Pepper
- Onions
- Garlic
- Tomatoes
- Zucchini
- Bananas
- Apples
- Grapefruit
- Peaches,
- Strawberries
- Blueberries
- Raspberries
- Lemons or Limes

HEALTHY FATS

- Natural Style Peanut Butter
- Olive Oil or Safflower Oil
- Nuts (peanuts, almonds)
- Flaxseed Oil
- Organic Virgin Unrefined coconut oil
- Avocado

DAIRY & EGGS

- Breakstone Low-fat cottage cheese
- Eggs
- Low or Nonfat Milk
- Sargento ™ Reduced fat cheese (they offer thinner slices and slim sticks for portion control)

BEVERAGES

- Water
- Crystal Light
- All kinds of tea
- POM Pomegranate Juice
- Fresh squeezed fruit juices

CONDIMENTS & MISC.

- Kraft Fat Free Mayonnaise
- Kikkoman Reduced Sodium Soy Sauce
- Reduced Sodium Teriyaki Sauce
- Balsamic Vinegar
- Salsa
- Chili powder/paste
- Mrs. Dash
- A-1 Steak Sauce
- Sugar-Free Maple Syrup
- French's Mustard
- Extracts (vanilla, almond, amaretto-almond flavor)
- Low-sodium beef or chicken broth
- Plain or reduced sodium tomato sauce, puree, paste)

ESSENTIAL FITNESS MODEL SUPPLEMENTS

- BSN's Lean Dessert Protein
- BSN's Syntha-6
- BSN's Sythan-6 RTD(Ready to Drink)
- BSN's Volumaize
- BSN's Atro-Phex
- BSN's N.O. Xplode
- BSN's Endorush
- BSN's Cheaters Relief
- Multi-Vitamin
- Emergen-C
- Vitamin B-12
- Calcium Supplement

JNL FITNESS MODEL FOODS TO AVOID

- Any kind of white bread, rolls, crackers
- Cookies
- Cornflakes
- Matzo
- White Pasta
- White potatoes
- Instant potatoes
- White Rice
- Canned Fruit, juice-packed
- Fruit juice
- Ice Cream
- Donuts
- Cake
- Pastries
- High-fat bacon
- High- fat sausage
- Movie theater popcorn

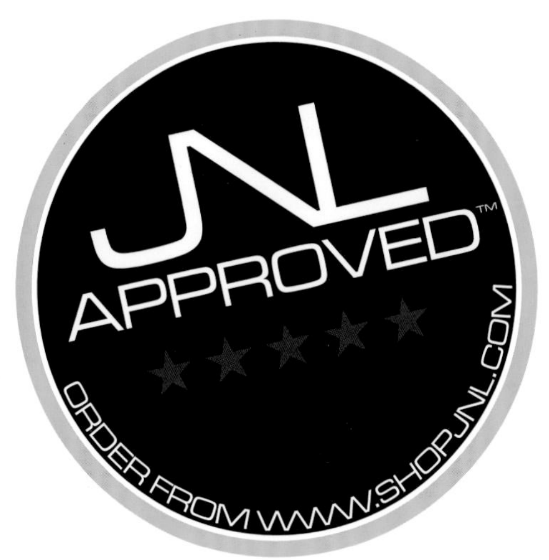

LIST OF JNL-APPROVED SUPPLEMENTS

"To be a super fitness model, you must supplement–plain and simple."

—JNL

As a specialist in sports nutrition and supplementation, I pride myself on knowing all supplements that are on the market. It's my job, as a leader in the fitness industry, to not only know them all, but to try them all, so I have personal experience with them and am able to rate them effectively. I'm kind of like a sommelier who professionally tastes wines, but my supplements are my wines! Many of you email me through my website asking me which supplements are my faves, so here are my answers. Remember, if you have a question for me, make sure to email my team and me through my website at www.JenniferNicoleLee.com.

JNL-APPROVED PROTEIN POWDERS

The #1 self-sabotaging behavior women do regularly is that they don't consume adequate amounts of protein. Protein is not only important for your muscle growth and maintenance, but it is the building block of life. It's essential for keeping your hair, skin, and nails healthy and strong. So make sure you get in enough protein to keep yourself strong and beautiful, from the inside out. I highly recommend BSN's Lean Dessert Protein when you want to "lean out," and Syntha-6 for a complete meal replacement

JNL-APPROVED PRE-WORKOUT IGNITER

If you want a little extra motivation before you get to the gym or begin your workout, I recommend BSN's N.O. Xplode

JNL-APPROVED ENERGY MANAGEMENT SUPPLEMENTS, AKA "FAT BURNERS"

If you choose the route of using an "Energy Maintenance Supplement" with your program, I highly recommend, from my own research, BSN's Atrophex.

JNL APPROVED ENERGY DRINKS

If you feel as though you need to use an energy drink with your program, I highly recommend these top brands:

- Endorush by BSN
- Volumaize by BSN

PG 128

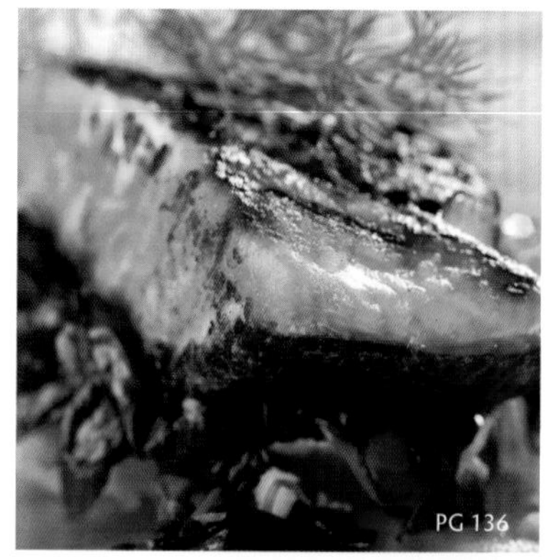
PG 136

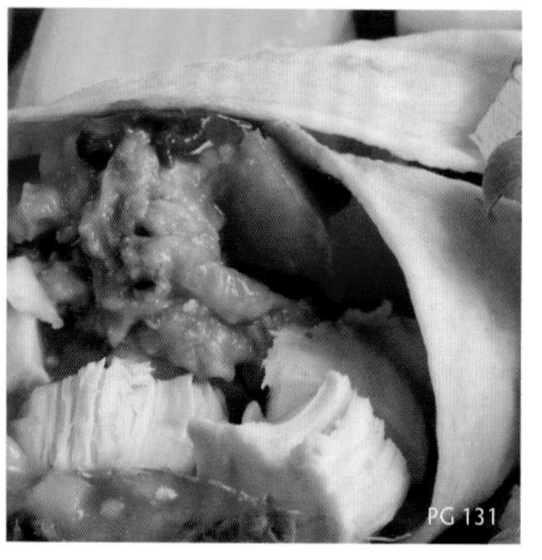
PG 131

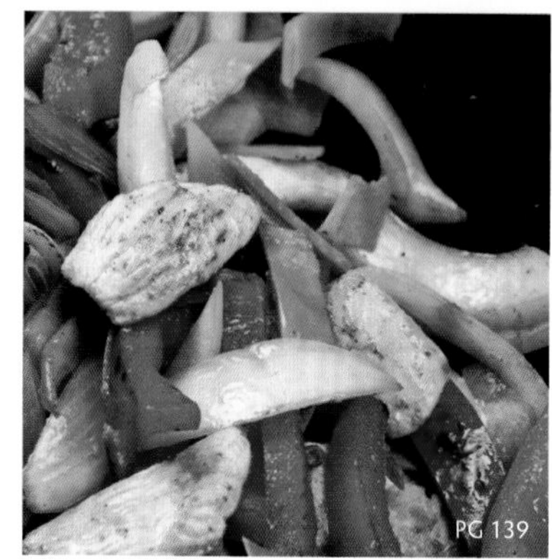
PG 139

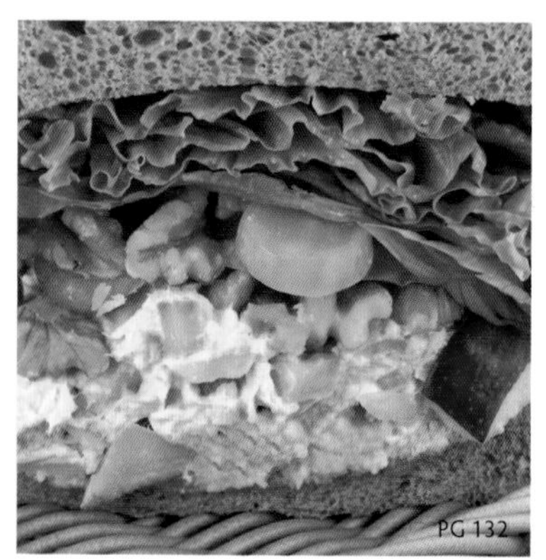
PG 132

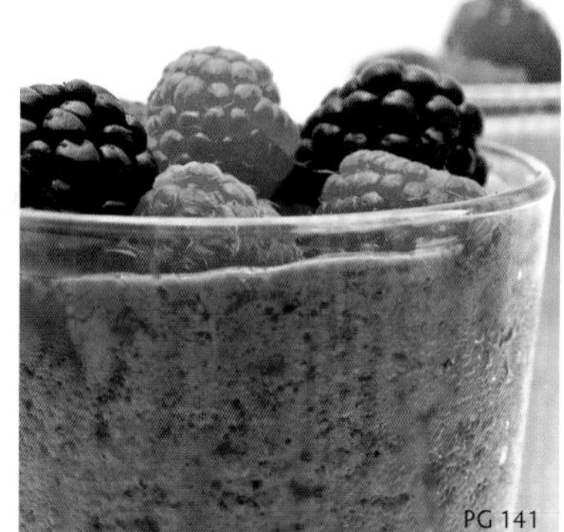
PG 141

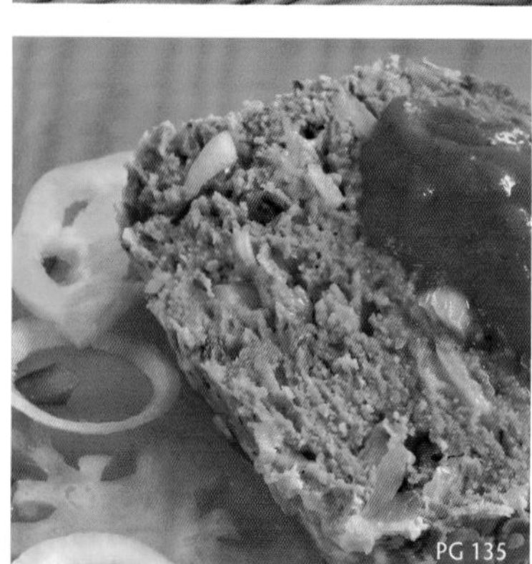
PG 135

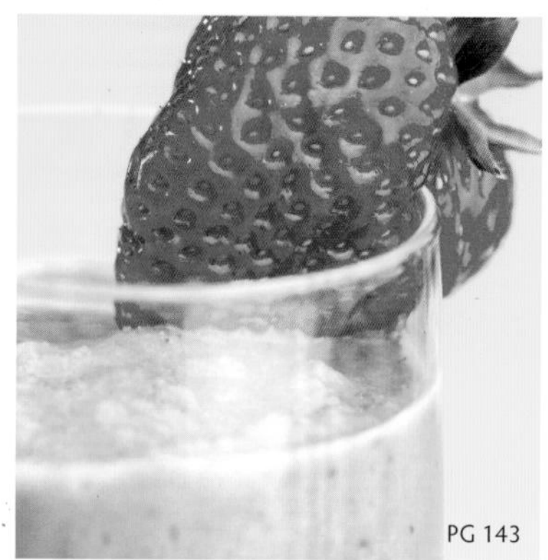
PG 143

JNL FITNESS MODEL FOOD PLAN

"People think that fitness models starve themselves, or only eat a diet of oatmeal and egg whites. Actually, super fitness models spoil their tastebuds and bodies with nutrient-rich, super healthy foods that are good for them. And their healthy bodies' show the benefits."

—JNL

Fitness models really don't "diet." Instead, they plan out their food and meals. That's why I call this the Fitness Model Food Plan. Below, you will find a day-by-day calendar that will give you a sense of how fitness models strategically plan their meals, so that they don't go too long without eating, and are always careful to eat high quality meals with a balance of protein, carbs, and healthy fats.

SUNDAY

Fitness Model Enchiladas

Fitness Model Protein Shake

Fitness Model Grilled Salmon

Spinach Salad

Fitness Model Protein Shake

Fitness Model "Muscle Loaf"

Fitness Model Protein Shake

MONDAY

Fitness Model Veggie Scramble

Fitness Model Protein Shake

Fitness Model Fajitas with Guacamole

Fitness Model Protein Shake

Fitness Model Grilled Salmon with Sautéed Spinach

Fitness Model Protein Shake

TUESDAY

Fitness Model Oatmeal Pancakes

Fitness Model Protein Shake

Fitness Model Apple Walnut Chicken Salad

Fitness Model Protein Shake

Fitness Model Stir Fried Chicken and Vegetables

Fitness Model Protein Shake

WEDNESDAY

Fitness Model 40 Second Omelet

Fitness Model Protein Shake

Fitness Model Thai Curry

Chicken and Grape Salad Sandwich

Fitness Model Protein Shake

Fitness Model Lettuce Wraps

Fitness Model Protein Shake

THURSDAY

Fitness Model Peanut Butter Chocolate Protein Oatmeal

Fitness Model Protein Shake

Fitness Model Chicken Caesar Pitas

Fitness Model Protein Shake

Fitness Model Shrimp Ceviche with Green Salad

Fitness Model Protein Shake

FRIDAY

Fitness Model English Muffin Melt

Fitness Model Protein Shake

Fitness Model Sirloin Cheeseburger

Fitness Model Protein Shake

Fitness Model Grilled Cajun Salmon with Lemony Sautéed Spinach

Fitness Model Protein Shake

SATURDAY

Fitness Model Breakfast Burrito

Fitness Model Protein Shake

Fitness Model Chicken Quesadillas

Fitness Model Protein Shake

Fitness Model "Hot Stuff" Goulash

Fitness Model Protein Shake

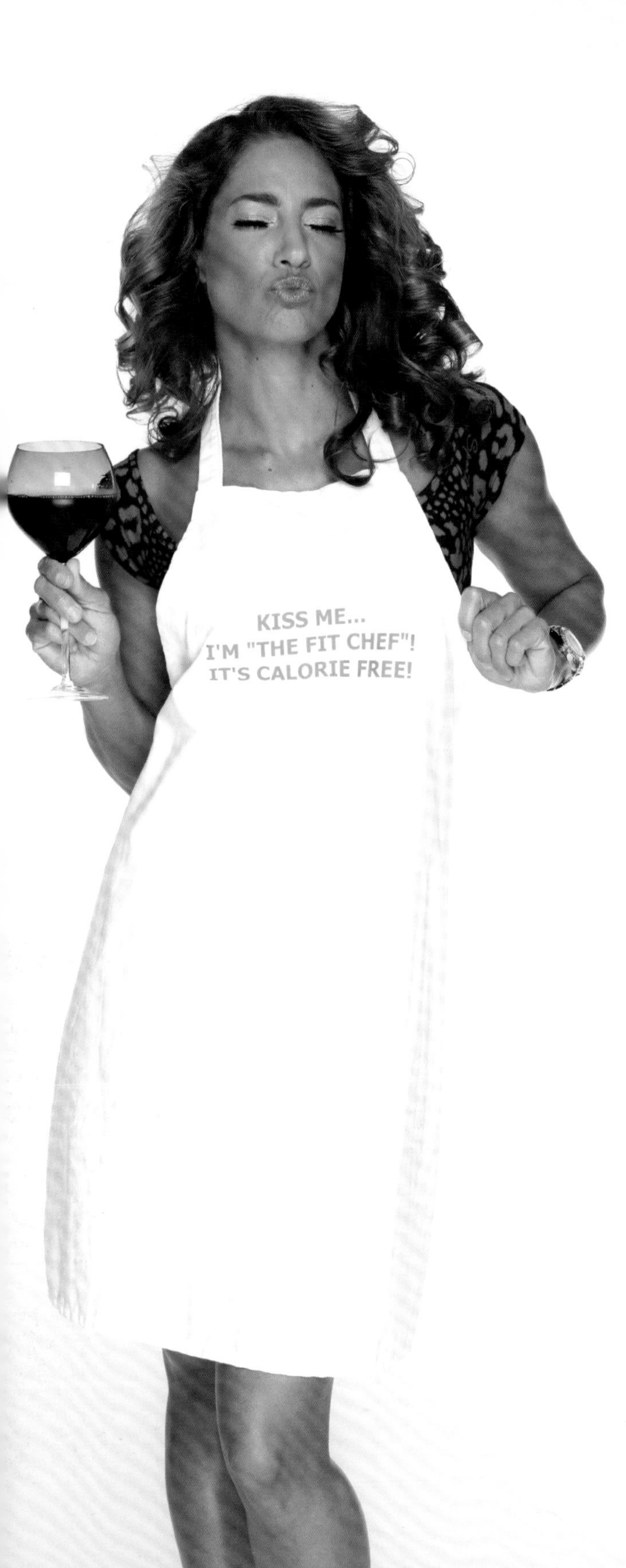

FANTASTIC AND FAST FITNESS MODEL RECIPES

BREAKFAST

FITNESS MODEL ENCHILADAS

Prep Time: 8 minutes

INGREDIENTS

- 1 whole egg, 3 egg whites
- 1 ½ Tbsp reduced fat shredded cheddar
- 2 wheat tortillas
- ¼ cup sliced avocado
- ¼ cup salsa

DIRECTIONS

- Lightly coat small nonstick skillet with cooking spray, and place over medium heat.
- Whisk egg and egg whites until blended, add shredded cheese, and scramble together
- Lightly dampen two paper towels and place wheat tortillas between them. Microwave for 30 seconds.
- Fill each tortilla with the scrambled eggs and cheese, then add a spoonful of salsa and a slice of avocado.

FITNESS MODEL VEGGIE SCRAMBLE

Prep Time: 15 minutes

INGREDIENTS

- 1 Portion of Diced Sweet Potato
- ½ Cup Frozen Vegetables
- 1 Vegetable Breakfast Patty
- 3 Egg Whites

DIRECTIONS

- Lightly coat a medium skillet with cooking spray over medium heat.
- Add diced potato and mixed vegetables to skillet.
- Crumble in thawed breakfast patty and sauté until heated through, and veggies are tender (about 5 minutes)
- In a small bowl, whisk egg whites. Pour into skillet and stir for about 3 minutes.

FITNESS MODEL OATMEAL PANCAKES

Prep Time 7 Minutes

INGREDIENTS

- ½ cup old-fashioned oatmeal
- ¼ cup low-fat cottage cheese
- 4 egg whites
- 1 tsp vanilla extract
- ¼ tsp cinnamon
- ¼ tsp nutmeg

DIRECTIONS

- Process the oatmeal, cottage cheese and egg whites, vanilla extract, cinnamon and nutmeg in the blender until smooth.
- Spray a nonstick skillet with cooking spray.
- Pour in batter, and cook over medium heat until both sides are lightly browned.
- Top with low-sugar syrup of your choice.

Enjoy!

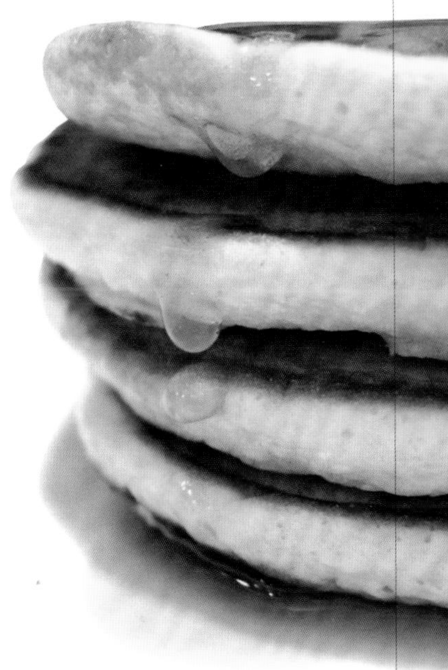

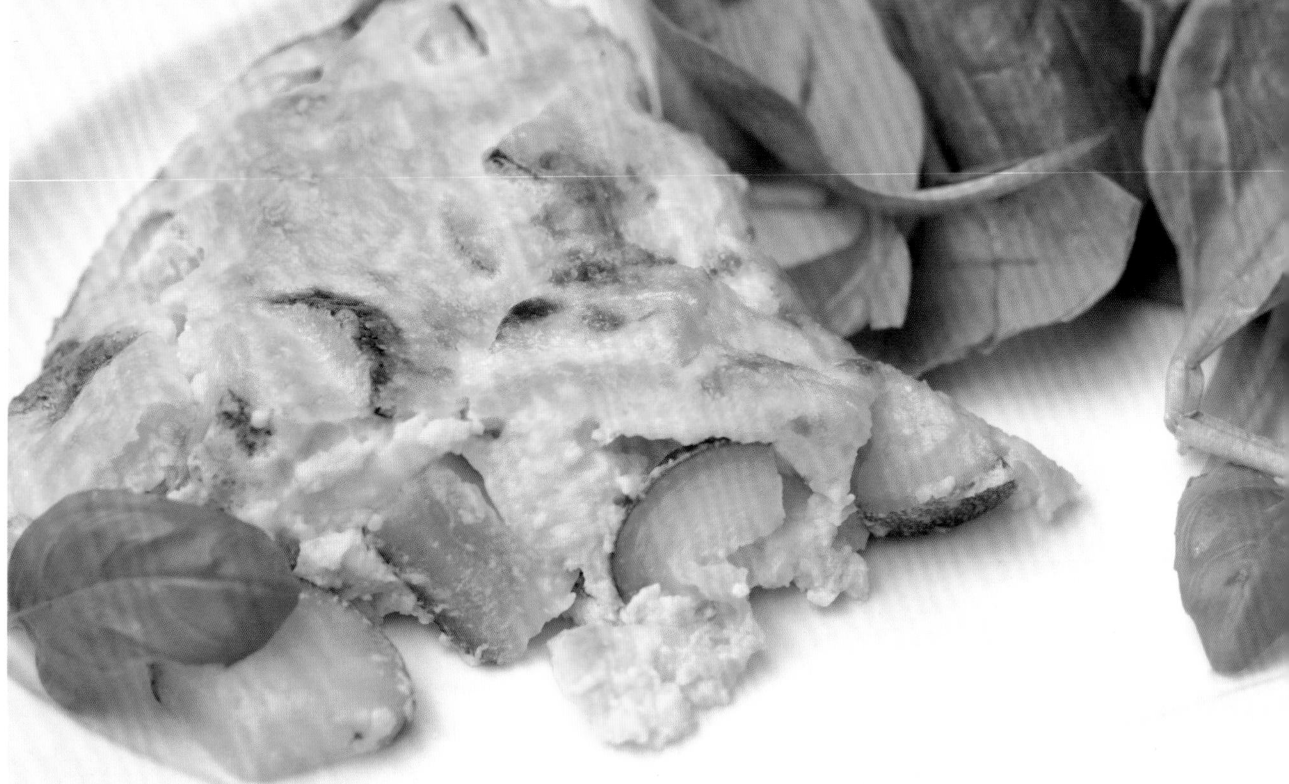

JNL'S FITNESS MODEL 60-SECOND OMELET

This breakfast recipe is excellent when you are short on time and long on hunger! I sometimes eat this for dinner, by taking out the side of oatmeal or whole wheat toast.

Prep Time: 60 Seconds

INGREDIENTS

- 4 egg whites, one whole egg
- Veggies of your choice (spinach, broccoli, mushrooms, green peppers, etc)

DIRECTIONS

- Whip eggs in blender
- Cook over medium heat in a skillet; add vegetables of choice
- Enjoy with a ½ cup of oatmeal, or a side of low-carb toast

FITNESS MODEL PEANUT BUTTER CHOCOLATE OATMEAL

Prep Time: 5 minutes

INGREDIENTS

- 1/3 cup uncooked wholegrain oats
- ½ cup water
- 1 scoop of BSN's Chocolate Fudge Pudding protein powder, or Syntha-6 Chocolate Peanut Butter
- 1 Tbsp natural peanut butter
- Splenda, to taste
- ½ cup skim milk

DIRECTIONS

- In a bowl combine oats, water and protein powder
- Microwave on high until oats are cooked (about 2 minutes)
- Stir in peanut butter and add Splenda to taste

Pour milk on top and enjoy!

FITNESS MODEL ENGLISH MUFFIN MELT

Prep Time: 15 Minutes

INGREDIENTS

- 1 Whole Wheat English Muffin, split
- 2 Thick Slices of Tomato
- 2 Slices of Reduced Fat Swiss Cheese

DIRECTIONS

- Preheat oven to 400 Degrees
- Place whole-wheat English muffin halves face up on baking sheet, and top with a slice of tomato, then layer with cheese
- Place in oven and bake for 35 minutes

"I love to eat, because I choose the foods that help me look and feel healthy, strong and beautiful."

—JNL

FITNESS MODEL BREAKFAST BURRITO

Prep Time: 10 Minutes

INGREDIENTS

- 1 whole wheat tortilla
- 1 whole egg, 3 egg whites
- 1 lettuce leaf
- 2 Tbsp fat-free refried beans
- 1 Tbsp fat-free shredded cheese
- ¼ cup salsa

DIRECTIONS

- Lightly coat a medium skillet with cooking spray and place over medium heat.
- Place tortilla on skillet and warm for 30 seconds, then turn and warm other side.
- Whisk the egg and egg whites together, then pour into warmed skillet and cook, stirring occasionally until set.
- While the eggs cook, place the lettuce leaf on the tortilla, and spread the refried beans over the lettuce leaf.
- Top the beans with cooked eggs, shredded cheese and salsa.

LUNCH

FITNESS MODEL GRILLED SALMON SPINACH SALAD

Salmon is low in calories, yet high in protein and the unique type of health-promoting fat, the omega-3 essential fatty acids. I love to grill it and eat it fresh right off the grill with a squeeze of lemon! And, knowing that its great for my hair, skin, nails and my body weight, I can even feel great eating it.

Prep Time: 10 minutes

INGREDIENTS

- 2 Tablespoons extra virgin olive oil
- ½ pound cleaned fresh spinach
- ¼ teaspoon salt
- 1/8 tsp freshly ground pepper
- ½ cup chopped yellow onion
- 3 fresh tomatoes (about 1 pound), peeled, seeded and cut into ½ pieces
- Grilled Salmon
- 1 Tbsp coarsely chopped flat-leaf parsley for garnish (optional)

DIRECTIONS

- In a skillet, heat 1 Tbsp. of olive oil over medium heat
- When hot, sauté spinach for ½ minute.
- Mix in the salt and pepper and divide the spinach into 4 servings
- Heat the remaining tbsp of oil in the skillet and sauté the onion and tomatoes over medium heat until the onion is tender (about 5-6 minutes)
- Grill salmon over medium heat for about 4 minutes each side
- Arrange the grilled salmon on the spinach, top with the tomatoes and onion

FITNESS MODEL APPLE WALNUT CHICKEN SALAD

This is a simple, yet completely satisfying, chicken salad recipe that I can make in under 5 minutes, which is full of heart-healthy walnuts, crunchy celery, and sweet raisins. One of my favorites!

Prep Time: 5 minutes

INGREDIENTS

- 5 oz cooked chicken breast, cut into bite-size chunks
- ½ cup chopped celery
- ¾ cup chopped apple
- 2 oz chopped walnuts
- 1 Tablespoon raisins
- 1/3 cup prepared low-sugar Italian dressing
- Bibb Lettuce

DIRECTIONS

- In a medium bowl, gently stir together the chicken, celery, apple, walnuts, and raisins.
- Pour the dressing over the mixture and toss gently to coat.
- Serve on a bed of Bibb Lettuce.

FITNESS MODEL FAJITAS WITH "HOLY GUACAMOLE"

Avocados are an essential part of the Fitness Model Program because they contain essential fatty acids, which are also great for your hair, skin and nails. An avocado also contains more potassium than a medium banana. I whip up a big batch of guacamole to share with some low-carb whole grain tortillas before our main fajita meal. My entire family loves it!

Prep Time: 15 Minutes

INGREDIENTS FOR FAJITAS

- 2 Chicken breasts, precooked and cut into fajita strips
- 4 Low-carb whole grain tortillas
- 2 tablespoons "Holy Guacamole"
- Lettuce
- Tomatoes, coarsely chopped

INGREDIENTS FOR HOLY GUACAMOLE

- 4 Haas avocadoes
- ½ cup of prepared tomatoes
- Juice of one lemon, juice of one lime

DIRECTIONS

- Mash the avocados and mix the tomatoes, lemon and lime juice in to make the guacamole
- Assemble fajita ingredients onto tortillas, add guacamole and enjoy!

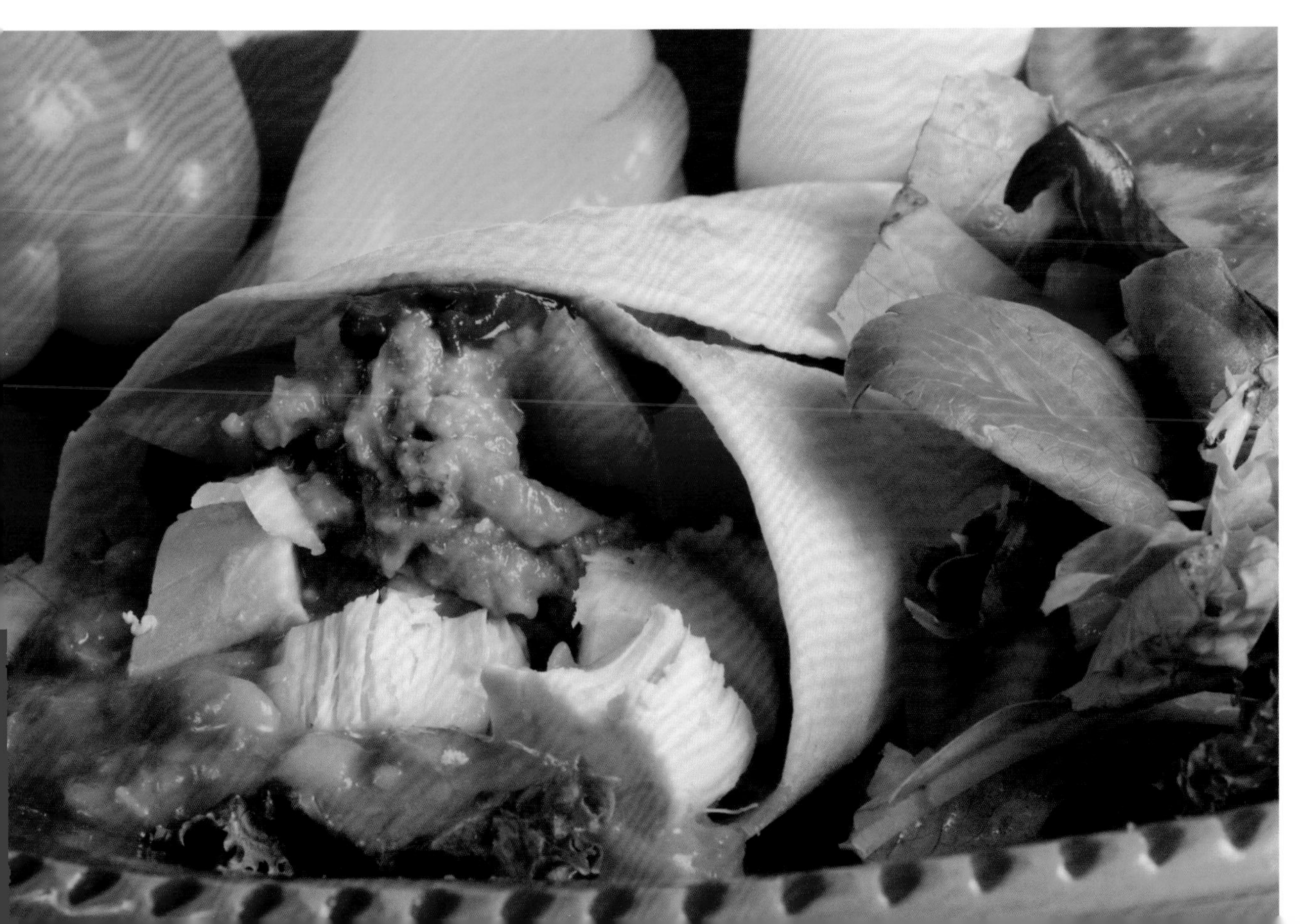

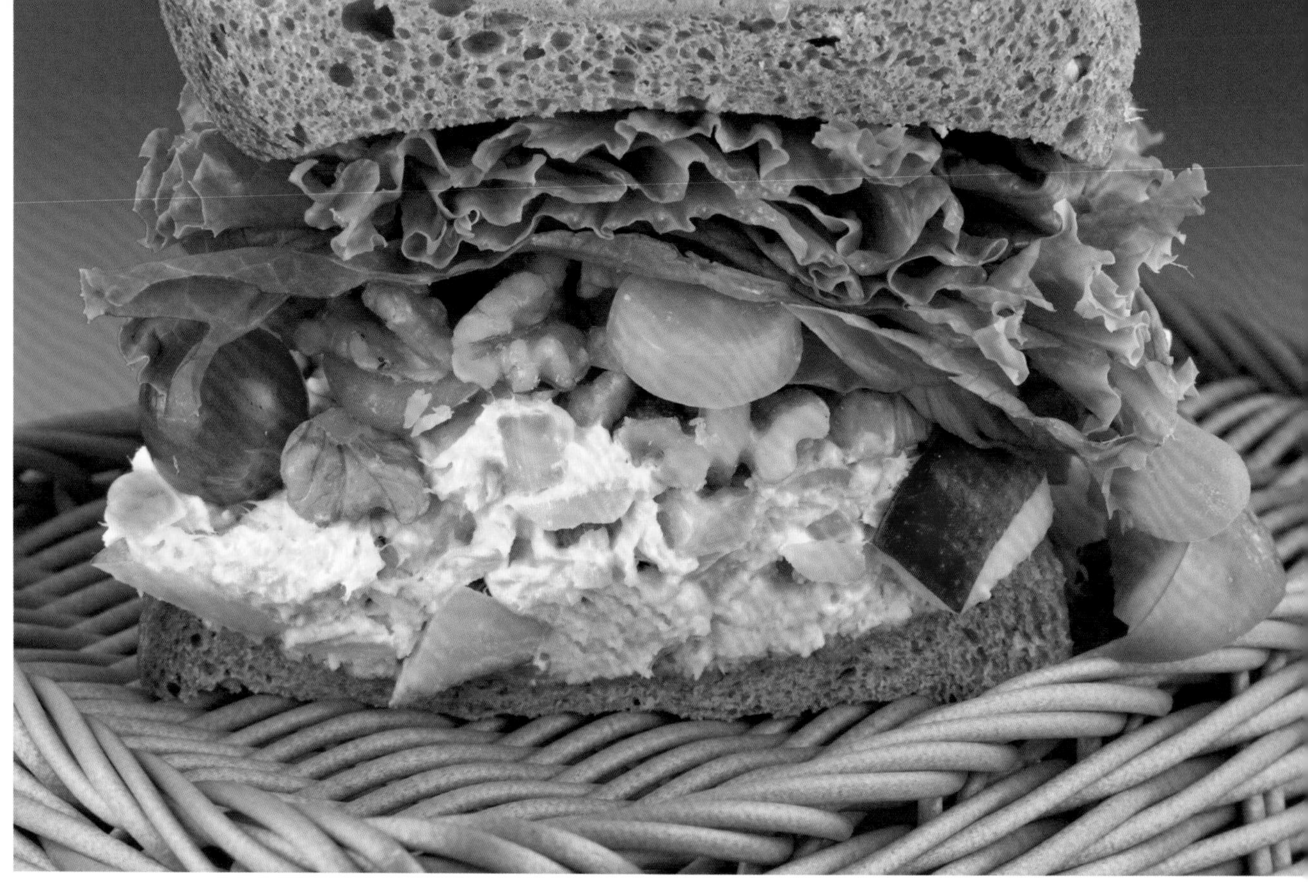

FITNESS MODEL THAI CURRY CHICKEN AND GRAPE SALAD SANDWICH

This is a meal that I prepare when all of my fitness model friends come over, and we all enjoy it outside by the pool, or its great right after our workout. I love the crisp sweet grapes and curry seasoning that add a lot of taste to this chicken salad recipe.

Prep Time: 10 minutes

INGREDIENTS

- 2 portions chicken breast, chopped
- ½ cup seedless red grapes, chilled, halved
- ½ cup green grapes, chilled, halved
- 1 apple cored and diced
- ½ cup fat free mayonnaise
- 1 lemon, halved
- 1 tsp. curry powder, to taste.
- ¼ tsp ground black pepper
- 2 cups baby romaine leaves
- 2 slices of whole wheat bread

DIRECTIONS

In medium mixing bowl, combine precooked and chopped chicken, chilled red and green grapes, apple, mayonnaise, lemon juice, curry powder, and black pepper.

Toast 2 slices of bread and place baby romaine on top along with chicken salad.

FITNESS MODEL CHICKEN CAESAR WRAP

This is an essential fitness model meal that can be made in minutes. Plus, I love that you can wrap it up, and eat it on the go, or brown bag it for lunch.

Prep Time: 10 minutes

INGREDIENTS

- I portion grilled chicken breast, sliced
- 1 cup romaine lettuce, cut into bite-sized pieces
- 1 Tbsp low-fat Caesar salad dressing
- 1 Tbsp reduced fat Parmesan cheese, grated
- One 10-inch spinach tortilla

DIRECTIONS

- In medium mixing bowl, toss together chicken, lettuce, Caesar dressing and parmesan cheese.
- Microwave tortilla for about 20 seconds to soften
- Spoon chicken mixture onto tortilla
- Wrap tortilla around filling and cut in half.

FITNESS MODEL OPEN-FACED SIRLOIN CHEESEBURGER

Cheeseburger on the Fitness Model Program, you ask? You bet! A cover girl needs her red meat, which packs the kind of protein, nutrients and vitamins, such as iron and B12, that poultry or fish will never have! The secret is in the quality of red meat you select. Aim for 4% ground beef that is antibiotic-free. It's a bit more expensive, but so worth it because it's leaner and also has no artificial growth hormone.

Prep Time: 10 minutes

INGREDIENTS

- ½ cup of 4% hormone- and antibiotic-free ground beef, patted into patty
- 1 slice of low-carb whole-grain toast
- Low-fat Swiss cheese
- Additional condiments such as alfalfa sprouts, low-fat hummus, tomatoes, or spinach. Dress your burger up as you like! Just stay away from full-fat mayonnaise

DIRECTIONS

- Heat up pan with a touch of olive oil.
- Cook to your liking.
- Top with the garnish of your choice.

JNL FIT TIP

If you do choose to top your burger with cheese, aim for low-fat Swiss. It usually packs a protein punch of 7 grams, with only 2 to 4 grams of fat and 60 calories.

FITNESS MODEL CHICKEN QUESADILLAS

Yes, I said quesadillas! They are allowed on my fitness model diet, because you are using reduced fat cheese and low fat sour cream, and adding no more unnecessary fat, calories, carbs or sodium. It's all the taste, without the fat!

Prep Time: 15 minutes

INGREDIENTS

- 2 portions uncooked chicken breast
- 1 cup salsa
- Two 8-inch low carb whole wheat tortillas
- ¼ cup reduced fat Cheddar cheese, shredded
- ¼ cup low fat sour cream

DIRECTIONS

- Lightly coat a medium skillet with cooking spray and place over medium heat.
- Slice chicken breast into half-inch cubes and sauté chicken and salsa until chicken is no longer pink (about 10 minutes).
- Lightly coat a large skillet with cooking spray and place over medium heat. Place a tortilla in the skillet and spread half the chicken mixture over the tortilla and top with the cheese.
- Fold tortilla over filling and cook until lightly browned (3-4 minutes).
- Remove from heat and set aside.
- Repeat with the remaining tortilla, chicken mixture and cheese.
- Cut quesadillas into wedges and place on small plates, put half the sour cream on each plate for dipping, and enjoy!

"Make sure that your dinner is your smallest meal of the day. Also, aim to have no carbs with your dinner. These two tips have helped me maintain my 80 lb-plus weight loss – and they work!"

—JNL

"Eat breakfast like a queen, lunch like a princess, and dinner like a pauper."

—JNL

DINNER

FITNESS MODEL MUSCLE LOAF

This is NOT your mom's meat loaf! I gave this boring and high fat meal a major fitness model makeover. My version is full of taste, high in muscle-toning protein, and low in fat. Enjoy!

Prep Time: 1 hour

INGREDIENTS

- 1 can no-salt-added tomato paste
- ½ cup dry red wine
- ½ cup water
- 1 clove garlic, minced
- ½ tsp dried basil leaves
- ¼ tsp dried oregano leaves
- ¼ tsp salt
- 16 oz. ground turkey breast
- 1 cup oatmeal
- 1 whole egg
- 1 egg white
- ½ cup shredded zucchini

DIRECTIONS

- Preheat oven to 350 degrees.
- Combine the tomato paste, wine, water, garlic, basil, oregano and salt in a small saucepan.
- Bring to a boil, then reduce the heat to low.
- Simmer, uncovered, for 15 minutes, and set aside.
- Combine the turkey, oatmeal, egg, egg white, zucchini & ½ cup tomato paste mixture in a large bowl and mix well.
- Shape into loaf and place into an ungreased 8′ x 4′ loaf pan.
- Bake for 45 minutes.
- Discard and drippings and pour the remaining ½ cup of tomato paste mixture over the top of the loaf and bake for an additional 15 minutes.
- Cool before slicing and serve remaining tomato sauce on the side.

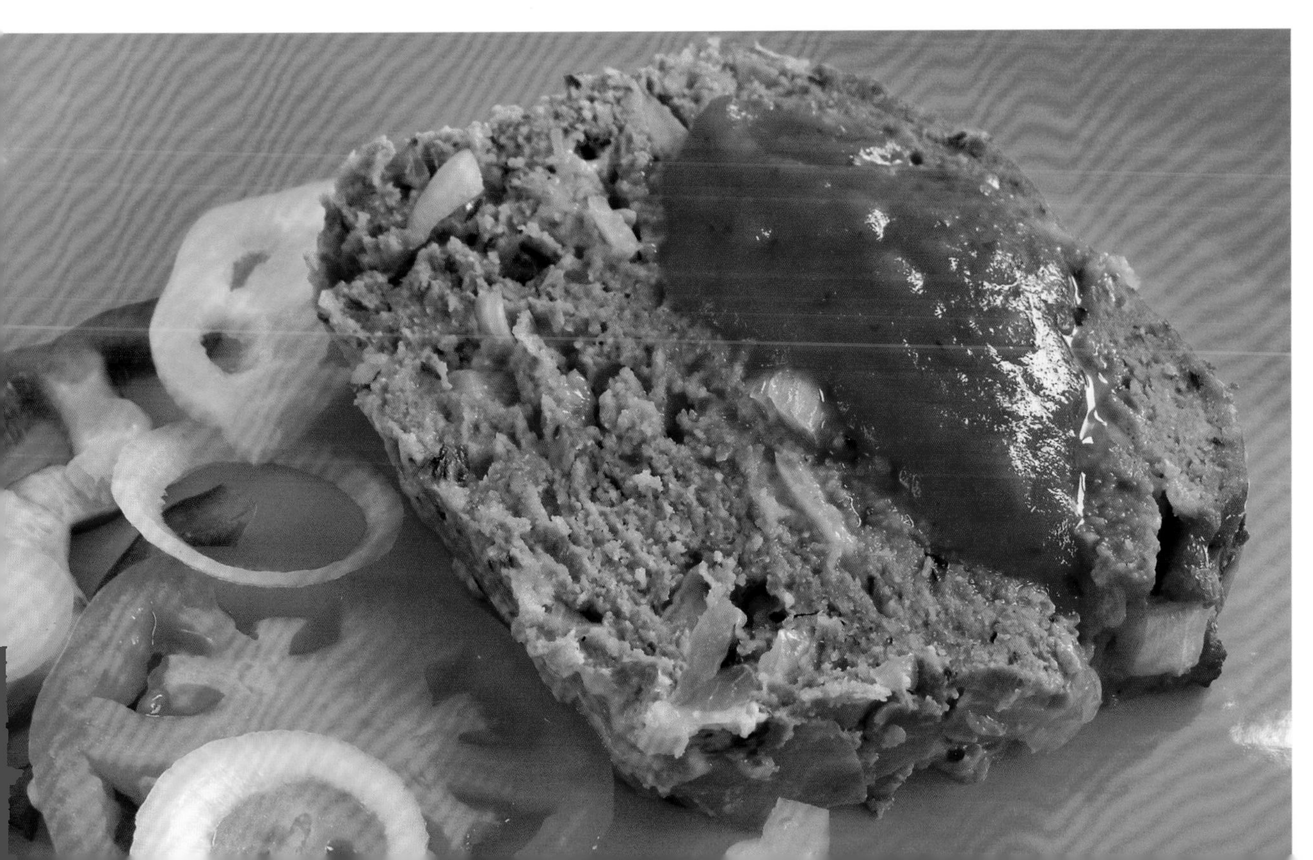

FITNESS MODEL SHRIMP CEVICHE WITH GREEN SALAD

Shrimp may be mini, but they are mighty! Yes, they are small, but they are big on protein and health benefits. Did you know that shrimp is the lowest calorie and lowest-carb food with the highest percentage of protein?

Prep Time: 10 minutes

INGREDIENTS

- 1 pound peeled and deveined shrimp, boiled and then rinsed and chilled.
- 1 cup of a combination of green peppers, onions, and tomatoes
- Juice of one lemon
- Juice of one lime
- 2 Tbsp of fresh-cut parsley, or a squeeze of parsley (From Gourmet Gardens Squeeze)
- 2 Tbsp of fresh-cut of cilantro, or a squeeze of cilantro (From Gourmet Gardens)
- 2 tablespoons of cold-pressed olive oil

DIRECTIONS

- Mix ingredients all together and enjoy!
- For lunch serve over a half-cup of brown rice.
- For dinner, serve with a side of steamed broccoli, asparagus, or a green salad.

FITNESS MODEL GRILLED CAJUN SALMON WITH LEMONY SAUTÉED SPINACH

A Fitness Model needs her Omega-3s for her shiny hair, strong nails, and her beautiful skin! Choose wild salmon over farmed because of the quality of fish.

INGREDIENTS

- 2 portions of salmon steaks, about 4 to 6 oz, lightly dusted with Salt Free seasoning.
- Salt-free Cajun Seasoning (try Mrs. Dash)
- One lemon
- 2 Tablespoons cold-pressed olive oil
- Bag of organic triple-washed spinach

DIRECTIONS

- Lightly coat broiler pan with cooking spray.
- Place salmon fillets on the broiler pan, and cook to your liking (tip: cooking your salmon to the well-done point will not take out any essential fatty acids)
- In another pan, heat the olive oil and add in the spinach.
- Cook until wilted, squeeze lemon over spinach, and serve!

JNL FIT TIP: If you are having this meal for lunch, feel free to add a half-cup of brown rice, or sweet potato. If for dinner, forgo the complex carb. This is always a Fitness Model's rule of thumb.

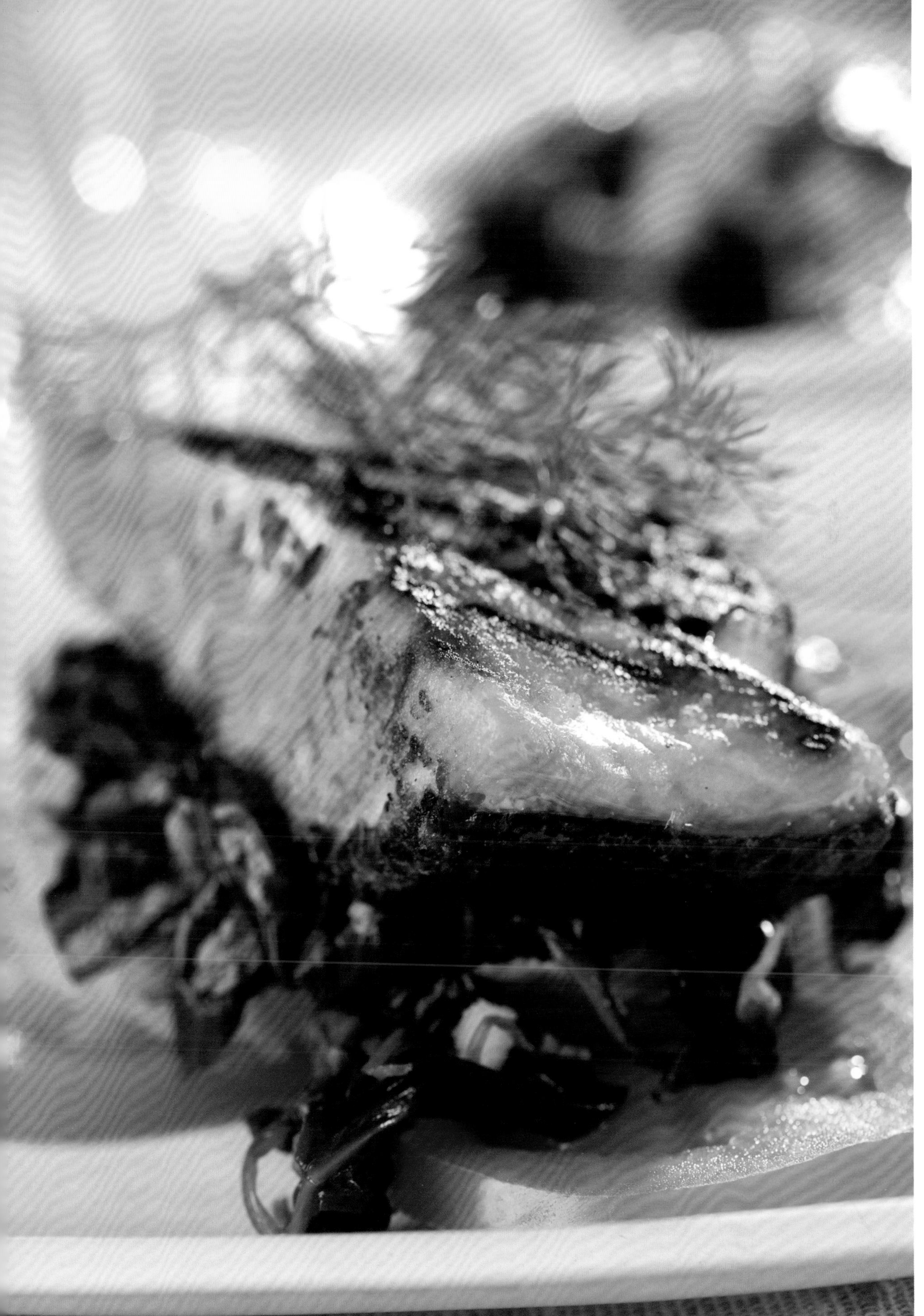

JNL FIT TIP: This recipe yields 4 servings, so this is a great one to store for left-overs for later in the week!

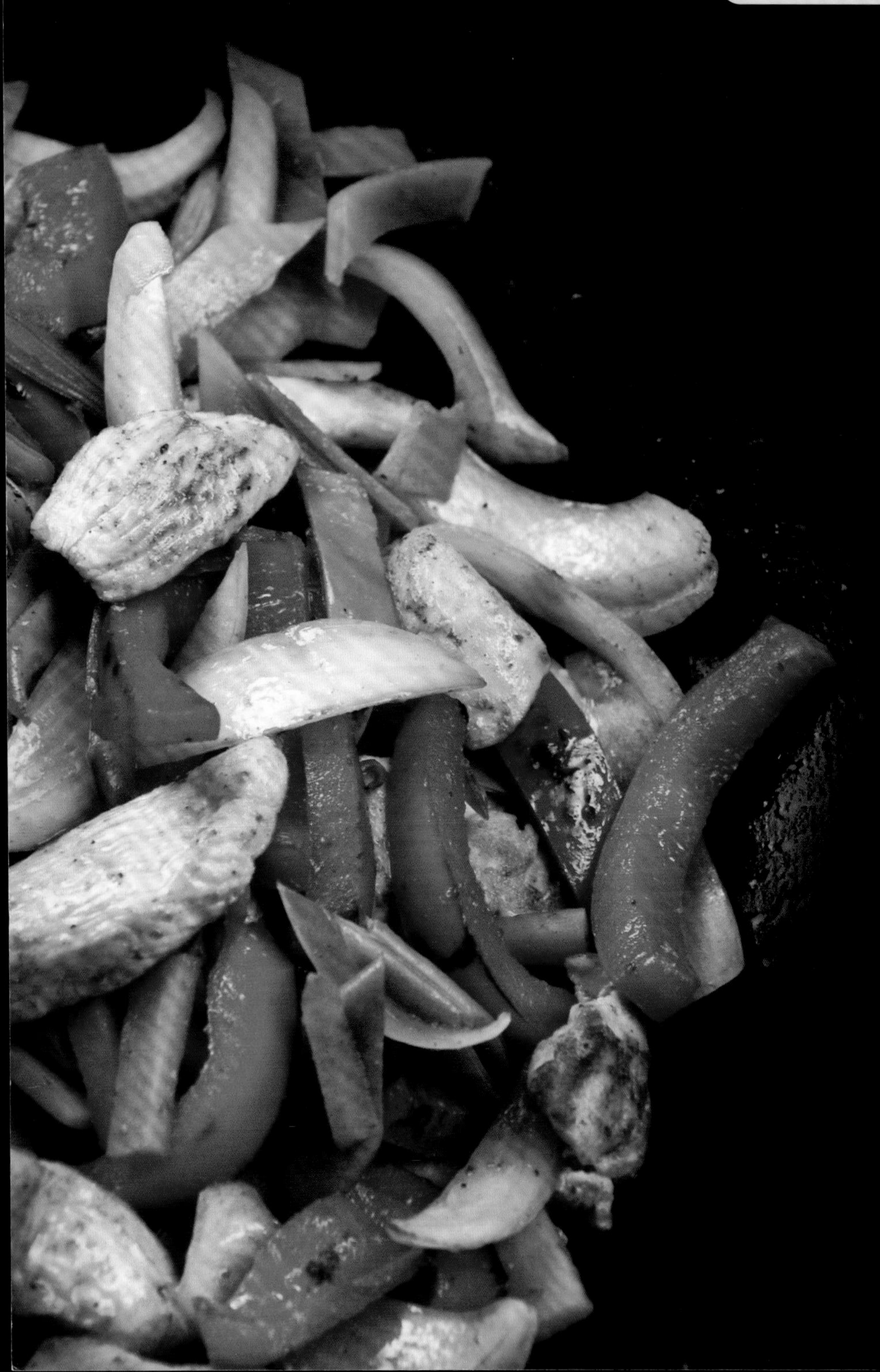

FITNESS MODEL STIR FRIED CHICKEN AND VEGETABLES

One of my top Asian faves, which I whip up in my wok. Add a touch of spice if you like your Asian stir-fries with a little kick!

Prep Time: 15 minutes

INGREDIENTS

- 3 Tbsp canola oil
- ½ pound cooked chicken breast cut diagonally into 1/8" thick slices
- 1 package of frozen vegetables containing broccoli, green beans, red bell peppers and mushrooms
- 2 Tbsp water
- 2 Tbsp soy sauce
- 1 package fresh spinach

DIRECTIONS

- Heat a large, heavy skillet or wok over high heat until water sizzles when dropped on the metal.
- Add 1 Tbsp of the canola oil and tilt the pan gently in all directions until the oil has coated the surface.
- Once the oil is hot, add chicken breast slices and stir-fry for 2 minutes.
- Remove chicken to a bowl.
- Add the remaining oil to the skillet and, once hot, add the frozen vegetable mix and stir-fry for about 4 minutes, until the larger pieces are cooked through.
- Return the chicken to the skillet and add the water and soy sauce to the pan, and steam over medium heat for 2 minutes.
- Add the spinach. Using tongs, turn the spinach once so that it heats evenly. Cover and steam for an additional 2 minutes.
- Remove the chicken and vegetables with a slotted spoon, and spoon the liquid into small bowls and serve as a gravy/dip

FITNESS MODEL "HOT STUFF" GOULASH

There's nothing like a hot home cooked meal. My mom made a fabulous goulash, but unfortunately it all ended up on my hips, buns and thighs. My version is lower in fat and extremely healthy for you. Enjoy!

Prep Time: 30 Minutes

INGREDIENTS

- 4 portions egg noodles, uncooked
- 1 chopped onion
- 1 red bell pepper, sliced
- 1 zucchini, sliced
- 4 portions lean ground turkey (about 1 lb)
- 2 cups tomato sauce
- 2 Tbsp fresh basil, chopped
- 2 Tbsp red wine

DIRECTIONS

- Prepare egg noodles according to package directions
- Lightly coat a large skillet with cooking spray and sauté chopped onions for 2 minutes over medium heat.
- Add bell pepper and zucchini to the onion and sauté for another 2 minutes; remove veggies from skillet and set aside.
- Add ground turkey to the skillet and sauté until no longer pink (about 5 minutes).
- Once turkey is done, return veggies to the skillet and add tomato sauce, basil, and red wine. Cook and stir occasionally for 5 minutes until heated, Place a portion of noodles onto each plate and top with a portion of turkey mixture.

FITNESS MODEL LETTUCE WRAPS

No boring egg whites here! Crunchy, crisp, cold and hot at the same time-plus high in protein and low in carbs. This is the perfect fitness model dinner that the entire family will all be glad you cooked!

Prep Time: 30 Minutes

INGREDIENTS

- 4 fresh shitake mushrooms
- 7 stalks Napa cabbage
- 1 lb lean ground turkey
- ½ onion, chopped
- 2 Tbsp hoisin sauce
- 1 Tbsp lite soy sauce
- ¼ tsp five-spice Powder
- One 8 oz can sliced water chestnuts, drained
- 12 large leaves of iceberg lettuce

DIRECTIONS

- Remove and discard stems from shitake mushrooms and chop the mushroom caps and Napa cabbage, keeping leaves and stems separate.
- Lightly coat a wok or skillet with cooking spray and place over medium heat.
- Add turkey and stir-fry until no longer pink (about 5 minutes).
- Remove turkey from wok and set aside
- Lightly recoat the wok/skillet with cooking spray; add chopped cabbage stems and onion, and stir-fry until tender (about 2 minutes)
- Stir in Hoisin sauce, soy sauce and 5-spice powder. Add cabbage leaves, mushrooms and water chestnuts, and stir-fry for about 1 minute.
- Add cooked turkey back into the skillet and stir-fry until well-combined and heated through (about 2 more minutes).
- Place 3 lettuce leaves on each of 4 plates and divide the stir-fry mixture into 4 portions. Then divide each portion into thirds and spoon into lettuce leaves

Serve and enjoy!

JNL FIT TIP: These wraps taste better when you add dipping sauces such as Chinese hot mustard, light soy sauce and chili sauce!

"Cheers to your fit and trim body! Sipping on protein shakes is a fitness model must-do to ensure your body is getting the essential amounts of protein, without the unnecessary calories and carbs, to keep it sexy, strong and sleek."

—JNL

PROTEIN SHAKES

FITNESS MODEL ULTIMATE BERRY BEAUTY BLEND PROTEIN SHAKE

INGREDIENTS

- 6-8 oz water
- 3 ice cubes
- 1 scoop of BSN Lean Dessert Protein Shake powder, Whipped Vanilla Flavor
- 1 tsp of unrefined organic virgin coconut oil
- 1 tsp flaxseed oil
- 1 tsp primrose oil
- 1 tsp of ground flaxseeds
- 1/2 cup of mixed berries

DIRECTIONS

- Put all ingredients into blender
- Blend until completely mixed

FITNESS MODEL ON-THE-GO PROTEIN SHAKE

I love this, because it's to the point, and it is the foundation of any great protein shake.

INGREDIENTS

- 6-8 oz water
- 3 ice cubes
- 1 scoop of BSN Lean Dessert Protein Shake powder, any flavor

DIRECTIONS

- Add water to the BSN protein powder in your portable protein shaker
- Shake well until powder has completely dissolved

FITNESS MODEL BLUEBERRY BLAST

Berries are great for boosting your immune system and your skin, so sip this protein shake knowing that it's a big deposit into your beauty bank.

INGREDIENTS

- 6-8 oz water
- 3 ice cubes
- 1 scoop of BSN Lean Dessert Protein Shake powder, Whipped Vanilla Flavor
- ¼ cup of orange juice or cranberry juice (optional)
- ¼ cup blueberries

DIRECTIONS

- Pour water into blender
- Add powder
- Blend on medium speed for 15 seconds
- Add blueberries, plus optional orange juice and/or cranberry juice.

Cheers!

FITNESS MODEL ICED CHAI PROTEIN SHAKE

Love Iced Chai Tea? Then you will LOVE my version, which is actually healthier for you because of the protein that your strong body will get.

INGREDIENTS

- 6-8 oz water
- 3 ice cubes
- 1 scoop of BSN Lean Dessert Protein Shake powder, Whipped Vanilla Flavor
- ½ cup of Chai Tea Concentrate
- 1 dash of cinnamon
- 1 dash of ground ginger

DIRECTIONS

- Pour water into blender
- Add powder, Chai tea concentrate, cinnamon and ground ginger
- Blend on medium speed for 15 seconds

JNL FIT TIP: You can usually find Chai Tea concentrate in the coffee and tea section of your grocery store

FITNESS MODEL COOKIES & CREAM PROTEIN SHAKE

Remember those fast-food frozen treats with the vanilla ice cream and chocolate cookies whipped inside? Well, my fitness model version won't give you a guilt trip afterwards!

INGREDIENTS

- 8 oz cold water
- 1 scoop of BSN's Syntha-6 Cookies & Cream Flavored Protein Powder
- ¼ cup Cool Whip Lite
- 6 ice cubes
- 3 chocolate wafer cookies

DIRECTIONS

- Pour water into the blender and add Protein Powder.
- Blend on medium speed for 15 seconds
- Add Cool Whip and ice cubes; blend for 30 seconds on high speed.
- Add cookies and blend on medium speed until mixed.
- Pour into a tall glass and enjoy

FITNESS MODEL STRAWBERRY BANANA SMOOTHIE

When you combine the Vitamin C-rich strawberries with potassium-rich bananas, you are giving yourself a power punch of a protein shake that your body will love you for!

INGREDIENTS

- 6-8 oz water
- 3 ice cubes
- 1 scoop of either BSN Lean Dessert Protein Banana Cream powder, or BSN's Syntha-6 Strawberry Flavor
- 1 small banana
- 3 strawberries

DIRECTIONS

- Pour cold water into blender and add Protein Powder. Blend on medium speed for 15 seconds.
- Add banana and blend for 30 seconds.
- Add strawberries and blend on high speed for 30 seconds more.
- Pour into a tall glass and enjoy.

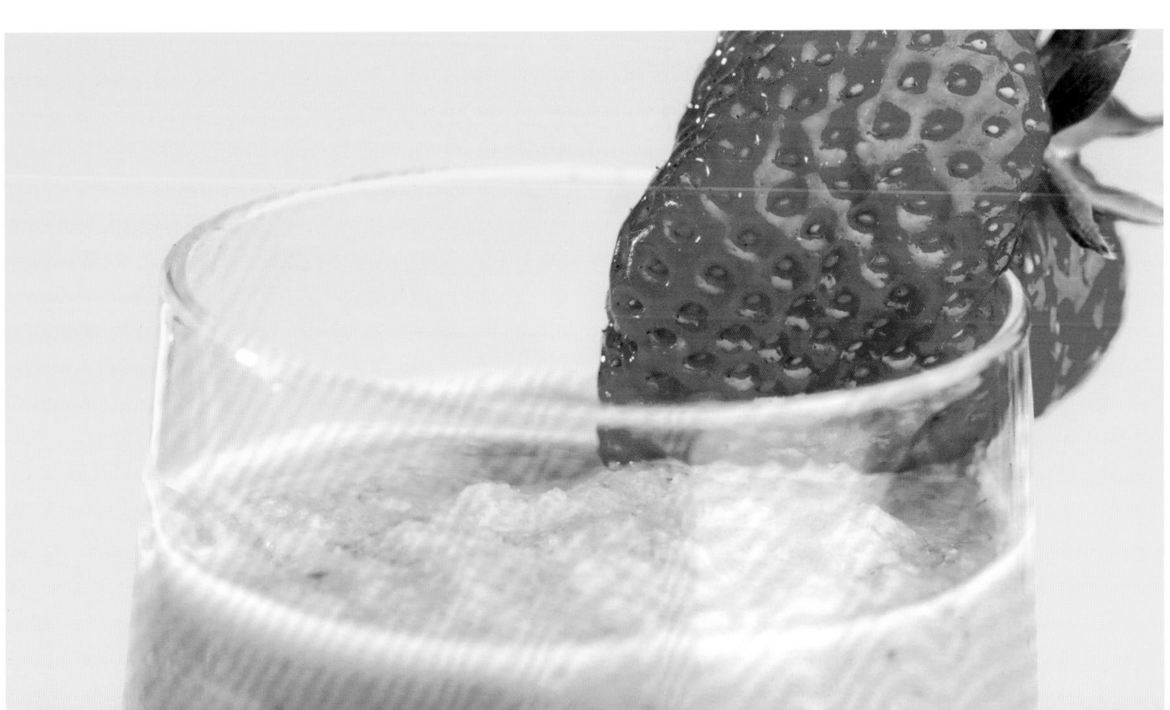

FITNESS MODEL CHOCOLATE PEANUT BUTTER PROTEIN SHAKE

To me, there is nothing more tempting or delicious than the lethal combination of chocolate and peanut butter. When I get the craving for a chocolate peanut butter candy bar, I make a smart decision and make this protein shake.

INGREDIENTS

- 6-8 oz water
- 3 ice cubes
- 1 scoop of BSN Syntha-6 powder, Chocolate Peanut Butter Flavor
- 1 Tbsp natural peanut butter

DIRECTIONS

- Pour water into blender add protein powder, and blend on medium for 15 seconds.
- Add peanut butter and blend for another 30 seconds, then add ice cubes and blend on high speed until smooth (about 30 more seconds).
- Pour into a tall glass and enjoy!

JNL FIT TIP: Portion out and freeze. This Sweet Potato dish does very well when thawed and reheated in the microwave.

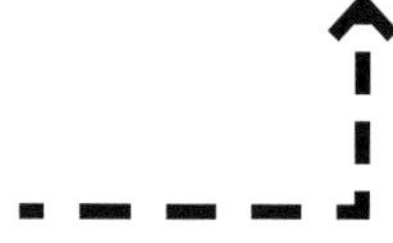

"What's life without all the extra sweet sides?"

—JNL

SIDE DISHES

FITNESS MODEL SWEET POTATO PECAN PIE

This is my healthy version of a pecan pie! Sweet potatoes are excellent sources of Vitamins A and C, and are rich in antioxidants, which fight off free radicals. Cinnamon is also known to curb the appetite. This is a delicious dish that you can have for breakfast or lunch as a side.

Prep Time: 1 hour 15 minutes

INGREDIENTS

- 2 large sweet potatoes, peeled and wrapped loosely in aluminum foil
- 1 cup of raw unsalted Pecans
- ¼ Cup Splenda Brown Sugar
- Dash of cinnamon

DIRECTIONS

- Bake sweet potatoes in aluminum foil in the oven for one hour at 350 Degrees
- Take out of oven, place in large bowl, and mash or whip until soft.
- Stir in pecans and brown sugar and cinnamon.

Serving Size: ¾ cup

FITNESS MODEL ASPARAGUS

If I had to choose between broccoli and asparagus, I would definitely choose the asparagus!

Asparagus is a MUST in the cover girl's food plan! It's a natural diuretic, allowing you to "pee off" those extra pounds. Fitness competitors and models will actually go out of their way to eat it a good week before their competitions or photo shoots, because it helps them to get really lean and cut by helping them to drop unwanted water weight. Always keep asparagus in your fridge washed and ready to steam.

INGREDIENTS

- One package of fresh organic asparagus, rinsed with the hard bottom stems snapped or cut off.

DIRECTIONS

- Steam over steamer until tender yet still crisp, or sauté in a pan until slightly cooked.

FITNESS MODEL BROCCOLI

Broccoli has many health benefits, such as being high in calcium and fiber. Plus, its 'fridge life is long. You can buy a big head of it, and it keeps for a while. It is a staple in the Fitness Model food plan because it can be steamed, added to stir-fries, omelets, or eaten raw with a side of fat-free dip.

INGREDIENTS

- One large head of broccoli, or a package of broccoli florets

DIRECTIONS

- Steam over steamer until tender yet still crisp, or sauté in a pan until slightly cooked.

FITNESS MODEL SPINACH

Spinach is an excellent source of fiber, iron, and powerful antioxidants which fight ovarian cancer. It's delicious in omelets, in soups, stews, or in a green salad. You can also steam it or sauté it for a quick healthy side dish that will complete either your lunch or dinner.

INGREDIENTS

One bag of organic triple washed spinach.

DIRECTIONS

Steam over steamer or sauté in a touch of olive oil until slightly wilted

CREATIVE GARNISHES FOR ASPARAGUS, BROCCOLI, AND SPINACH SIDE DISHES

Feel free to top with any of the following garnishes to make your side dishes a bit more satisfying without blowing your calorie budget!

- Drizzle with olive oil
- Sprinkle with slivered almonds
- Garnish with a squeeze of fresh lemon
- Dust lightly with parmesan cheese
- Lightly top with low-fat feta cheese
- Raw unsalted walnuts
- Crumbled whole grain crackers
- Pecans
- Low-fat hollandaise sauce

CHAPTER 7:

TIME

How to Strategically Budget Your Time to Achieve the Fitness Model Look

"To be your best you must honor your time, respect your priorities in life, and take the time to schedule in your successes and achievements."

—JNL

THE FITNESS MODEL TIME MANAGEMENT PLAN

True, she makes it all look too easy! Balancing work, workouts, and errands, preparing her meals, and doing it all with style, grace, strength, and ease! The Fitness Model is a "make it happen" kind of woman who gets things done, on time and on schedule.

Goal setting is very important in becoming a Fitness Model or just looking like one. If you don't know where you are headed, you will just go nowhere fast, like a gerbil on a wheel, getting caught up in the here and now. Set goals, use a journal, and set your sights high!

HOW TO "CREATE" TIME BY SETTING YOURSELF UP FOR SUCCESS

One of the keys to achieving the Fitness Model™ Look and mastering the program is learning how to efficiently budget and schedule your time. Too many times I have heard the excuse "But I just don't have enough time to exercise or prepare my meals!" I am here to say, "Yes, you do and I will show you how!"

First of all, it starts with your mindset. Give yourself an instant attitude adjustment by improving your mindset towards exercising, eating healthy and making time for yourself, from "Ugh! I HAVE to do this" to "YAY! I GET to do this!" Change your "I HAVE to's" to "I GET to's" and you will gain a whole new paradigm towards taking care of yourself! Look at exercising as a GIFT. You GET to give fresh blood and oxygen to all of the cells in your body! You will be a healthier and happier person and a better wife, girlfriend, daughter, mother, worker, and best friend to those around you.

OLD ATTITUDE & BEHAVIORS	NEW ATTITUDE & BEHAVIORS
Diet Food is expensive so I will go through the drive-through instead	Eating out every day ends up costing more than preparing your meals
It takes too much time to prepare my meals, so I will grab whatever I can find	I am worth the 5 extra minutes it takes to prepare my meals for the day, thus setting myself up for success.
I love socializing with my co-workers at the local restaurant.	I can still enjoy the company of others that share my new healthy mindset
The instant comfort that I get from food soothes me.	Emotional eating is something that I can control. Food does not help solve my problems.
It takes too long to work out- I don't have 2 hours a day to waste on training.	I have learned that I only have to train 45 minutes a day 4 times a week to achieve my fitness goals- I am healthier and happier.

People always start to hate on me when I begin losing weight. It's as if they are jealous that I am starting to feel and look better. I choose to only surround myself with positive supportive people who want me to be fit and happy. I will take a deep and honest look at those who are in my life and see if they truly want me to be fit. If not, I will weed them out of my life. If I can't weed them out, I will learn to live with them and not allow them to steal my joy, while staying committed to my fitness goals.

"Put yourself on your to do list!"

—JNL

HOW TO ELIMINATE TIME ZAPPERS WHICH DILUTE YOUR MOMENTUM AND FOCUS

Just as an accountant audits accounts, you must take an audit of your personal, professional, and spiritual situations/relationships. I urge you all to get real with the circumstances, situations, and people whom you choose to have in your life.

Ask yourself this very empowering question:

> *"Does this person, place, thing or idea help me or hinder me in achieving my personal goals?"*
>
> —JNL

If the answer is "hinder" when you're considering a particular person, you must do whatever is in your power to release that person from your life.

I coached one lady by the name of Barbara whose mother, despite her best intentions to help her daughter reach her fitness goals, actually hindered her, with constant, destructive nagging and complaints. Although Barbara's mother wanted the best for her, she lacked the expertise to help Barbara increase the momentum in her life and end her self-sabotaging behaviors.

I coached her to take a "mini-vacation" from her mom for at least 14 days, so that she could get more in touch with herself, rediscover her passions, and unveil her hidden potential, without being distracted by white noise.

YOU ARE ONLY AS GOOD AS THE PEOPLE YOU SURROUND YOURSELF WITH

Think about Barbara's story, take a good look at the inner circle of people who surround you, and ask yourself these questions:

1. Do they have the same goals as you do?
2. Are they moving forward in their lives, or standing in the same place?
3. Have they made personal achievements comparable to those that you wish to make?
4. Do you feel that you are, at times, compromising your own belief system and allowing yourself to become "brainwashed" by their low standards and mediocrity?
5. Do you honestly feel, deep down inside, these people are helping you to move forward in life? Or are they hindering you, by stagnating your life?

Honest answers to each of these questions it will make it easier for you take the initiative in weeding out people who weigh you down. Surround yourself with those who share the same goals and objectives. It's the law of metaphysics that, when you surround yourself with those who share your interests and goals, results are produced and you accomplish more!

TOP FITNESS MODELS TIPS AND TECHNIQUES FOR TIME

"If you fail to prepare, you might as well forget being successful."

—JNL

"Use the power of anticipation, as it's what separates the winners in life from the losers."

—JNL

PREPARATION IS KEY

Set yourself up for success by doing small, yet very meaningful, everyday practices. Creating and enforcing these powerful habits will pave the way to victory on your quest to a Fitness Model physique!

"By failing to prepare, you are preparing to fail."

—BENJAMIN FRANKLIN

FOOD PLANNING

Always designate at least one official grocery shopping day per week. Make sure to go prepared with your grocery list. Try to schedule your grocery shopping at a time when the store is not crowded, so you can focus on getting what you need as quickly and efficiently as possible. Mine is early Sunday morning before church. It's the best time because no one is there, and I can get in and get out!

Always designate one or two days a week as your food preparation days. Measure, cook and store your food in microwavable or Pyrex containers for the days ahead. Stack neatly in your refrigerator, so you can grab & go. Dry foods such as nuts and cereal or whole grain crackers, can be measured out and stored conveniently in zip-lock bags.

Always carry a few highly portable snacks, such as fruit or a protein bar, in your purse/gym bag, so you never go hungry.

Keep a food journal- this will help keep you on track by reminding you of how far you have come.

Make a weekly food planning chart for each day of the week. Map out your week and plug in the meals you plan on eating each day. Although you may not follow this plan to a T, you will go into your week with a game plan.

Take a "Before" photo and refer to it daily for constant motivation!

FITNESS MODEL WEEKLY FOOD PLANNER

MEAL	SUNDAY	MONDAY	TUESDAY
Breakfast			
Mid-Morning Snack			
Lunch			
Mid-Afternoon Snack			
Dinner			
Pre-bedtime Snack			

WEDNESDAY	THURSDAY	FRIDAY	SATURDAY

Use a copy of this Weekly Food Planner to schedule your Fitness Model meals.

THE JNL FITNESS MODEL FOOD JOURNAL

MOTIVATIONAL QUOTE OF THE DAY: ______________________________

DATE: ______________________________

BREAKFAST: ______________________________

____

MID-MORNING SNACK: ______________________________

LUNCH: ______________________________

____

MID-AFTERNOON SNACK: ______________________________

DINNER: ______________________________

____

MID-EVENING: ______________________________

SUPPLEMENTS: ______________________________

THOUGHTS/REFLECTIONS: ______________________________

____

____

____

____

____

Use a copy of this Food Journal to keep track of your Fitness Model DIet.

JNL-APPROVED SUPER FITNESS MODEL TIPS FOR EXERCISE PLANNING

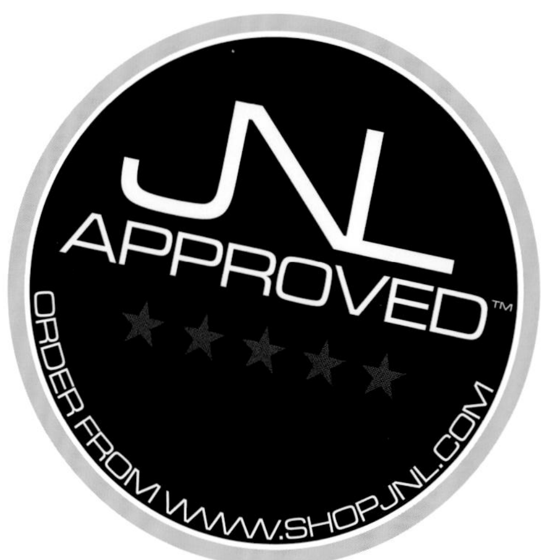

1. Have a gym bag packed in the back of your car/trunk for the impromptu workout at your local park/gym.
2. Always know what body part(s) you are training the next day so you can get yourself mentally prepared.
3. Always have your workout clothes set out and ready to go the night before. Put them in a designated space, where you know where they are, to put on after your morning shower, or first thing in the morning when you change out of your pajamas. This is a success anchor to make sure you don't skip your workouts.
4. Designate a certain area in your home as your personal exercise area, where you keep your Fitness Model program tools/equipment. This needs to be a special place, allotted for your workouts. I suggest having it near a television, stereo, or a window where the natural sunlight can shine through to motivate you! Again, don't put it in a dark, dirty basement! This will be your workout zone. Honor that space by using it only for working out, and you will!
5. Schedule and plan your workouts, like appointments in your agenda. If you reserve ahead for a good solid hour to work out, you will be just that much more likely to work out.
6. Pick out 3 workout outfits, and have them ready in your closet, so you can grab and go to get dressed for working out.
7. Purchase portable plastic protein shake tumblers so you can use them on the run!
8. Pick a time at the gym when there are fewer people there, so that you can focus and move more easily from one piece of equipment to the next.
9. Invest in at-home equipment, like my Ab Circle Pro, which you can see at www.JNLAbCirclePro.com. I love this machine, because you get more results in less time!

FITNESS MODEL ON THE GO

"A great thing about living a super fitness model lifestyle is that its action packed, you are always on the go, and you lead an active, robust life that is worth celebrating!"

— JNL

Learning how to healthfully eat on-the-go is part of mastering the Fitness Model Diet. With the increasing amount of "healthy food" options which most fast food chains are now offering, there are no more excuses!

SUBWAY	▪ Any six inch sandwich on whole wheat bread from their "7 under 6" menu (forgo the cheese, mayonnaise, oil and salt, and load up on the veggies!) ▪ Turkey Breast ▪ Roasted Chicken Breast ▪ Sweet Onion Chicken Teriyaki ▪ Roast Beef ▪ Tuna Salad made with low-fat mayonnaise
WENDY'S	▪ Southwest Chicken Caesar Salad ▪ Mandarin Chicken Caesar Salad ▪ Southwest Taco Salad (forgo sour cream) ▪ Chicken BLT Salad ▪ Grilled Chicken Sandwich (no mayo or cheese, top bun off, and opt for lettuce & tomato) ▪ Grilled Chicken Wrap (no mayo or cheese, top bun off, and opt for lettuce & tomato) ▪ Side Salad with Low-fat Honey mustard ▪ Diet Lemonade or Bottled Water ▪ Small Chili and Side Salad

JNL FIT TIP: toss the top bun of your sandwich, so you are only eating the bottom bun. This little fitness model tip will help you to eat less carbs, yet still enjoy the sandwich.

MCDONALDS	▪ Southwest Salad with Grilled Chicken ▪ Asian Salad with Grilled Chicken ▪ Premium Bacon Ranch Salad with Grilled Chicken ▪ Premium Caesar Salad with Chicken ▪ Snack Size Fruit & Walnut Salad ▪ Grilled Chicken Classic (no mayo or cheese, top bun off, and opt for lettuce & tomato) ▪ Grilled Snack Wrap (ask for no cheese, add lettuce & tomato)
TACO BELL	▪ Soft Tacos ▪ Steak or Chicken Al Fresco (no cheese, no sour cream or Guacamole; just made with lettuce and tomatoes) ▪ Crunchy taco Fresco style ▪ Beef or Chicken Soft Taco ▪ Ranchero Chicken Soft Taco Fresco Style ▪ Bean Burrito Fresco Style ▪ Chicken Burrito Fresco Style ▪ Steak Burrito Fresco Style
BURGER KING	▪ Chicken Caesar Salad ▪ Shrimp Caesar Salad ▪ Chicken Garden Salad ▪ Shrimp Garden Salad ▪ Plain hamburger (no mayonnaise; opt for lettuce and tomato instead) ▪ Grilled chicken (no mayonnaise; opt for lettuce and tomato instead) ▪ Veggie Burger

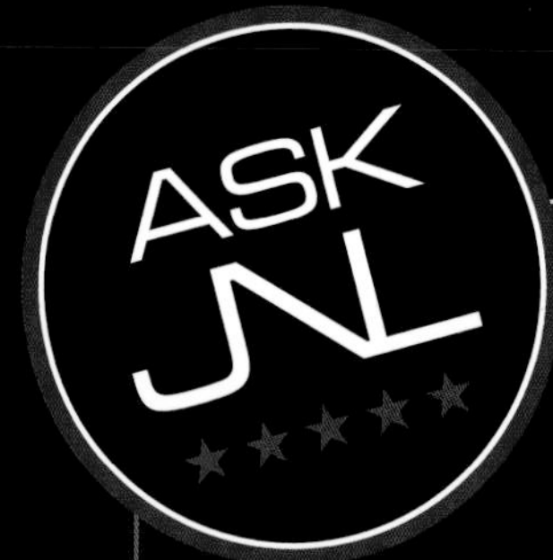

CHAPTER 8:

FREQUENTLY ASKED QUESTIONS

This chapter is dedicated to YOU, and all of the amazing questions that you all have emailed to our offices. It's my mission to provide you with the latest cutting-edge information to help you achieve your fitness goals. If you have a burning question to ask my team of professionals and me, simply drop us an email at www.JenniferNicoleLee.com

Q: JNL, How much protein do I need?

A: 0.8-1.0 grams of protein per pound of body weight. Example: if you weigh 130 pounds you need 104 grams to 130 grams a day of protein. I round up to 1 gram of protein per pound of body weight, to keep it simple.

Q: In your opinion JNL, what type of protein is the best?

A: The #1 most bio-available form of protein is egg whites. Your body assimilates them into the muscles the quickest. The next most important form of protein is whey protein, which is your BSN Lean Dessert Protein powder. You can also get lots of protein through chicken, fish, or lean red meat.

Q: What is the major "roadblock" keeping some away from achieving their fitness goals?

A: The #1 self-sabotaging behavior that I see women doing is failing to take in adequate amounts of protein. Protein is not only important for your muscle growth and maintenance, but it is the primary building block of life! It's essential for the health and strength of your hair, skin, and nails. Make sure that you get in enough protein to keep yourself strong and beautiful, from the inside out!

Q: JNL, How much cardio is enough?

A: It really depends on your fitness goals. However, the common Fitness Model rule of thumb is no less than 25 minutes, to no more than 45 minutes. If you refer to your Fitness Model exercise program, you will see that the emphasis is not on cardio, but on weight training. This is the key; if you find yourself with only 45 minutes to work out, I cannot stress enough how important it is to choose weight training over cardio. Your weight loss results may not be instant, but they will be long-term, with the power of weight training. Perform no more than 25 to 45 minutes on Wednesdays and Saturdays after you perform your ab exercises.

Q: Do I do weights before cardio?

A: This is a resounding, absolute, always, never-changing YES – always perform your weight training routine before cardio! Working with weights, you are burning fat and calories as you get your metabolism revved up. Plus, you're focusing your freshest energy where you need it most, on the weight training rather than the cardio, After you have done your 45-minute cycle of weight training, your body is already in the fat-burning zone. Finish strong with even more fat-blasting cardio in your 65-75 percent target heart rate!

Q: Help me, Jennifer! How do I get rid of this stubborn cellulite on my butt, hips and thighs?

A: This has got to be one of the most frequently asked questions, along with "How do I get rid of stretch marks?" Cellulite is a sign of toxic build up within the body. Therefore, detoxing at least monthly is very important. Weight training improves the inner architecture of the body, thus helping to diminish the appearance of cellulite. Coupled with fat-blasting cardio, and combined with a low-fat food plan as described in this book, you will certainly see an improvement. I thank the beauty industry for helping us women who suffer from cellulite, by providing us with supplements, topical lotions, creams and oils that can be applied to the skin externally to help diminish (if not eliminate) the appearance of cellulite.

The most effective way to treat severe cellulite and get visible results is the little-known medical spa procedure known as Endermologie. For more information on this "top secret" beauty procedure, please visit www.ShopJNL.com and click on my Audio Seminars.

Q: How do I get rid of stretch marks?

A: Getting rid of stretch marks can be simply accomplished through the use of certain lotions, oils and creams which help to diminish and eradicate them. In addition, you can also use tanning to help lessen their appearance. For a list of my top topical lotions, creams and oils, please visit www.ShopJNL.com and click on my Audio Seminars.

Q: What is the best way to achieve that Fitness Model™ Tan? The tanning bed or sunless tanning lotion?

A: Always opt for a sunless tanning lotion! My motto is "Fake it, don't bake it". Tanning beds and sun baking have many disadvantages, such as premature aging, burning, and skin cancer. Always choose sunless skin lotions over tanning. To learn how to achieve the perfect Fitness Model glow, please visit www.ShopJNL.com and click on my Audio Seminars.

Q: How do I safely get rid of water weight?

A: There are many ways to safely get rid of water weight. First, I urge you to utilize the power of food. Asparagus is a natural diuretic, allowing you to "pee off the pounds." In the Fitness Industry, asparagus is a staple among figure and fitness competitors, who always eat it days before stepping onto the stage.

Other ways to minimize water weight include doing cardio while wearing comfortable layers of clothing, allowing your body temperature to rise and helping you to sweat more. Also, if you refrain from eating foods high in sodium, you will notice a difference in about 3 days (no salt, so soy sauce, no canned foods, no deli meats; choose salt free seasonings such as Mrs. Dash).

For an extreme method of helping your body release trapped water in the system, many fitness models and competitors rely upon watershed pills. These water-shedding pills are to be used sparingly, and only when truly needed — for special occasions such as a pool party, wedding, photo shoot, or after getting off a long flight, or before a fitness or figure competition. To learn about my favorite watershed pills in my top picks along with other high quality supplements, please listen to my instant downloadable audio seminar on Supplements by visiting www.ShopJNL.com

Q: Are soy products good for me?

A: Well, not exactly. You see, contrary to what you hear and read, soy products such as edamame, tofu and soy milk may not be as beneficial to your health as the media and marketing make them out to be.

Soy products are scientifically proven to raise the level of estrogen in the body. Just as birth control pills raise your estrogen level in order to "fool" your body into thinking it is pregnant, soy bloats you around your pelvic area, abdomen, hips, buns & thighs. Soy products can also interfere with your normal thyroid function

Q How do I get rid of that kangaroo patch and flabby skin under my belly?

A: It's a combination of a lifestyle program consisting of everything in your Fitness Model Program. The lifestyle program includes exercise (specifically on my Ab Circle Pro, which you can see here at www.JNLAbCirclePro.com), food planning, and other beauty secrets including endermologie. Endermologie not only eradicates cellulite but also helps break down that very thick or thin layer of fat found on most women's abdominal area. For more on endermologie, please visit www.ShopJNL.com and click on my Audio Seminars.

"Follow the guidelines and principles in this Fitness Model Program and, with patience and persistence, you will safely lower your body fat."

Q: Will running help me look like a Fitness Model?

A: Absolutely not! If you want to look like a Fitness Model and not a runner, than don't run! From my extensive research, I have discovered that most fitness models, competitors, and/or body builders do not run because it actually "eats away" at the muscle. Most runners have a higher body fat percentage than fitness models. We in the Fitness industry call them "skinny fat people." Yes, they may be thin; however, their body fat percentage consists of more fat than muscle.

Q: How do I lower my body fat safely?

A: Follow the guidelines and principles in this Fitness Model Program and, with patience and persistence, you will safely lower your body fat. Use this program — do not let it collect dust!

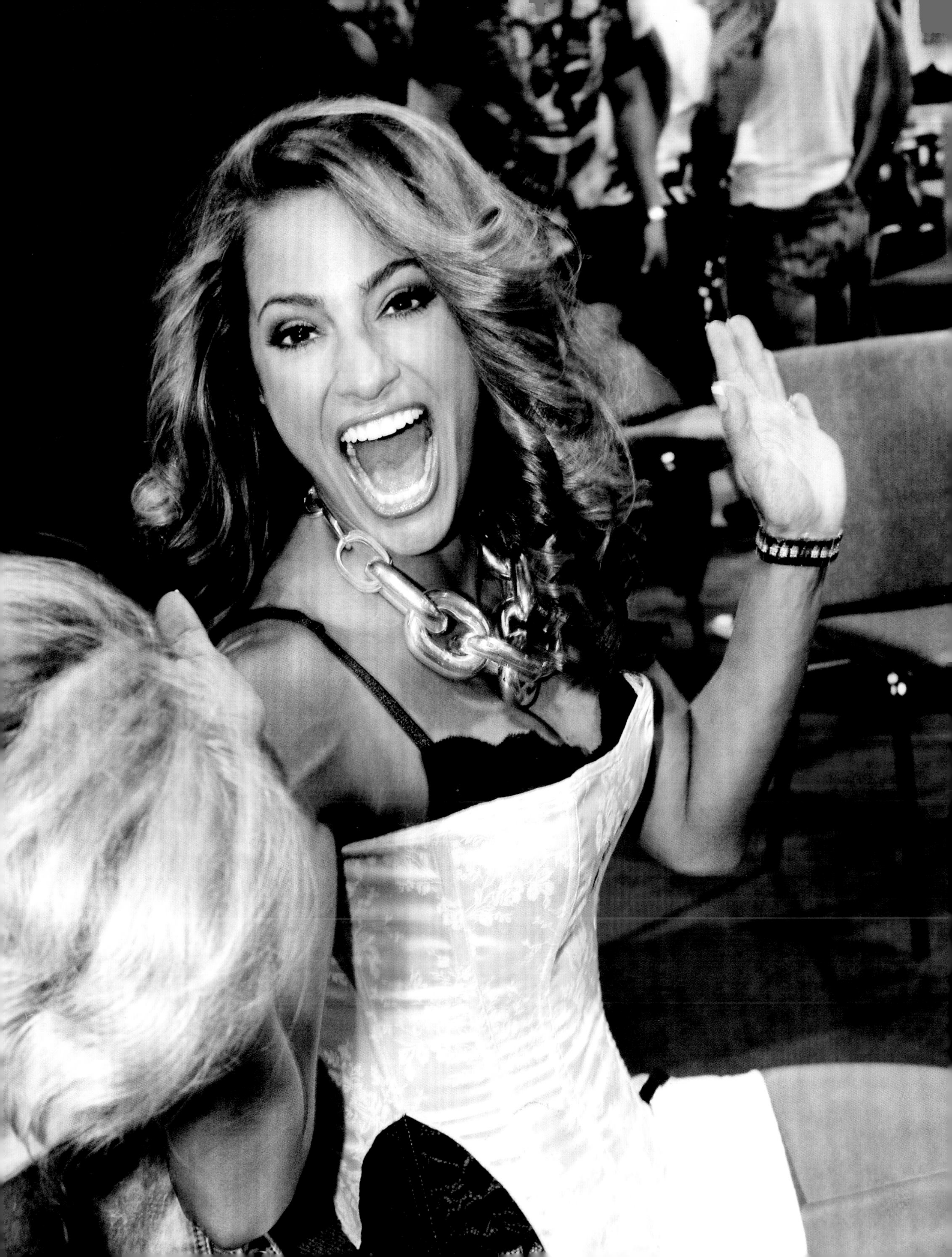

CHAPTER 9

HOW I SURVIVED MY FITNESS MODELING YEARS

And How I Become a Leader in the Industry

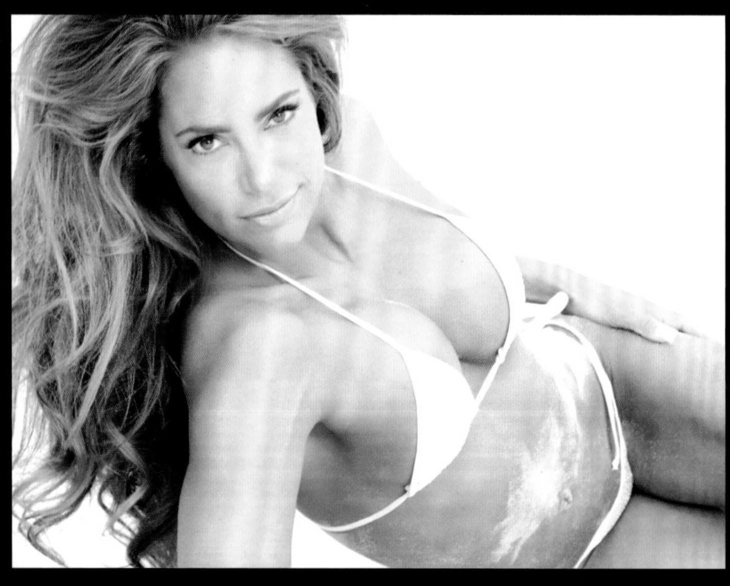

I have a really great career! Modeling has taken me to far, exotic places – places I had never dreamed of going. But I have always remembered my humble beginnings, and where I came from. And, to be honest, I know that I have survived my fitness modeling years, and am still surviving them, not because I'm the best, but because I am one of the hardest working, most driven, and truly focused.

HOW I BECAME A SUPER FITNESS MODEL

I started at the bottom of the bottom in the fitness modeling industry. I wasn't part of some inner-girl clique, or some boot camp where all the hot girls went every year to network and be seen. I didn't know the top coaches, or fitness publications, or competition prep camps. I was never an athlete, didn't know any other fellow fitness models, and had no "in" with the industry. I was the definition of "beginner"! I was a stay-at-home mom who had suffered a miscarriage with her first pregnancy, got pregnant 3 months later, and then after my first baby turned one, got pregnant again. For a period of about five years, I was either pregnant, breast-feeding or fat, or somewhere in between! Then I took action and got myself in super fitness model shape.

It was really due to the urging of my friends and family, who pushed me to go and compete at a local fitness competition, because they were so proud of my new-found fitness level and physique. With their support, I enrolled into the competition. And to my disbelief, I ended up placing first-runner-up!

So, when I came onto the fitness modeling scene, I was a nobody, and no one knew who I was. I kind of came out of nowhere. But I didn't let all of these strikes work against me. I was hungry to be successful at fitness modeling, so I did what I could do.

I broke down a lot of barriers in the fitness modeling areas. I started in my late 20's, had not had a gymnastics or dance background, had never worked out with weights and was never in shape until after my children were born. For someone who was in her late 20's, who had once weighed over 200 pounds, who was a devoted wife and mother, with no fitness modeling background whatsoever, to become one of the world's most accomplished fitness models, is nothing short of a miracle. You see, it's not about being perfect, but about being persistent.

"Always ignore your haters. Nothing annoys them more."

—JNL

HOW TO DEAL WITH THE NEGATIVES AND TURN THEM INTO POSITIVES

Instead of being ashamed of having been obese at one time, I used this to my advantage. I shared my weight loss success story, and the courage it had taken to face my weight problem, to inspire others and motivate them to be their best, too. My story got around the fitness industry, and that led to key media appearances, and to getting booked for magazine covers, editorial spreads, endorsements, and ad campaigns.

I celebrated me being different, and not going along with the crowd or being a part of some inside clique. Instead, I let my true personality shine through when I went on go-sees, or met with the editor in chief of a magazine, and was polite to all the people I met. Today, this is my personal mission; to show young women how important their inner beauty and personality are.

REJECTION AND NOT BEING (FILL IN THE BLANK) ENOUGH

What's the one thing that you will receive a lot of from the fitness modeling industry? Rejection. But you will also receive tons of joy and pleasure if modeling is your true passion in life. So, my advice to you, in order to keep your eye on the prize and to keep steadfast towards achieving your career goals, is to learn how to deal with rejection.

When you meet very important individuals in the fitness modeling industry, you will have to deal with rejection, and I have had my fair share of it. But you must be thick-skinned, and not let it penetrate your spirit, or break you. When I began fitness modeling I had so many photographers, stylists, hair and makeup artists point out flaws in me that I didn't even know that I had, or be straight-out rude to me, even treat me like something less than human. But did I let these negative experiences stop me? Never!

This is why your passion and drive must be stronger than any negativity that comes your way. You've got to be ready to stand up for yourself. This is where your strong ego must kick in and come out!

My nickname and the name of my alter ego is "La Tigra," which represents the fearless, fierce, and feisty personality that comes out when I'm tested, challenged, or unfairly attacked. So I urge you to reconnect with your inner female fighter spirit who will keep you strong, focused, and fuel your determination when the times get tough and challenging.

OUTSMARTING THE HATERS & SABOTEURS

Yes, there is a stereotype that fitness models are catty, negative, bitter, self-absorbed divas. And yes, I have met those kinds of fitness models, and they do exist. But these women were miserable and unhappy with themselves from the inside out. And most of them are nowhere to be found today. I was always friendly with the models who were nice to me, and had no ulterior motives. But at times, those lil' divas made it very hard for me to be successful, and for me to be efficient in my profession, I had to outsmart them. I had to be strong inside, and stay super-focused on my dream. I told myself every day that I would not let anybody or anything stand in the way of my dreams, especially a shallow, desperate wanna-be fitness model. So, instead of allowing them to intimidate me, I went toe to toe with them and would call them out. I treated fitness modeling as a business, and they were obviously treating .it as a gossip forum.

There are negative, sabotaging enemies in all professions, and sometimes we all have to deal with those "hatas". But my expert advice to you, if you really want to make it into the fitness modeling industry, is to stay focused on your goals, and not allow these saboteurs to drain you of your energy. Always "keep your side of the street clean," by not engaging in negative gossip. Frequently revisit your goals, and re-write them out, to keep yourself super-charged by asking yourself empowering questions like "Where do I want to be in one year? In two years? In five years?" Remember the old adage "You are only as good as the people who you surround yourself with"? Well, that is the truth! So make a commitment to yourself to only surround yourself with true friends and family members, who love and support you. Rely on them when the times get tough. And sometimes you've just got to keep away from the catty girls!

> *"Rejection is just a part of living a super fitness model lifestyle. Those who have been able to outsmart and silence the critics will always end up being successful in their career and in their life."*
>
> —JNL

> *"Hating, to me, is just a form of flattery."*
>
> —JNL

HOW I REDEFINED THE FITNESS MODELING INDUSTRY

Many people thought that fitness modeling was "mindless" and easy to do, that you simply had to look hot in a bikini. But it is an art form, and to be an amazing fitness model, you must practice, train, go to the best workshops, and perfect your craft.

I helped to redefine the fitness modeling industry by showing that women today are very multi-dimensional, and that we today wear many hats. Women today are not just "superficial" beings, with one side. We are moms, students, wives, best friends, entrepreneurs, and we deserve to have it all!

I was one of the first true, proud moms to show up on the scene. When I broke into the industry, not many models were being open about their families or having children, and it was taboo to even speak of your kids. But I was proud of the fact that I was a mom, that I ballooned to up over 200 pounds while pregnant, and that I had the mental strength to lose the weight. I made fitness modeling my art form, my profession, and my passion, and showed the world that to be the best fitness model, you must be articulate, intelligent, and trustworthy. I showed many health companies that, to really be considered a force, you must become a triple threat. Today, to be a super fitness model, not only do you have to be in ultra-fit shape, you must also be able to do interviews, charm the media, be well spoken, and be prepared at all times. To make it big, you must study who is who, and be in–the-know as to who the big names and important editors are at the best magazines. Being savvy is an major piece in building your career.

KNOWING WHEN TO MAKE YOUR GRAND EXIT-AND YOUR GRAND ENTRANCE

You must also know when to bow out, and leave the fitness modeling industry at the right time, to allow your career to evolve into the next profession and move it in the right direction. I'm now executive producing, writing books, branching out to TV and commercials, and leaving my fitness modeling years behind me. I've made my grand exit from modeling, and my grand entrance into other fields of the entertainment and wellness industry.

I have seen way too many examples of fitness models who have hung onto their modeling days too long, and failed to cultivate the other gifts that God gave them. I have seen women cling onto their fitness modeling bookings like an old security blanket that they just can't let go of, because they didn't dare be bold enough to test themselves in other areas of the industry. So, my advice to you is to aim at always learning something new, making a new contact and nurturing new passions along your journey, so that one day you can close one door to walk through ten more.

My fitness modeling career led me to a crossroad of "Well, do I keep modeling? Or do I expand my brand, build upon my gifts and talents, and challenge myself by pushing myself to the next chapter?" And I boldly accepted the challenge, and allowed the natural progression of my career, where I made the leap from fitness model to mega-mogul.

CHAPTER 10:

JNL'S LEAP: FITNESS MODEL TO MEGA-MOGUL

"Confidence is 50% of what you are about, and 50% what people think you're about."

—JNL

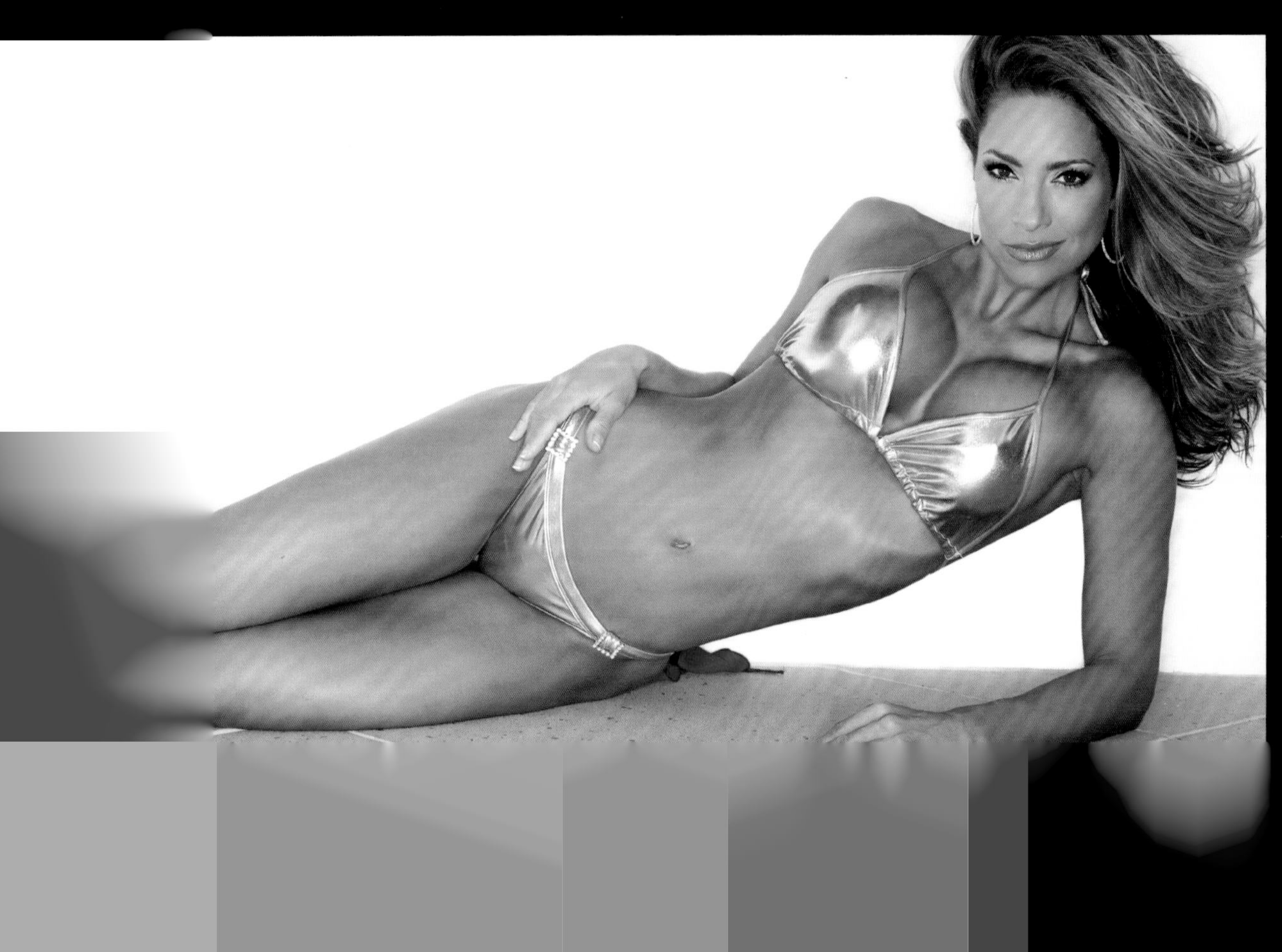

It's been a long journey, but it's nice to know that now, today, I am not just a fitness model but a mega-mogul. I don't say this because I think that I'm all that. But I share this with you to show you that you can make your dreams come true, and that you should never stop dreaming. Becoming a high-profile leader in the fitness, entertainment, and wellness industries is all the result of my hard work, focus, and dedication. It's also because I treated fitness modeling with sincere respect as a profession, not just a hobby.

I loved fitness modeling so much that I asked myself this empowering question: "How can I turn my passion into a profession?" The answers didn't come to me instantly, but rather, since I had my "antennae" up ready to receive, the answers came to me over a period of time. I collected all of my answers and then created a successful global business. I knew that I could not be truly successful as just a fitness model, so I made contacts with the right people, and learned as much as I could. I knew that in order to be extremely successful, I would have to branch out of fitness modeling, and into producing, product development and marketing, and go global. With my infomercials appearing in over 100 different countries on TV, and my voice being dubbed into over 20 different languages, I am proud to say that I am now a household name around the world. My Ab Circle Pro machine is currently ranked as the number one best-selling exercise product to date, with sales around the world. You can visit www.JNLAbCirclePro.com for more information.

But I looked to my own mentors to guide me in my businesses. I recently created another company in addition to my JNL, Inc. My new company is called JNL Worldwide, Inc., which focuses more on my global presence, and is about helping to bring the power of fitness to different countries around the world. I loved how Kathy Ireland, Cindy Crawford, Tyra Banks, and Christy Brinkley all knew when to exit the modeling world and enter new phases of their careers. They created brands around their names and images, licensed out their names to endorse products, and became bestselling authors, producers, and creative directors. I look up to these super-strong, powerful and beautiful women, and admire them for being powerful role models – and not only models.

I structured my JNL Worldwide, Inc. to maximize my global presence, so that I could generate sales of my innovative digital products, exercise equipment, infomercials, and books anywhere, at any given time, allowing me to enjoy a residual income from marketing to every corner of the world.

"A smart, intelligent superfitness model is an excellent role model."

—JNL

"Compete only with yourself, by pushing yourself always to the next level, and one day you will be looking over your own empire."

—JNL

THE FUNDAMENTAL BUSINESS GOALS OF A SUPER FITNESS MODEL

As you can see, I have been able to achieve a lot in a short time, just under 5 years. But it was still a long journey, in which I learned a lot along the way. I learned what do to, and what must be done, to make a name for yourself in the business. The fundamental business goals that you must achieve in order to make sure you have a long, prosperous career in the fitness modeling are the following:

1. Create a website that is your name. Your name represents YOU, and it's YOUR brand.

2. Create a logo that is based on your name, so people will remember you, your logo, your brand, and what you stand for in the industry.

3. Define what your niche market is. My niche market is the real-life working mom who wants to look like a fitness model, even if she isn't one. So ask yourself, who your market is – and make it a point to become friends with them!

4. You must train to look your absolute best. This is part of the game; working out so that your body is your business. It's your billboard, marketing you. So treat your workouts as important business meetings that you cannot call in sick for, cancel, or not show up to, with the most important person in the world – you!

5. Create products. This is a must! Write digital products, e-programs, or e-books that will help you to enjoy a constant stream of residual income.

6. You must be a triple threat to have "stickability" in our industry. Practice speaking in front of a mirror, take acting lessons, work at being well-spoken. If big fitness companies see that you can read from a teleprompter, connect with the video camera, speak well on TV, and that the media loves you, they will book you time and time again.

7. Have a store on your website. In order to really have longevity in your career as a fitness model, make sure you have an online shop at your website. Sell your autographed 8 x 10s, your calendars, your exercise DVDs, and all of your memorabilia. This will not only make you money, but will put your products into the hands of your fans.

8. Make appearances! Your fans want to see you, chat with you, and meet you in person. Every month, aim to be at a fitness convention, and promote this date to your fan base.

9. Collect emails! On the homepage of your website, make sure that you have an email opt-in box. When people visit your website, make sure that they leave their email address so that you can market and sell to them in the future.

10. Lastly, aim to get endorsement deals from supplement companies, from exercise equipment companies, exercise clothing lines, swimsuit lines, and health-related companies. Send them your press kit, email them your info, and let them know that you are interested in being a part of their company.

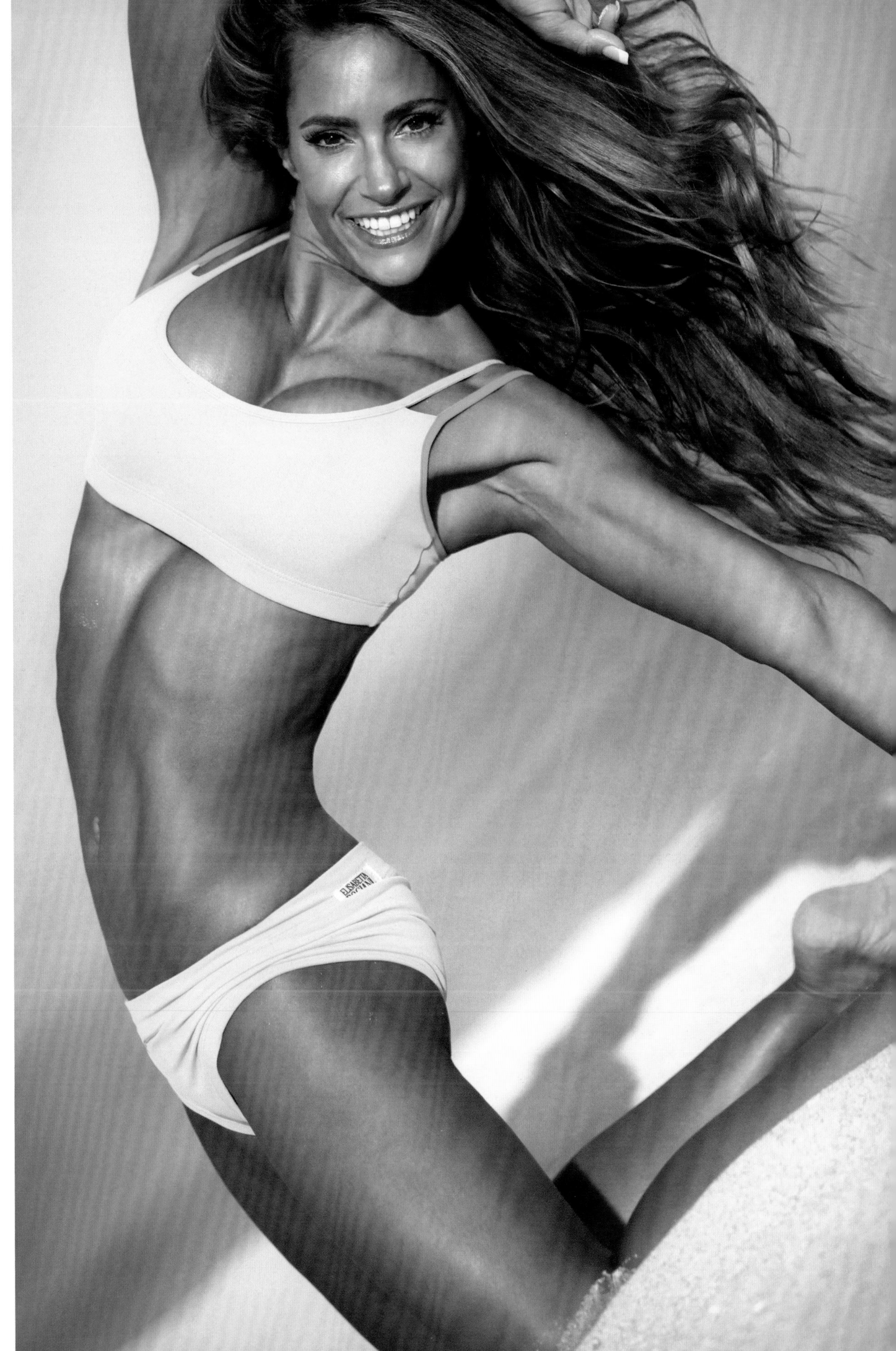
ELISABETTA

CHAPTER 11:

TIPS FOR A SUCCESSFUL FITNESS MODEL PHOTO SHOOT

"Looking sexy, fun and fit in the roughest, toughest conditions with other people you don't know, in distant far away places in tiny, almost invisible outfits isn't easy—it's an art form, and one that I'm darn good at."

—JNL

"If I go a week without doing a photo shoot, I have serious withdrawals. It's my passion, and my art form that I am dedicated to. I am always perfecting my craft."

—JNL

I'm here to banish the myth that fitness modeling is easy. It's not! It is one of the hardest art forms and professions to perfect, and can be downright grueling at times. First of all, fitness models live such a strict, dedicated super fit lifestyle, and this alone can be extremely challenging at times. Then add a 12 hour-long photo shoot to the mix with a super diva photographer, and you will definitely discover just how hard being a super fitness model can be!

For instance, I remember one of my first photo shoots, where I was stuck out in the cold ocean water for hours on end, and I had to pretend to feel healthy and fit, and to look like I was having fun. But the truth of the matter was that I was miserably cold, tired of being wet, and sick of pretending to look like I was enjoying myself! So just remember that fitness modeling is tough at times, but here are my top tips to help you to have successful photo shoots.

CREATE YOUR FITNESS MODEL MINDSET

When in front of the camera, use your "fitness model" mindset. Think of the person who will be looking at this photo of you. What feeling do you want to project to them? Use your eyes, your face, your body to express this message, and then penetrate the camera lens with this energy.

MAKE THE CAMERA YOUR BEST FRIEND

Look right into the cameras lens, and imagine that the lens is a person. When I realized this trick, my photos became much more moving, and evoked more emotion from the viewer. Instead of thinking of the camera as just a camera, think of it as one of your favorite people in the world, and "warm" up to it.

PREPARE, PREPARE, PREPARE!

Be prepared! If you fail to prepare, be prepared to fail. This means, do your research on the photographer, know exactly where the location is beforehand, have your own personal outfits picked out and packed, and also always pack your own hair and makeup kit, even if there is a makeup artist on set. I have gone to photo shoots where the stylist on set didn't have anything that really made me look my best. I learned the hard way to always bring back-up outfits that accentuate my positives while down playing my weaknesses. Also, I have had horrific experiences with professional makeup artists, so I now always pack my personal makeup and hair essentials, and am always ready to do my own if needed.

PRACTICE IN FRONT OF THE MIRROR

Practicing in front of the mirror will help you to learn new poses, work your angles, and see which side is your best side. This is a workout in its own right. Posing in front of a mirror will help you to understand your body better, and help you to be able to "turn it on" when in front of a camera.

STUDY PHOTOGRAPHY & OTHER FITNESS PHOTOS

I'm not saying you've got to go to college for photography, but at least open up a fitness photography book! Learn the fundamentals of photography, such as lighting and some of the terminology. This will help your relationships with the photographers who you work with, thus helping to generate better photos. Select some top fitness magazines, and study some of the poses in these magazines. Create a file of your favorite tear sheets, and always bring them to photo shoots with you. You will have access to your instant library of poses when you are on location. And believe me, when you are in front of the camera, it's easy to freeze up. Taking a glance at your tear sheet collection before and during your photo shoots will help you to warm up in front of the camera, stay fresh in your poses, and keep your energy creative.

UNDERSTAND THAT FITNESS MODELING IS AN ART FORM

When you truly understand that fitness modeling is an art form, you give it 'way more respect, and this energy will show up in your photos. Your super-fit body and its lines, your face and your poses, become much more than just a subject for a photo. It becomes a piece of art, and the photograph will exude this aura!

BE YOUR OWN WORST CRITIC

When you are brutally honest with yourself, and take time to critique your own photographs, you will learn to become better at your craft. Take a really close look at your wardrobe, the styling, the hair and makeup, the athletic level of your body, and be totally real with yourself. What can you do better? How can you work your strengths more effectively? How can you improve your poses? Your energy? Your connection with the camera?

STUDY!

Know who everyone is in the fitness industry, and connect with them! Knowing them a bit better will help you to have more confidence when it comes to camera time. Having some kind of personal bond with the photographer, the publication, or the manufacturer of the swimsuit company that you are being booked with, will help you to understand their company more and what they stand for, and how you can project this in your photos.

BE CAMERA-READY – ALWAYS!

One way to make sure that you are always booked is to stay in shape, and always be camera ready. Publishers, editors, and photographers are always on deadline, and they will need a model at the last minute. Anticipate this, and be ready to say YES when they call! Be ready from the top of your head, to the tips of your toes! Have your hair, toes, and nails all in tip-top condition. Make sure your teeth are whitened, to give you that million-dollar smile that lights up a room! And always stay within 3-5 pounds of your ideal weight, never allowing yourself to go over by five pounds.

ALWAYS KEEP A POSITIVE ATTITUDE

When it rains at an outdoor shoot, when the water you are modeling bikinis in is freezing, and when the photographer is a loud-mouthed diva, STAY POSITIVE! There ARE tons of fitness models out there ready, willing, and able to replace you. And at the end of the day, it's your reputation that will either make you or break you.

KNOW YOUR LIMITS, AND STICK TO THEM!

Sadly enough there are some seedy, ruthless pervert photographers out there. So always go to a photo shoot with someone. Never go alone! Also, know your limits before-hand, and let the photographer know them from the start. I have been at photo shoots where, at the end of our shoot, the photographer wanted me to strip it all off, and do nude shots, I kindly told him "no, thank you" and stuck to my guns. Luckily I had brought my best friend with me, so I was not alone. But this should never happen to you, so I urge you to do your homework on the photographer beforehand and make sure that he is someone who is solid and trustworthy in the industry.

HAVE FUN!

Last but not least, HAVE FUN! Enjoy this time in front of the camera, and show the entire world just how amazing you are! Think about all the time you put into training, eating right, and preparing for the photo shoot. Make your hard work worth it in front of the camera, by shining as bright as you can, and having fun.

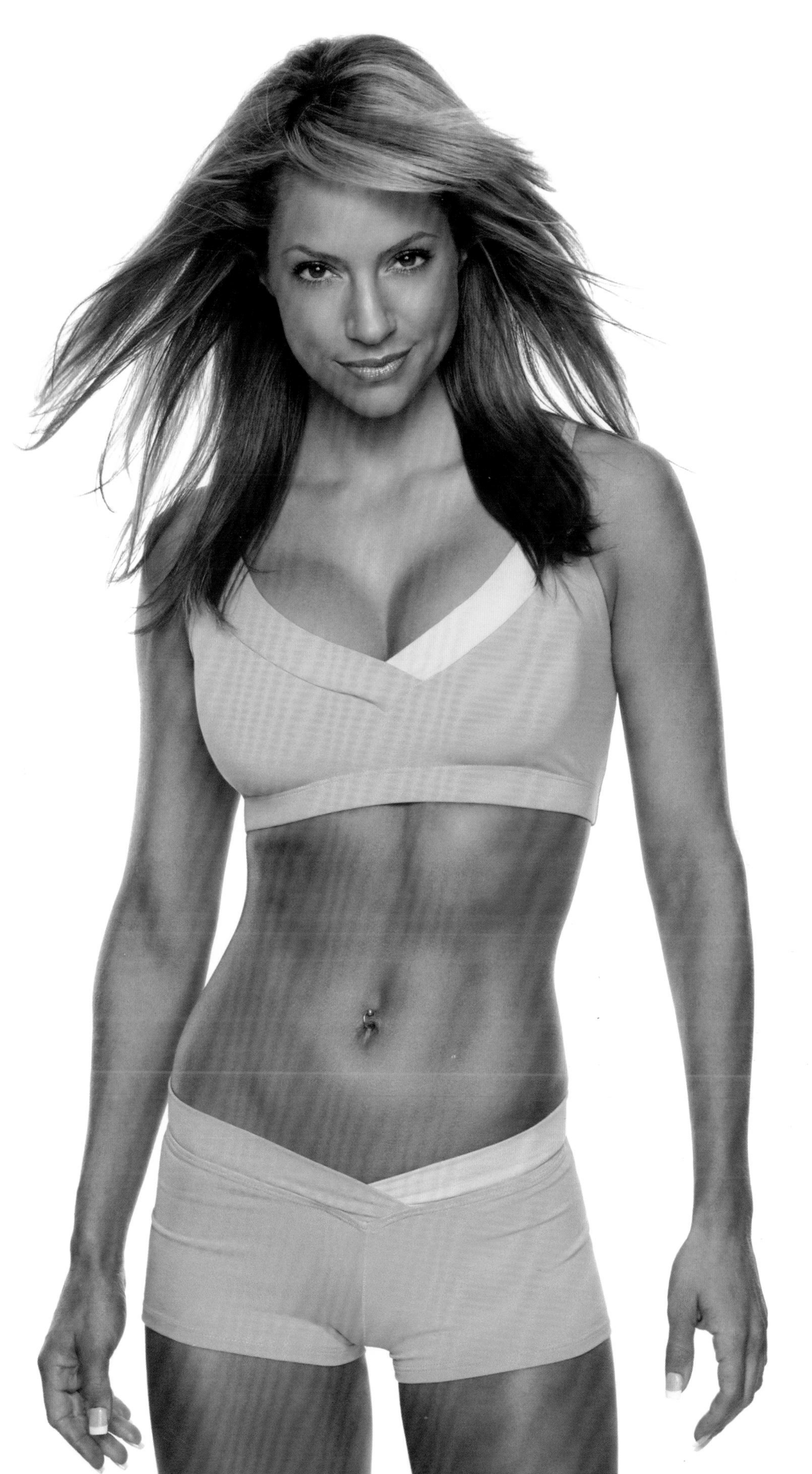

CHAPTER 12:

A WEEK IN THE LIFE OF JNL CHRONICLED

"If you want to really know that a week in the life of a super fitness model is like, just take a look at my calendar, if you can keep up!"

—JNL

FRIDAY SEPTEMBER THE 18TH 2009:

After months of dialed-in training in preparation for my return to the competition stage to defend my WBFF title as Miss Bikini Diva, I am flying to Toronto, Canada. Tomorrow is the competition, and I don't like to get out of my comfort zone too early. I always love to fly last minute to an event, show up and do my thing, and then leave. I'm flying with my best friend and executive assistant, Marli. She has been packing for weeks, making sure I have all that I need for the competition and the photo shoots. Last minute consults, telephone interviews, and a meeting with my stylist for all future shows—DONE!

We land, check into our hotel, and get ready for registration. My really great friend, Berns of Passion Fruit Designs, comes to my suite and sees me for the first time in my "Golden Python Suit," and we take a bunch of photos and video. We then head to registration, where I run into everyone who is a major player in our fitness industry. I see Rodney and Ocean of *Status Fitness* Mag, I also see David Ford, the photographer of the event. I see Allison and Paul Dillett, the co-founders of the WBFF, who are amazing people. I register, take some photos and then get back to my hotel suite to get some R&R for tomorrow's big day. Even though I can't sleep I focus on not moving my body, even though my mind is going a mile a minute — I have got to rest my body. I have no right being on that stage with 18 year old women when I'm 34, "God help me shine!"

SATURDAY SEPTEMBER THE 19TH 2009:

I wake up, and it's a beautiful day here in Toronto. I get ready, and get packed to head over to the competition headquarters. Preliminaries go pretty well, and I have fun seeing all of my fitness model friends and fans. I then leave to go back to the hotel to eat some lunch and get ready for my photo shoot, scheduled in between the prelims and finals. I meet with Coach A, whom I have known for years, and who is a real professional and always produces some great shots.

I then head back to the hotel suite to get ready for the big night, the finals!

The anticipation is building in the air, and everyone is excited and nervous. We go back on stage first with our competition suits on, and I still can't believe how beautiful Passion Fruit Designs has made my swimsuit. Then we switch to the evening gown round. I got my one-of-a-kind dress on South Beach. It was handmade in Italy, and it took a month to make. It's so beautiful that I want to wear it on my 10-year anniversary with my husband when we go back to Venice.

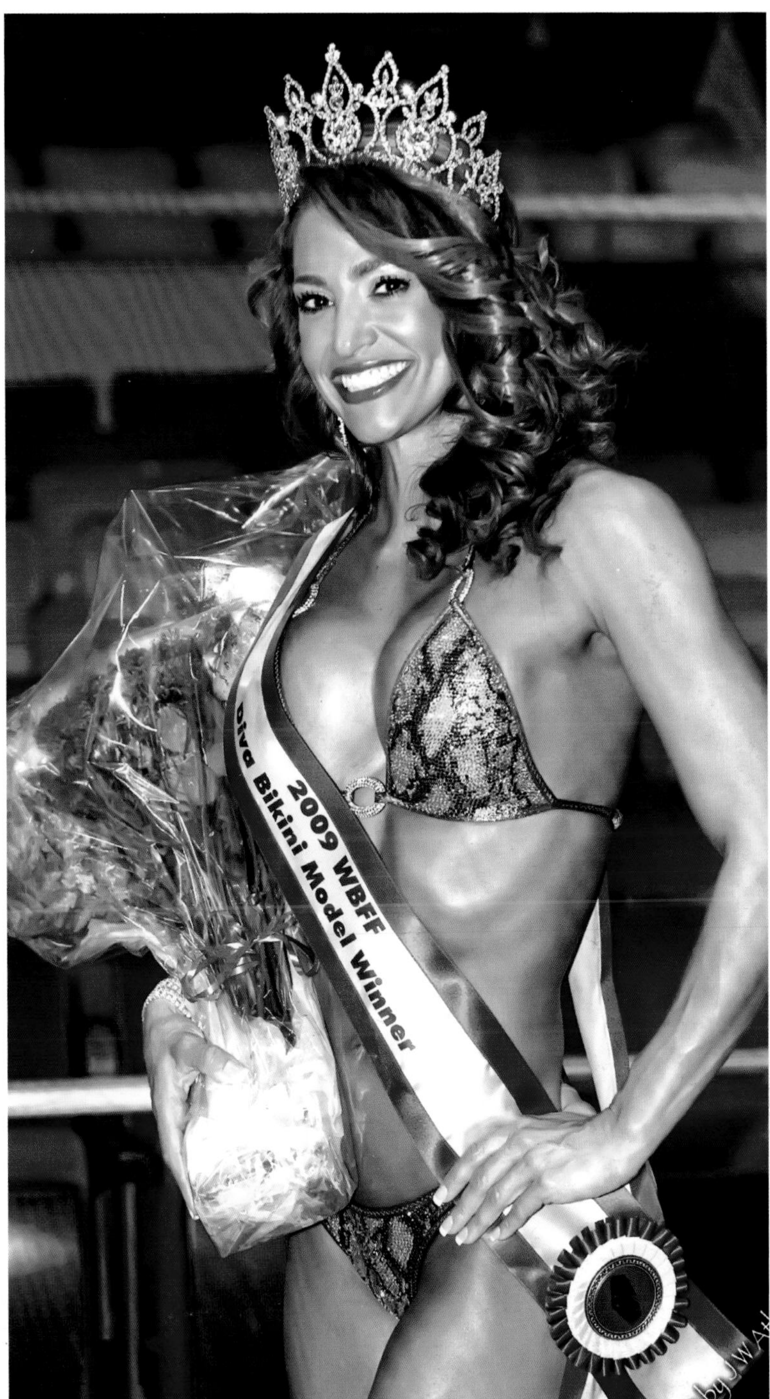

Well, I can't believe it. Thoughts do become things. All of my hard work, focus, and dedication has paid off, and I was crowned the WBFF Miss Bikini Diva for the second year in a row. I also could not believe the size of the crown! What bling!

I also was awarded with a $10,000 check from Paul Dillett of the WBFF as the cash prize, the biggest purse I have ever seen for a fitness competition. I go back to my suite on cloud nine for the super successful outcome. And I have an *Oxygen* photo shoot tomorrow morning, so I must get my beauty sleep. No partying for me!

SUNDAY SEPTEMBER THE 20TH 2009

Another beautiful day in Toronto. I wake up, have my coffee, my fresh-squeezed fruit juice, egg-white omelet and oatmeal with banana. My team in Miami called me from the JNL, Inc headquarters. CBS wants to do an interview, and Dr. Joe Vitale just finished writing my foreword to my other book, *The Mind Body and Soul Diet*. I'll have to deal with all of that when I get back to Miami, and back in the office, as I got to focus on my photo shoot and being in the zone here. I'm fueled and ready for the *Oxygen* photo shoot. I meet with Stacy Kennedy, Editor in Chief of *Oxygen* magazine there, and we do a quick interview before hair and makeup. We also go over wardrobe and the basic styling elements of the photo shoot. I see Paul Bucetta, *Oxygen*'s main photographer, and give him a hug. He was the photographer who shot my second *Oxygen* magazine cover, and he's a great dad and husband as well. He is a true talent and very creative. I also got to meet their new Creative Director, Stacy, who was super-nice and informative.

The photo shoot goes well, producing fun, joyful photos—I have worked with this team before, but its always a bit nerve racking, but I just focus on having fun and being my best, and letting that energy shine through.

Since my flight for Miami leaves at around 2:00, I have to make a mad dash to my last photo shoot before I head to the airport. I stop back at the hotel, to their main conference hall, where *Status* magazine is doing a large group photo shoot. David Ford is set up shooting models, and he takes a quick break to give me a hug. He finishes up with his photo shoot, and then gestures to me to pop in front of his camera. Rodney of *Status Fitness* Magazine is there also, doing video. We get some great shots in, and then I do a quick change, and go back to my suite to pack up my last-minute things, then go downstairs to check out and head over to the airport. On my way out, I hear "La Tigra!" and it's none other than Bob Kennedy of RK Publishing. He owns and runs *Oxygen* magazine, *Eat Clean* Magazine, and also *MuscleMag International* and is married to the lovely Tosca Reno. He hugs me and congratulates me on my win. It's nice to have seen him before I head out. He is a great guy and knows this industry from the inside out.

I check in to the airport and off I go back to Miami. I get in, unpack and head out to a much-needed family night with my husband and sons. We go out to dinner and a fun family movie to celebrate mommy's big win! But my greatest accomplishment is my family, and I am so lucky to be able to share these moments with them.

MONDAY SEPTEMBER THE 21ST

Nice to be back in Miami and in my office to tie up some loose ends after the Miss Bikini Diva competition, and before I head out to Las Vegas to make an appearance at the BSN booth at the Mr. Olympia. I leave on Thursday for Las Vegas, so I have tons to focus on before I leave my family again. Today, I am in the gym again with my coach, "Wicked Willie." He never fails me. I may be jet-lagged, tired, exhausted, and drained, but he always seems to pull the best out of me, giving me a reenergizing workout. He is a faithful friend and confidante, and he always kicks my butt.

After my training session, I drink my BSN Lean Dessert Protein shake (Banana Cream is my favorite) and take a shower. Then I make my way to my office, and sit down for a briefing with my secretary. Some producer in LA called, asking me to do a reality TV show about being a Super Fitness Model. The show idea sounds interesting, and I have a lot of ideas of my own to offer on this topic, so I tell my secretary to put the producer on the line. We chat and hit it off instantly. We make an appointment for a follow-up call after my Mr. Olympia appearances in Las Vegas, and also my HSN appearance for my Ab Circle Pro. I can't wait to get into HSN mode, and show the entire United States just how amazing my "treadmill for your abs" is.

I go through my mail and emails, and do a consult with a great friend of mine who lives in the Arab Emirates. She is down 20 pounds with 10 more to go. Boy, I love my job!

Five o'clock gets here sooner than it should, and my boys come home from school and tell me all about their very exciting day. I hear about what they did in Science club, who won in Chess club, and how sports went, too. I make my family dinner, then we throw the football in the back yard and even go for a swim. I make it a point to live an active lifestyle with my family, and we have fun doing it.

TUESDAY SEPTEMBER THE 22ND

I wake up, cook breakfast for my family, take my BSN Atrophex and get ready to go to my home away from home – the gym!

Another great day in the gym working out, focusing on legs and glutes. We kick off our training with 5 minutes of speed rope, and then go straight into my Quadruple Threat Lower body routine. Boy, that one always gets me!

Home, BSN protein shake, shower, and then back to the office. I have a meeting with my best friend and executive assistant, Marli, as we need to finalize my outfits for the Mr. Olympia, as well as the photo shoots that I have planned there. She brings in a rolling rack complete with tops, dresses, skirts, shoes, boots, and jewelry to match. She loves fashion and so do I, so we always have fun creating my next look and outfits. She encourages me to try new and different things to keep my image fresh and interesting. We decide on our outfits, and wrap up the fitting.

My secretary tells me that my entertainment lawyer is on the phone and is wondering about the TV producer in LA, and what the current situation is. I tell him that I would be consulting with her after I get back from my next whirlwind trip, and also invite him to call her to "sniff" her out, to see if she is a flake or the real deal. You can never tell in our industry who is legit or who is a big talker. So he calls her and starts the investigation.

My sons get home and I switch into super mommy mode! We review homework, eat dinner, and go over the details of a play date that we are hosting at our house next week. They want to order pizza, play sports outside with their friends and also swim. I check their homework and see that they both made 100% on their spelling tests. I could not be more proud!

My massage therapist comes to my house, and we do a 60-minute neuromuscular massage with active stretching exercises to loosen me up and get me limber and ready for the super hectic weekend. I take a bath and tuck my sons in after I read them a book. One last BSN Lean Dessert Shake before I go to bed to help lock in my gains today – beauty rest is a must. 'Night night!!!

WEDNESDAY SEPTEMBER THE 23RD

Last day before I fly out to Las Vegas for Mr. Olympia. I go over last minute details and agendas with my team. And since I am following my own Fitness Model Diet workout guide, I do abs and then cardio at home to save time.

My publisher emails me with exciting news about my "The Mind, Body & Soul Diet" and how it will be ready by October, no later than November. The endorsements from Jack Canfield of *Chicken Soup for the Soul* and Marci Shimoff, a featured teacher in *The Secret* and also the foreword being written by Dr. Joe Vitale, best-selling author of *The Attractor Factor*, all added a lot of value to my book, and my publisher was happy about that. I admire all of these people and to have their names on my book is just nothing short of a miracle.

My other lawyer calls me and tells me that my royalty statement from my Ab Circle Pro deal looks pretty good. We make an appointment for next week.

I go over all of my websites and domains with my webmasters and tech team. All is running well, and my www.SHOPJNL.com online store is doing very well. And it looks like my www.FitnessModelProgram.com is at the head of all my sales, making it my #1 top-selling baby. My secretary lists off about 50 other emails that are from fans, telling me how much they love www.FitnessModelProgram.com and the great results they have gotten from my other products, exercise equipment, and even exercise DVDs. Very fulfilling!

I get an email from a great photographer, Mike Brochu, who tells me that his plans of coming to Miami have solidified, and to be ready for at least four to five days of solid photo shoots. We need to shoot for BSN, for my book cover, inside workout photos, back cover, and also some fun fashion shots. It's always great to work with him, as he is a true genius, very talented, super-creative, and easy to work with. I put a call in to my stylist to let her know the dates of our photo shoots and to make sure that she is on board.

It's my last night before I leave town again, so my husband decides to take us all out to dinner for a fun family night out on the town of Miami. We drive to the beach, have dinner on Ocean Drive, and get some light frozen yogurt to celebrate with. I'm truly blessed to have the most supportive husband and loving kids in the world. The three men in my life (hubby and two sons) give the best hugs and kisses!

THURSDAY SEPTEMBER THE 24TH

I wake up and jump out of bed with a spring in my step! It's my last workout before I fly to Las Vegas for Mr. Olympia, and then over to Tampa for two days to be on Home Shopping Network for my Ab Circle Pro. I make breakfast for my family, kiss my sons good bye for school, and then head to the gym. We do a Total Body Circuit just to keep my entire body tight for the next flight over to the other coast.

I do the regular last minute checks before I head to the airport. Check into first class, and fly the friendly skies to LV!

I check in to my hotel, and get a good night's sleep. I had plans of going to the *Oxygen* Party at Bliss, but I have to pass as my body is screaming "SLEEP!" and it's going to be a long weekend. That's my "fitness model" mentality kicking in — always choose sleep over partying! Your body will end up thanking you and your energy will show up better in photos and in appearances.

FRIDAY SEPTEMBER THE 25TH

I wake up and Katie B, one of the best makeup artists ever, comes to my suite and does my hair and makeup. She is so sweet and extremely talented. She did my *Iron Man* magazine cover and editorial spread, and she is one of the best, if not the best. Her entire line of mineral makeup rocks, and so does her personality. The funny thing is that I met her exactly one year ago, when I was researching celebrity hair and make-up artists and found her. I had never met her before, but something told me to hire her, and just go with it. We ended up becoming great friends, and she is a true, genuine sweetie. I'm trying to get her to come to my birthday bash in Miami, and also be on set for my next infomercial deal so we are going to work out the details.

The convention is amazing! BSN always goes above and beyond, building a little city in the convention center. I do a bunch of interviews, photo ops, and meet/greet my fans. I know that I have the best fans in the world, and every time I meet them they are so loving and kind. I love seeing everyone in our fitness industry at these huge fitness conventions. The energy is super-electric, and my fellow team BSN athletes are so great to work side by side with. They are a real "class act" group of people.

At the end of the day, I'm pooped, and all I want to do is take a long hot bath, and sip a glass of red wine to calm me down from a super-successful, yet full day!

SATURDAY SEPTEMBER THE 26TH

FULL DAY! Another day at the expo, then I'll do a photo shoot and interview before I head back to the airport to take the red-eye back to Miami.

BSN ends up getting 8 awards from the Bodybuilding.com awards, and I end up going on stage to receive the awards with the Director of Marketing. One the third award, I finally ask for the microphone to say a sincere "thank you" for all the support our BSN consumers give us. I could not allow the moment to pass without saying "thank you" to the entire industry.

Events are over, and I fly back to Miami and land around 7:00 am.

SUNDAY SEPTEMBER THE 27TH

Waking up in Miami after sleeping all night in an airplane seat is not easy. But the show must go on! In tough times, I reflect upon just how blessed and lucky I am to have opportunities like these, and why I am doing all of this — for my fitness friends and fans. I get home, shower and go to church with my family. I spend some time with the family sharing our latest and greatest updates, squeeze in a quick workout, and then head back to the airport for a 3:00 flight to Tampa to appear on live TV in front of 100 million households on HSN with my Ab Circle Pro.

I love appearing on HSN, as it's the number-one at home interactive shopping channel and the energy there is so amazing! I end up selling over 20,000 units in only two days, and my appearances on live TV are a big hit, making records and breaking records with our sales.

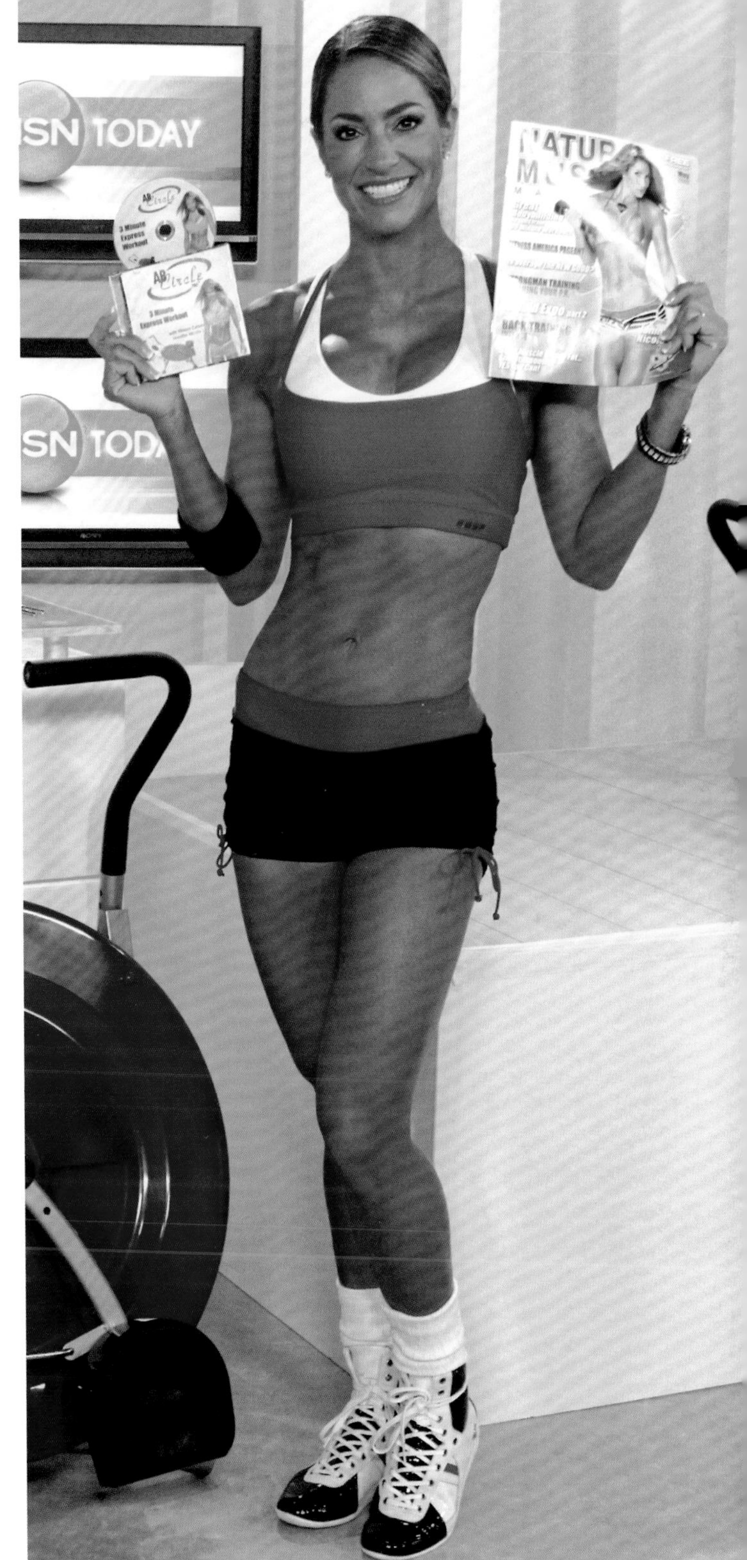

IN: on set at the Home Shopping Network

CHAPTER 13:

JNL'S EXCLUSIVE COLLECTION OF PHOTOS

"We all have an inner genius that we either choose to express or not. Leonardo DeVinci painted the Mona Lisa, Alexandros of Antioch carved the Venus De Milo, and Andy Warhol was famous for his Campbell Soup can paintings. My fitness modeling and photography captures my inner genius and are in sense a form of masterpiece."

–JNL

I have so many thousands of photos to choose from, however these have been my favorites. I have taken the time to chose them wisely, as there are many deeper meanings that lay behind the photo, that if you look close enough, you just may grasp them. Enjoy, and know that for more photos, you can always go to my gallery at www.Jennifer-NicoleLee.com!

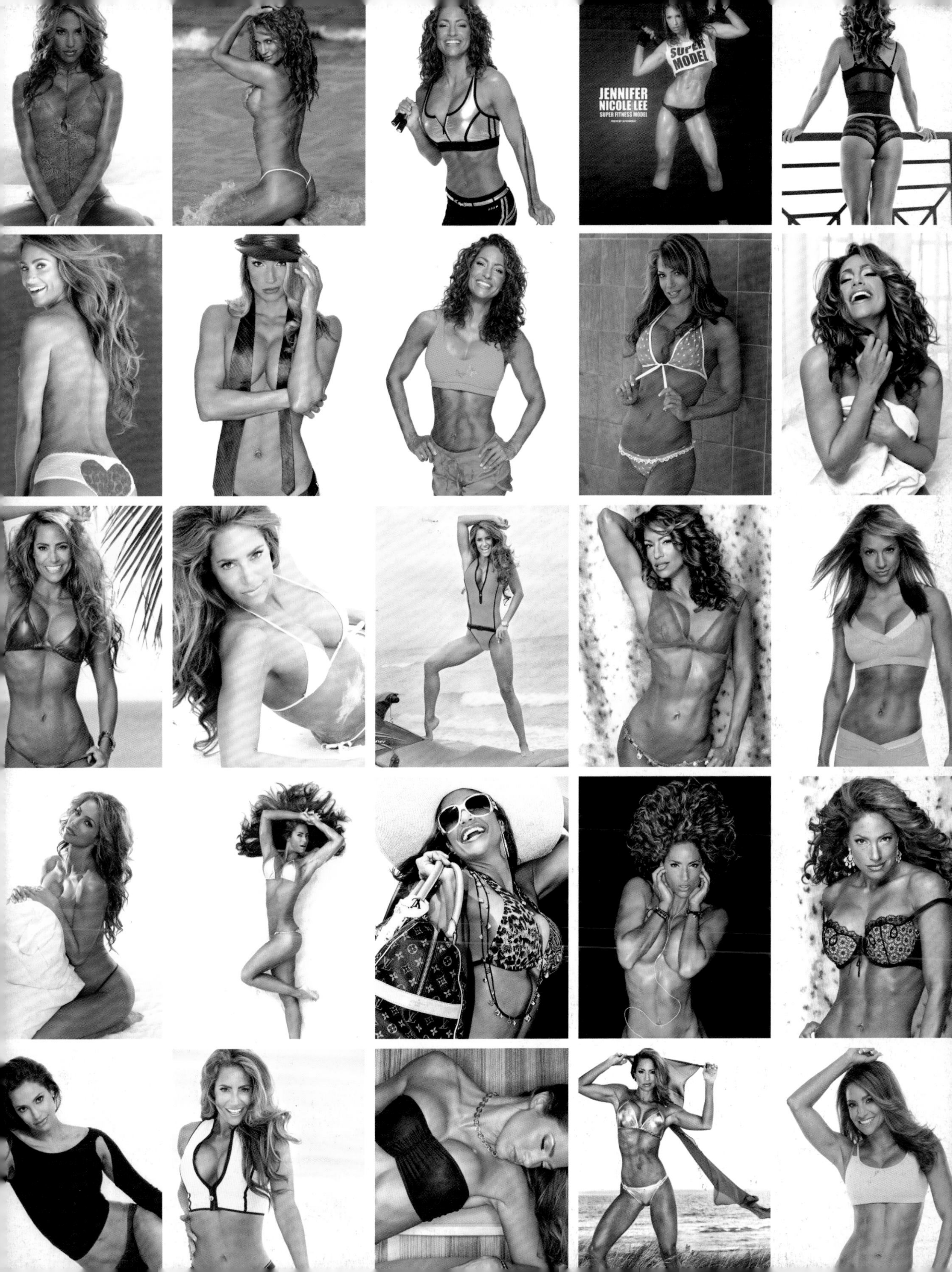
SUPER MODEL
JENNIFER
NICOLE LEE
SUPER FITNESS MODEL

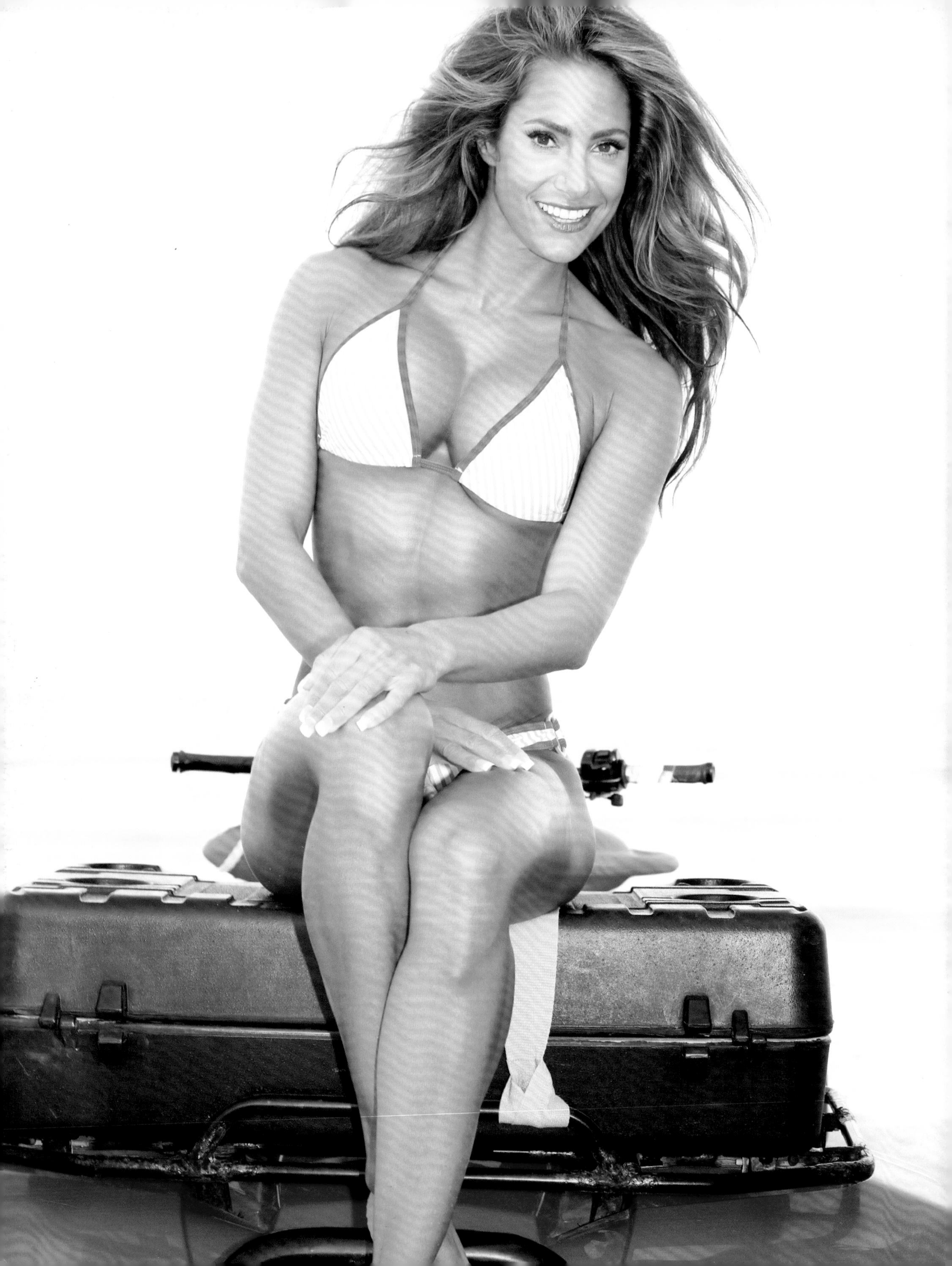

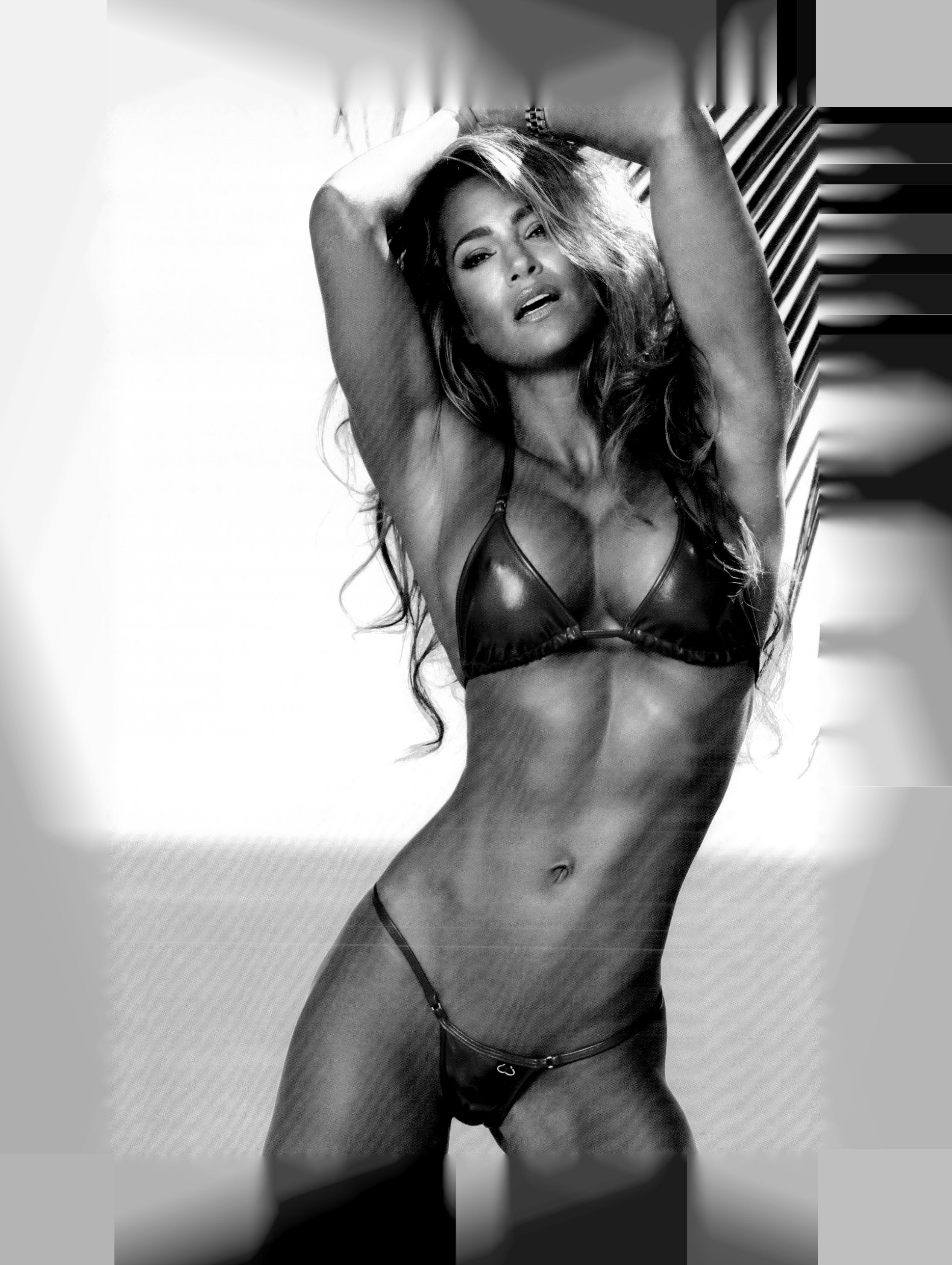

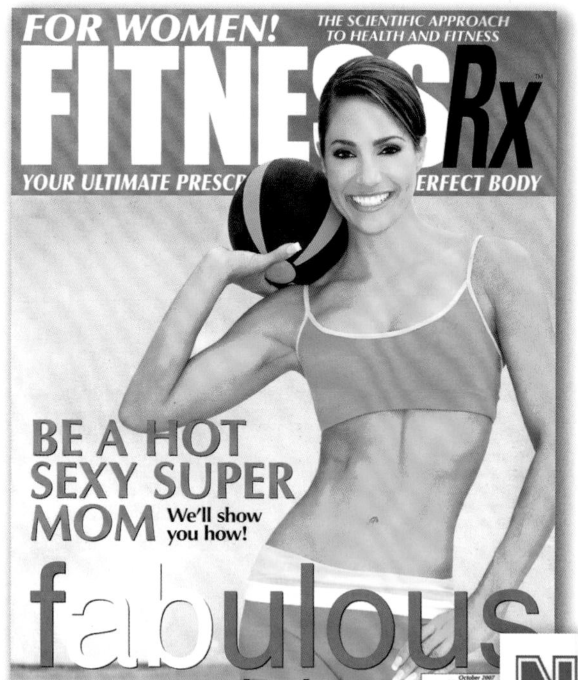
FOR WOMEN!
THE SCIENTIFIC APPROACH TO HEALTH AND FITNESS
FITNESS Rx
YOUR ULTIMATE PRESC
ERFECT BODY
BE A HOT SEXY SUPER MOM
We'll show you how!
fabulous
Get Lean, Shed Fat
Show Off Your Abs!

NATUR
MUS
MAGA
FREE
Pick one up!
May 2009
Skip La Cour's
TOP 10 TRAINING TIPS
HITTING A PLATEAU IN THE GYM
RFC
REVENGE OF WARRIORS
PERK IT UP IN THE PARK
THE TOP 7 MASS BUILDING/FAT BURNING EXERCISES ON THE PLANET!
DUMP THE PUMPS
FLIP-FLOPS & BALLET SLIPPERS ARE NOT THE ANSWER.
JENNIFER NICOLE LEE
BREAKING THE RULES TO FITNESS

THE NEW ANABOLIC FAT-BLASTING DIET

IRON MAN™

Jennifer Nicole Lee

How She Shed 70 Pounds to Become a Fitness Icon (Her Ab Circle Pro Is a TV Hit!)

Kid Kong

Amazing 21-Year-Old Powerhouse

Shocking Protein Power

Researcher Reveals New Mass-Building Discovery

All-Dumbbell Workouts

Pack On Muscle at Home

DECEMBER 2009

www.IronManMagazine.com
Please display until 12/1/09

PLUS:

- Sergio Oliva Jr.
- "BenchMonster" Benching Tips
- Squat to Grow

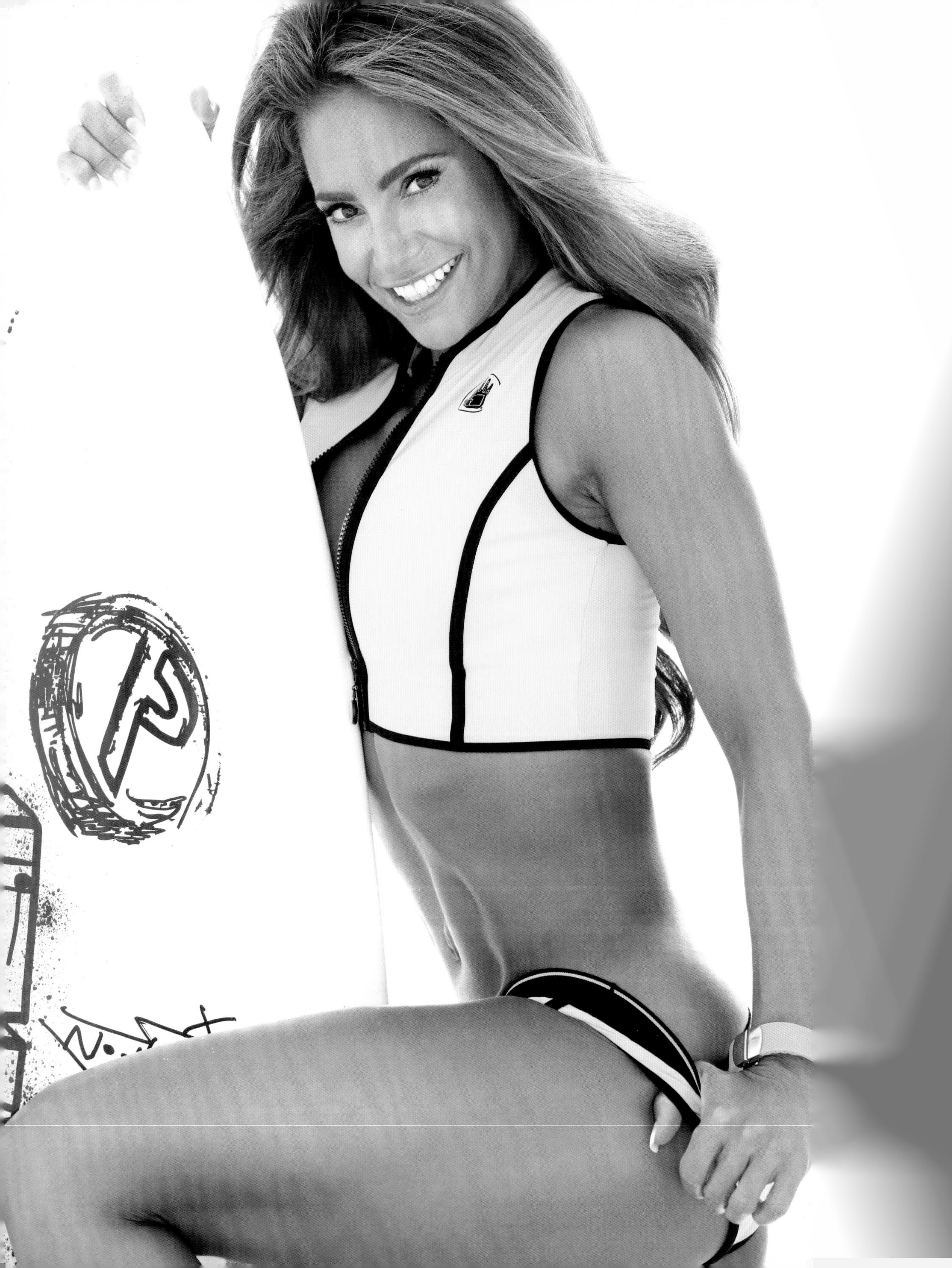

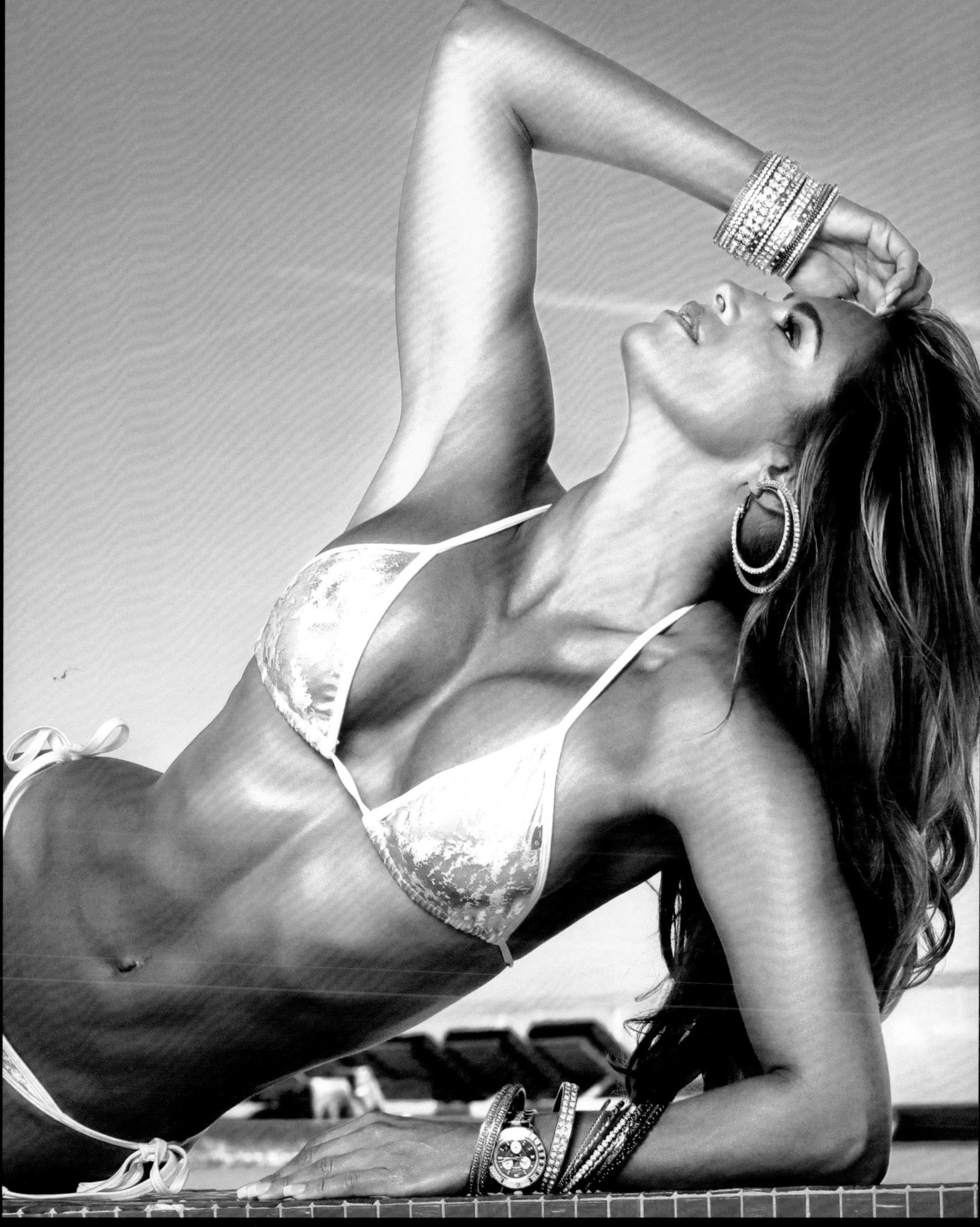

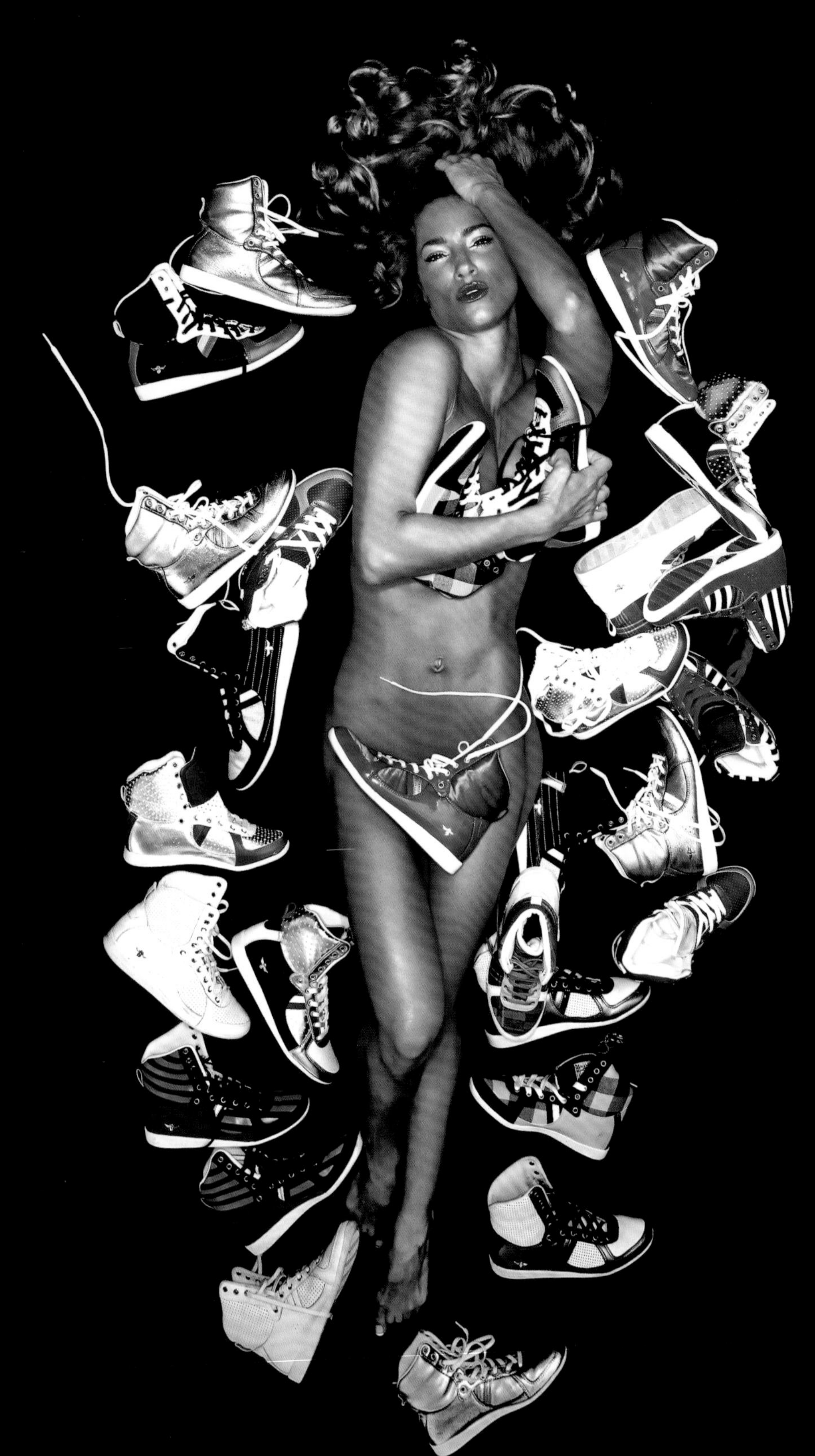

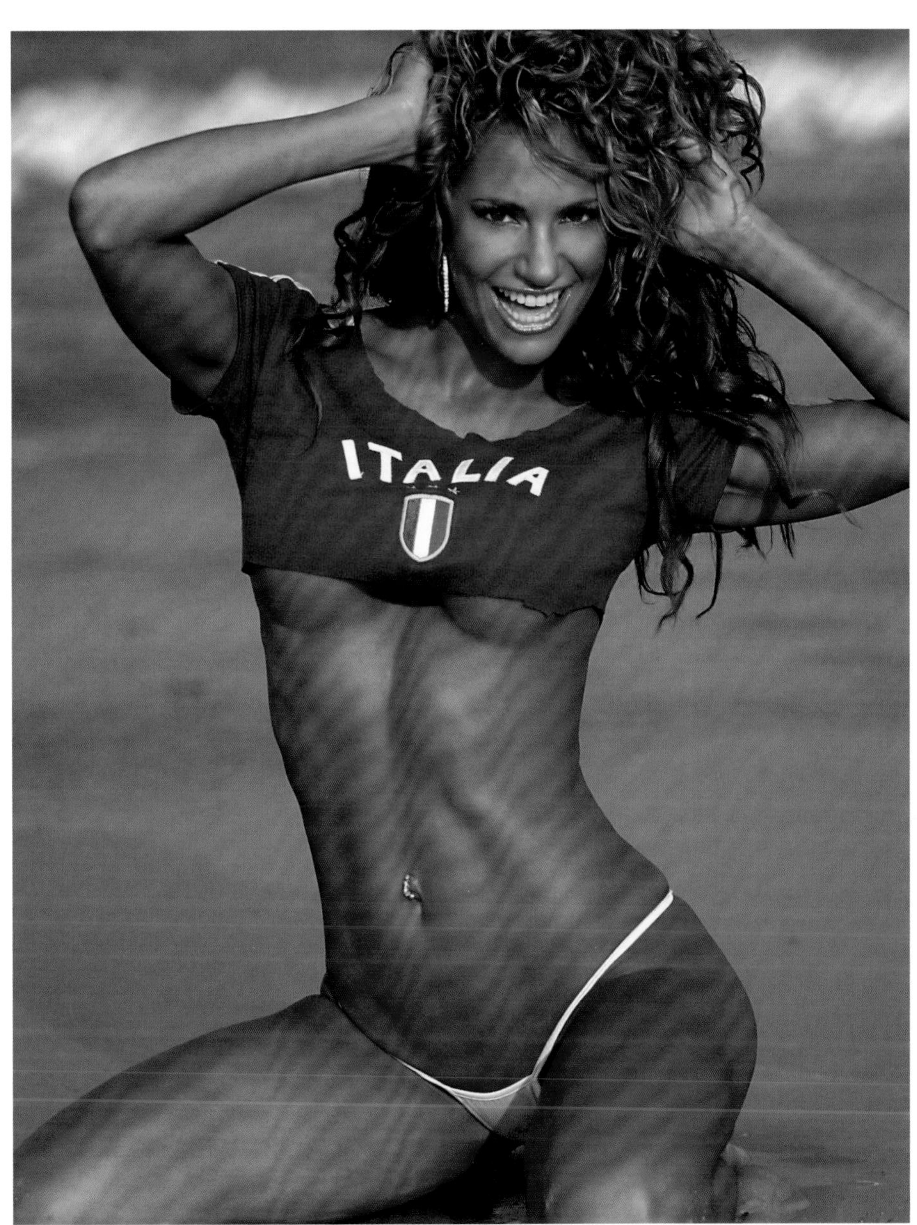
ITALIA

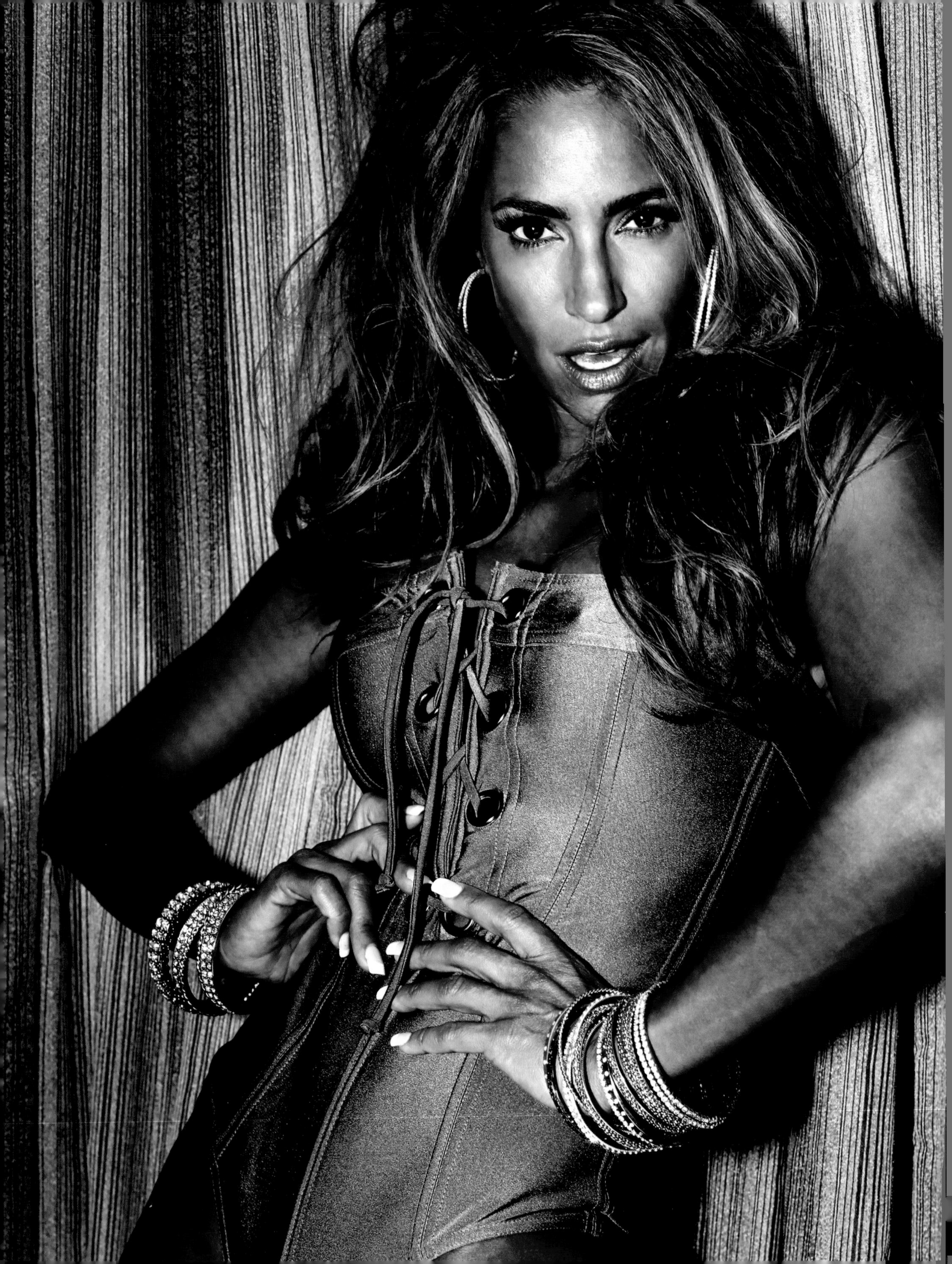

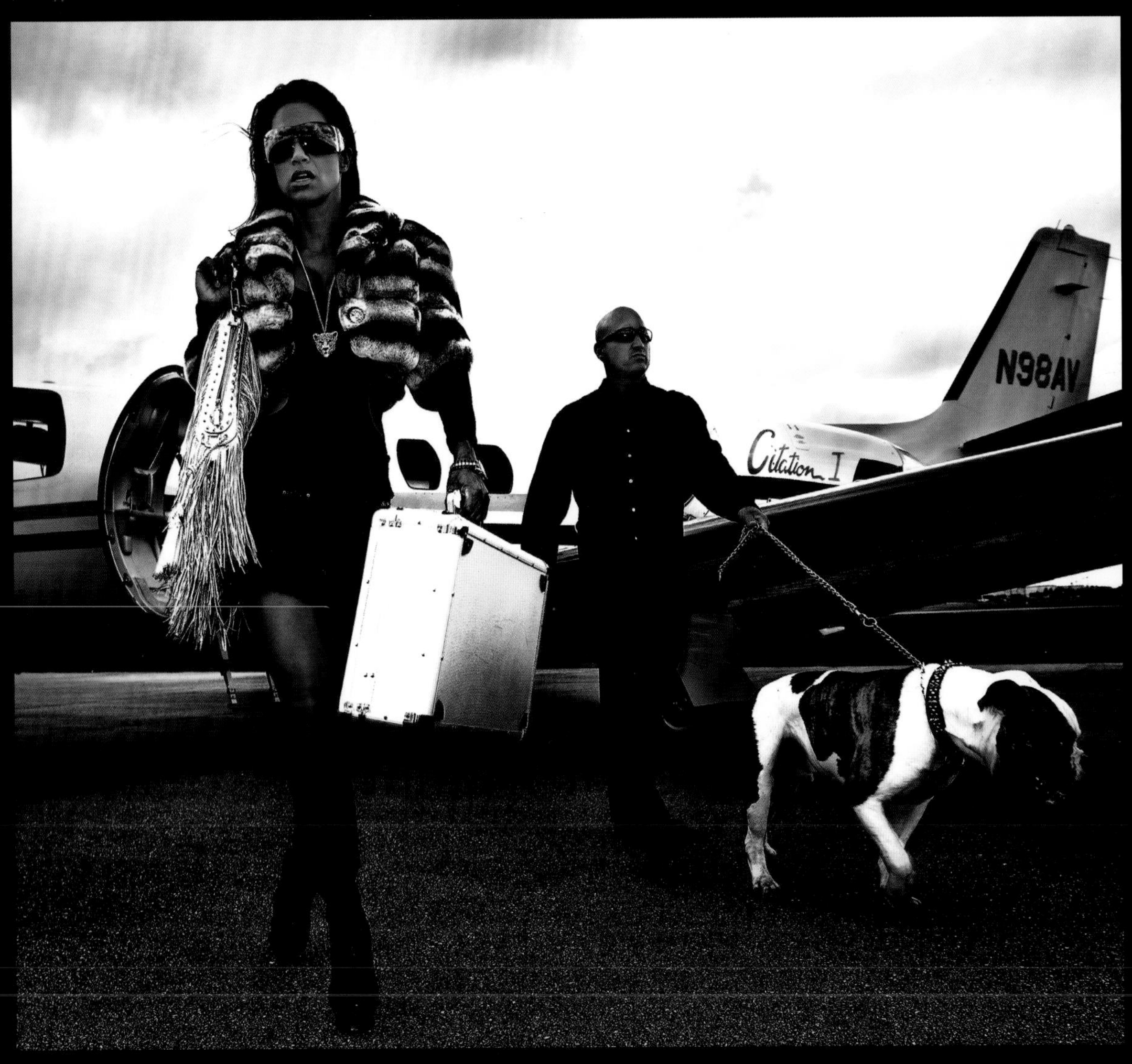
N98AV
Citation I

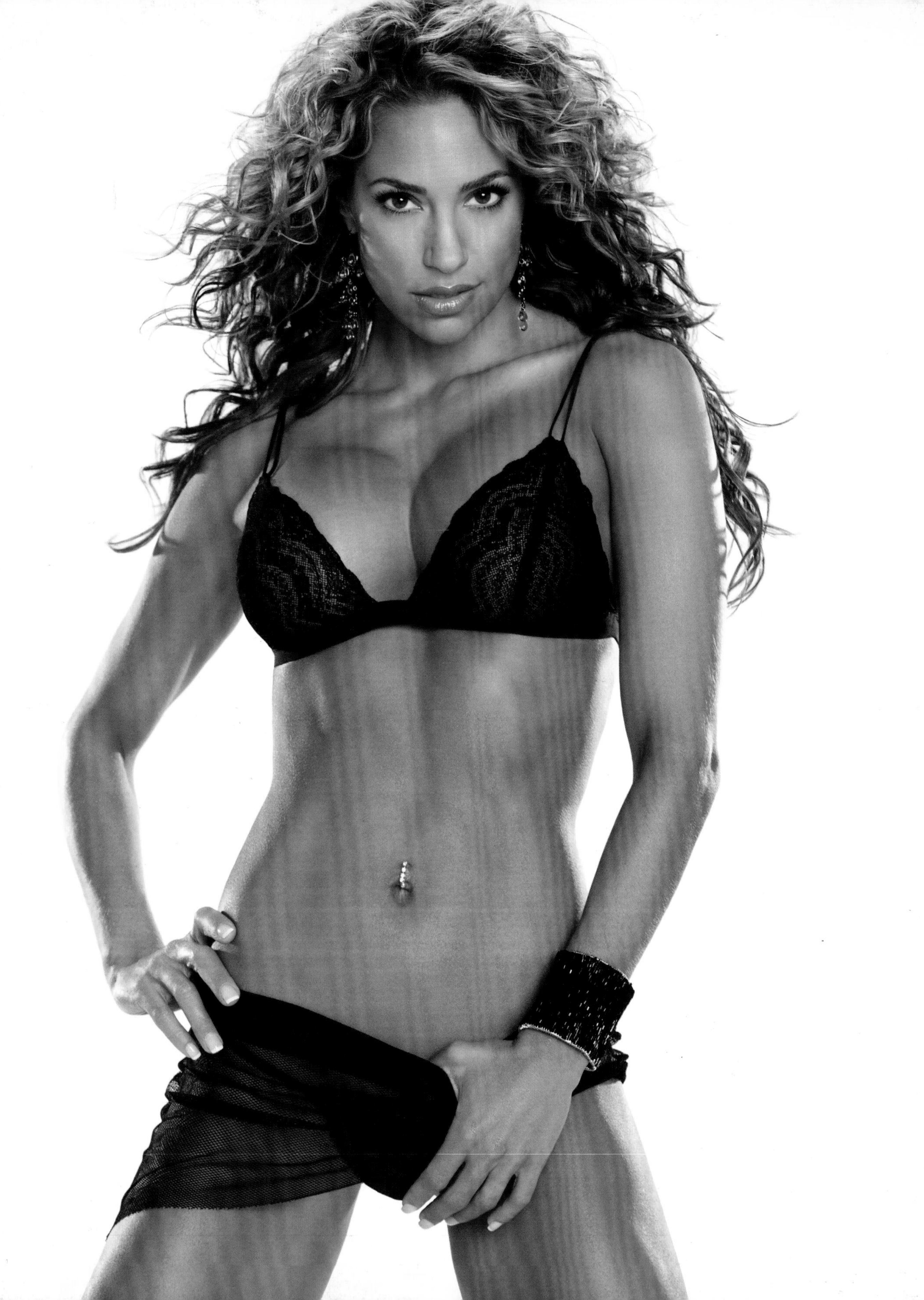

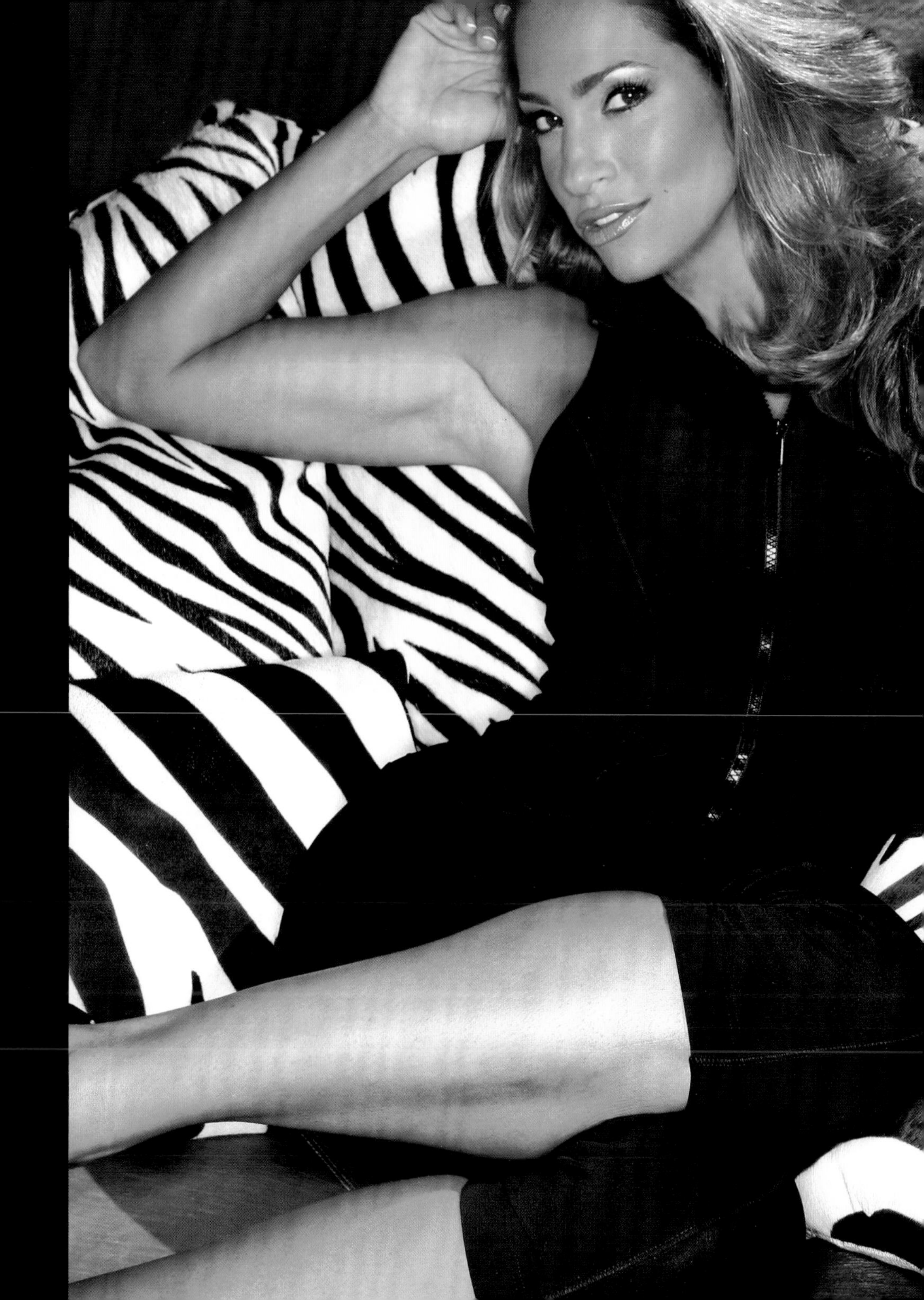

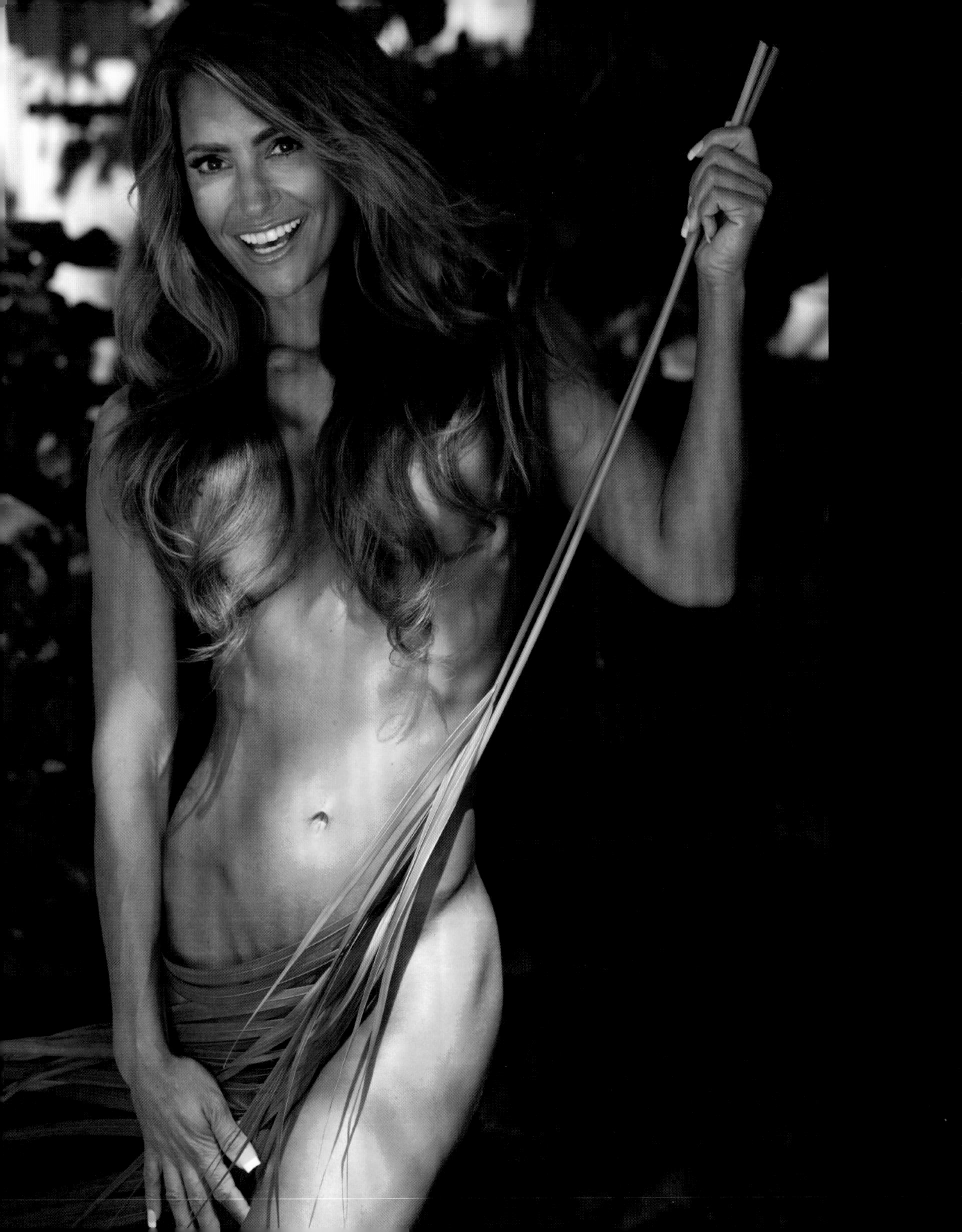

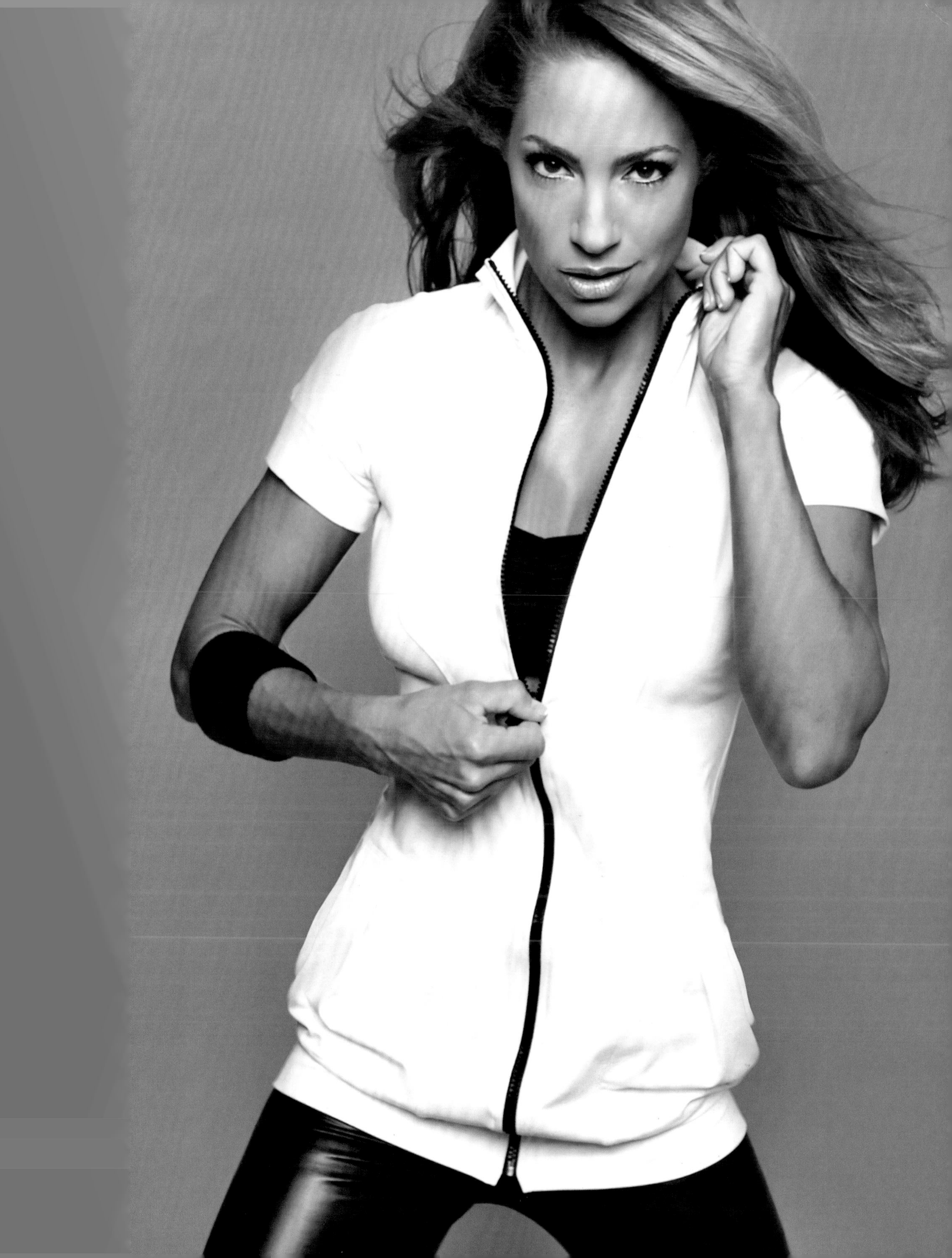

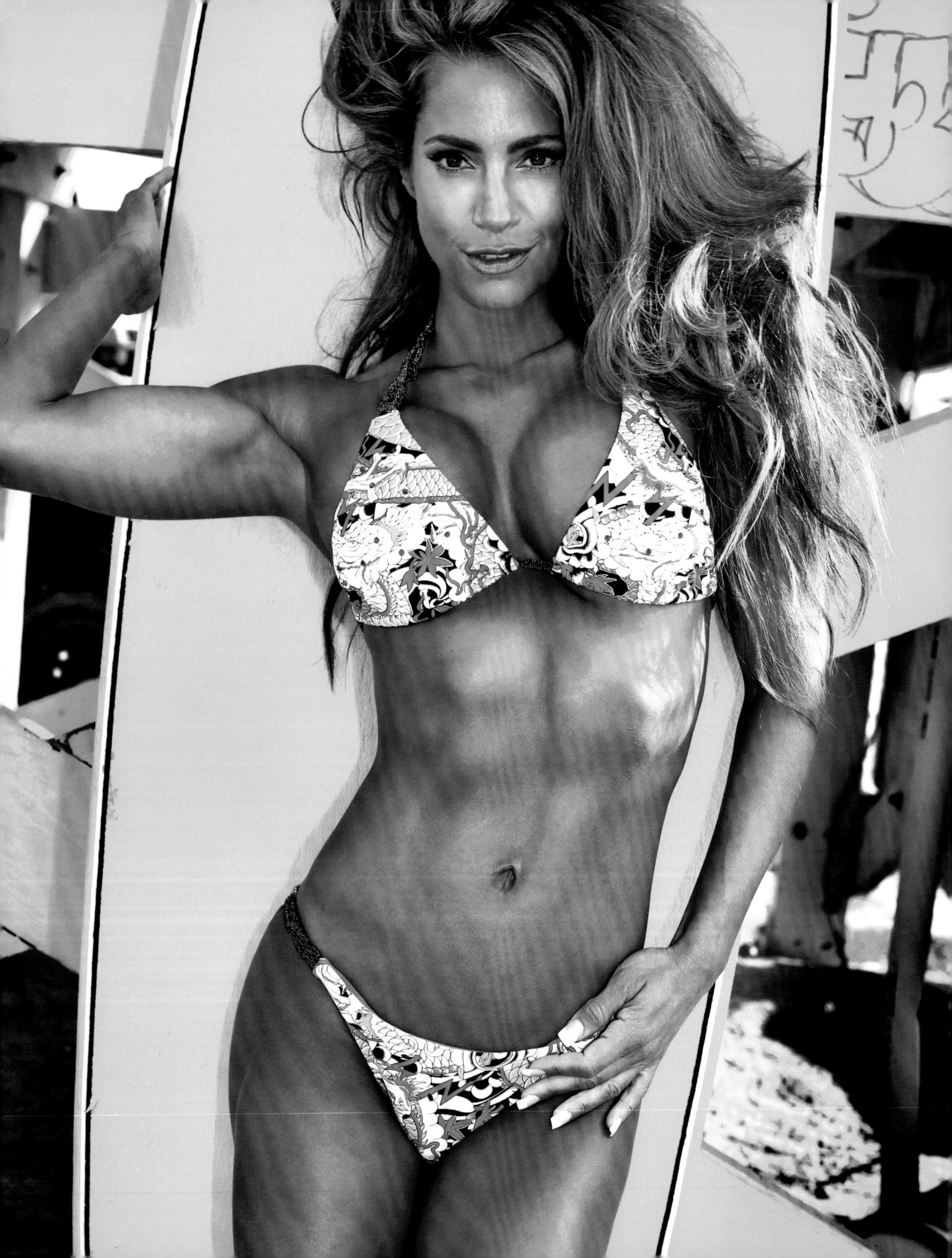

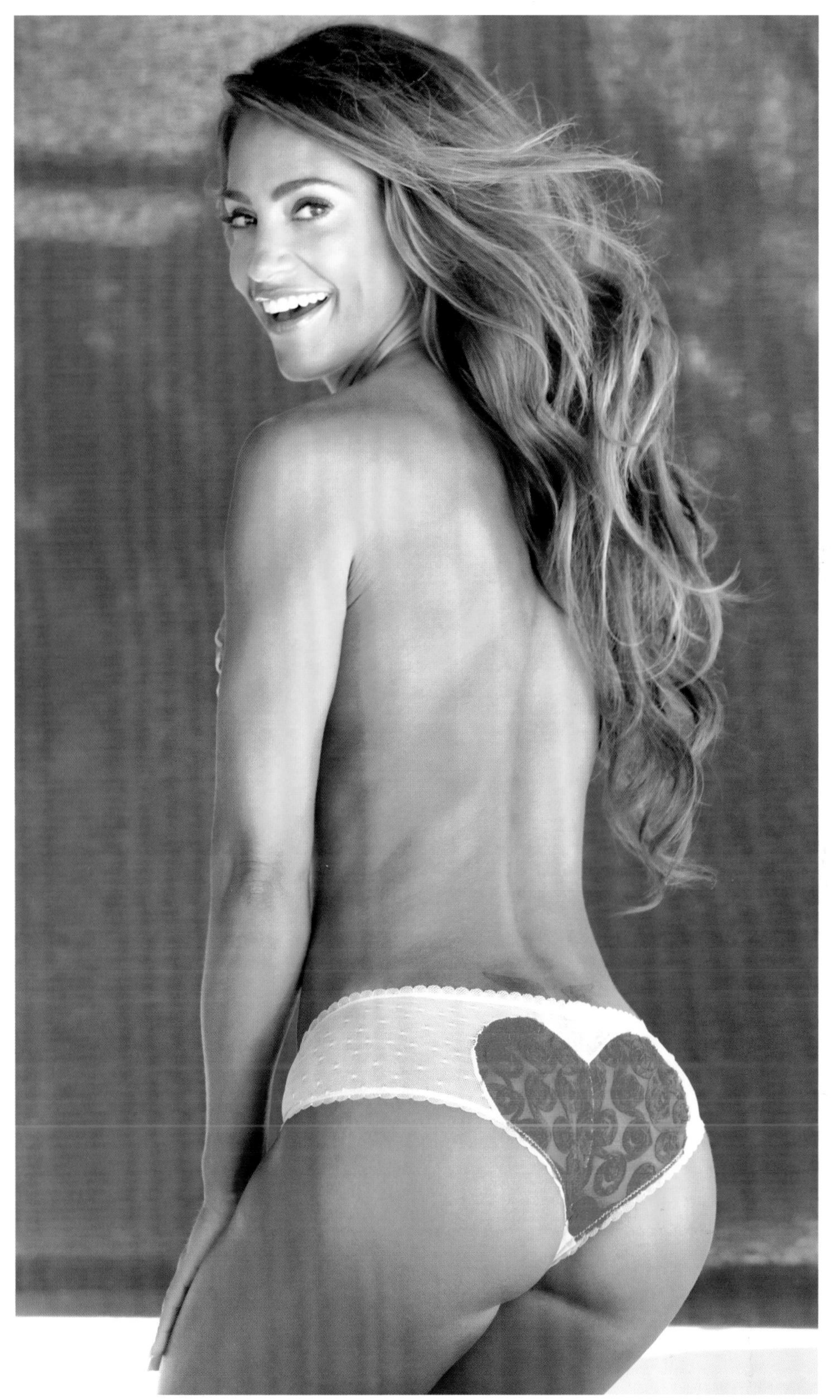

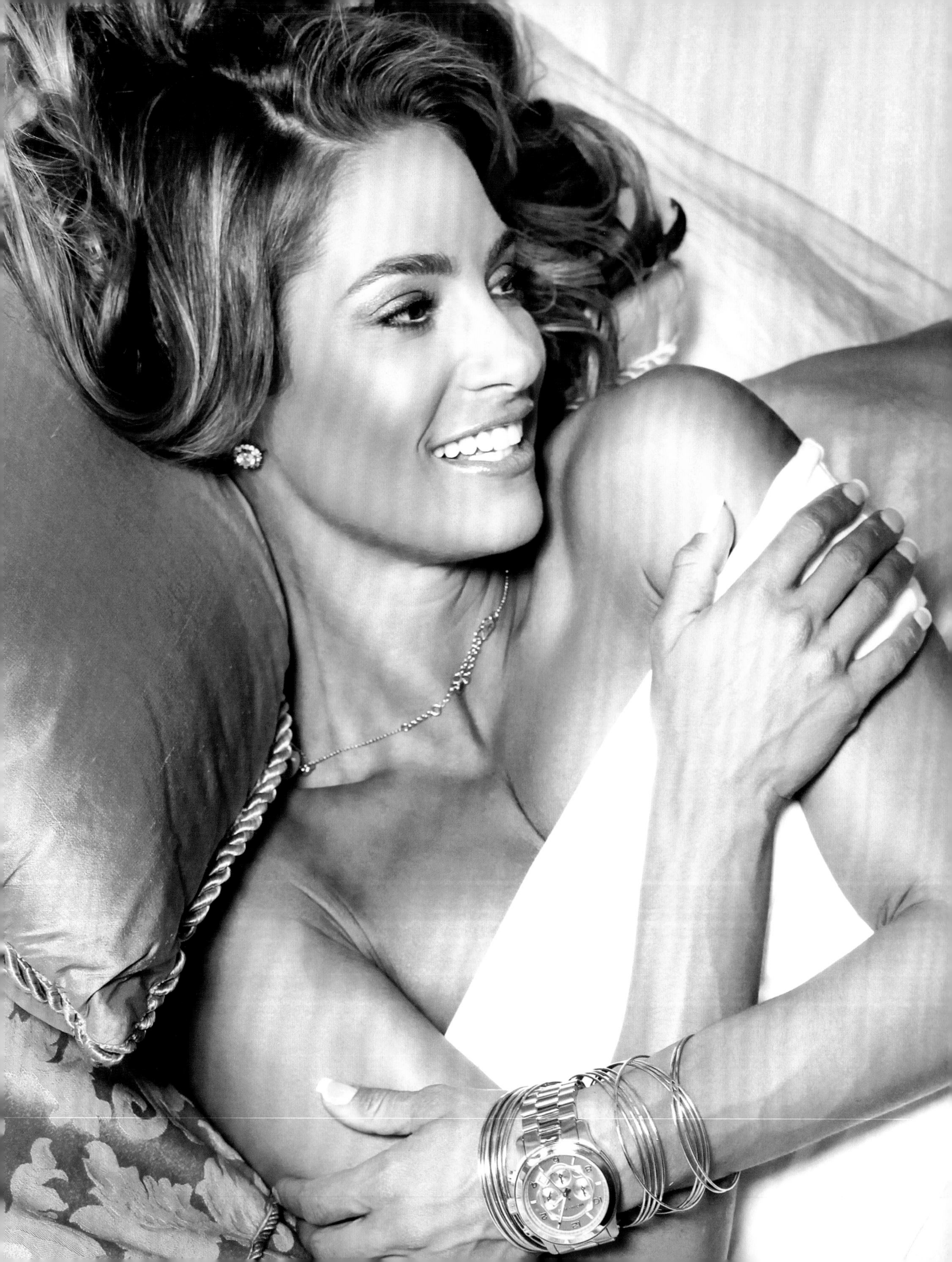

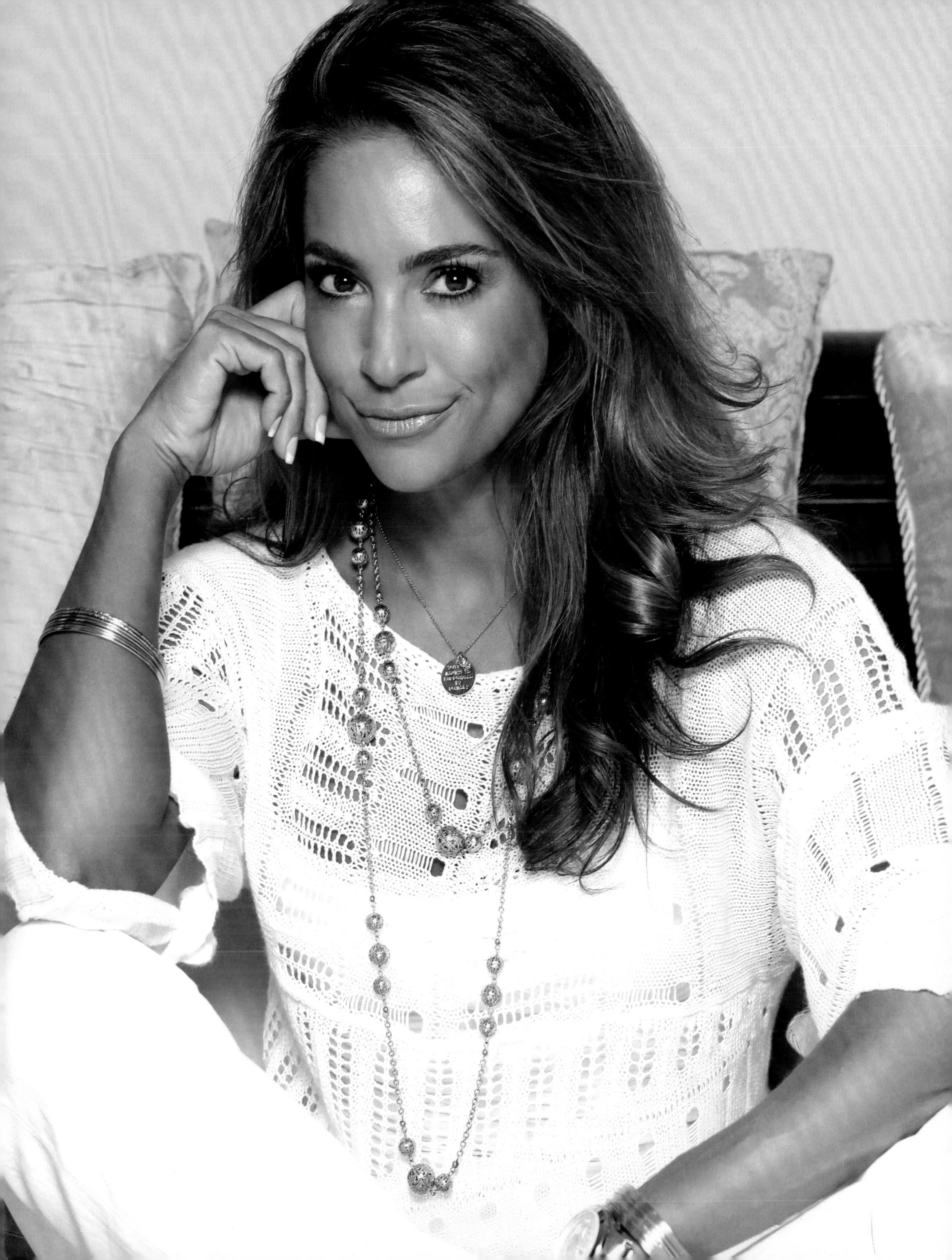

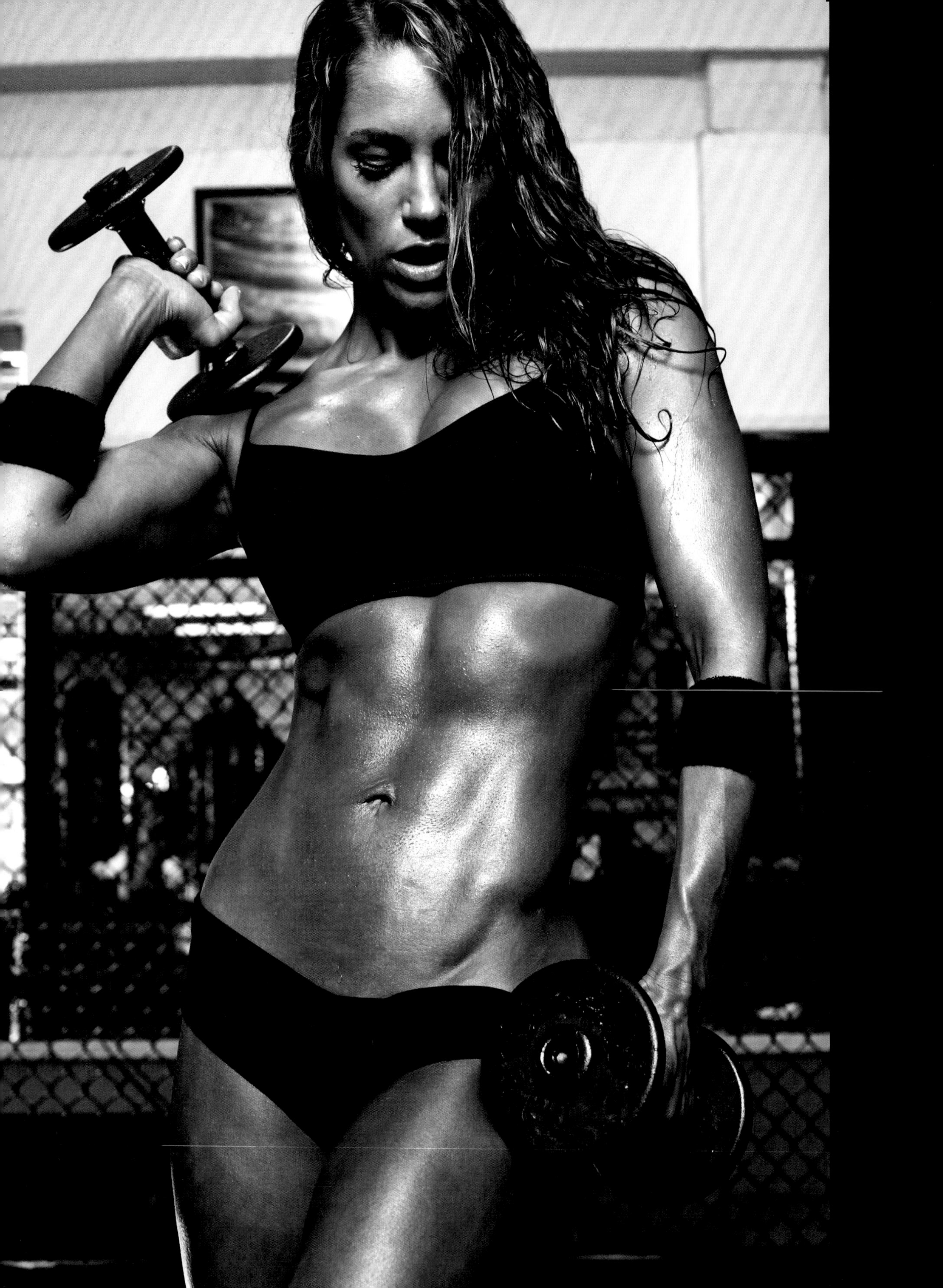

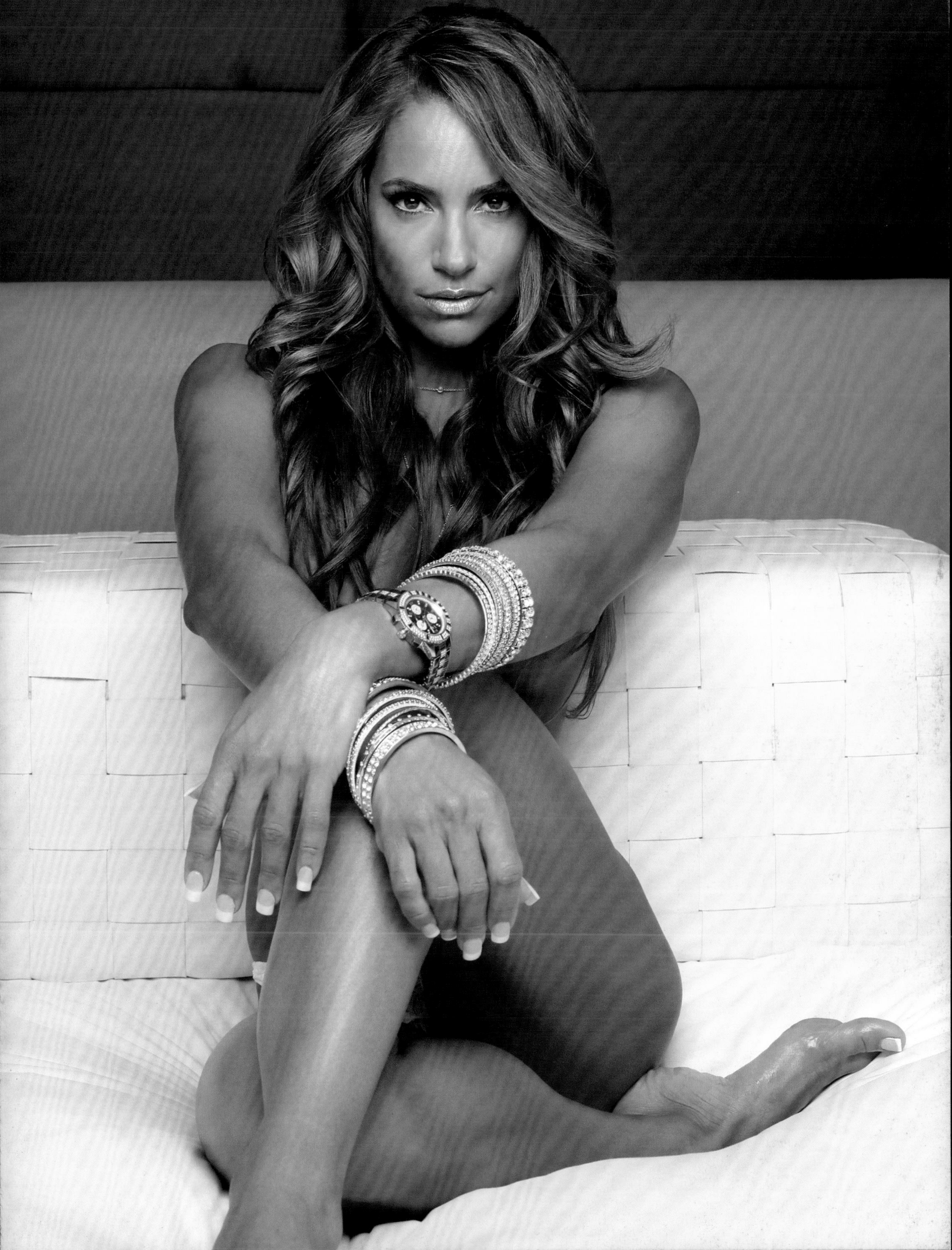

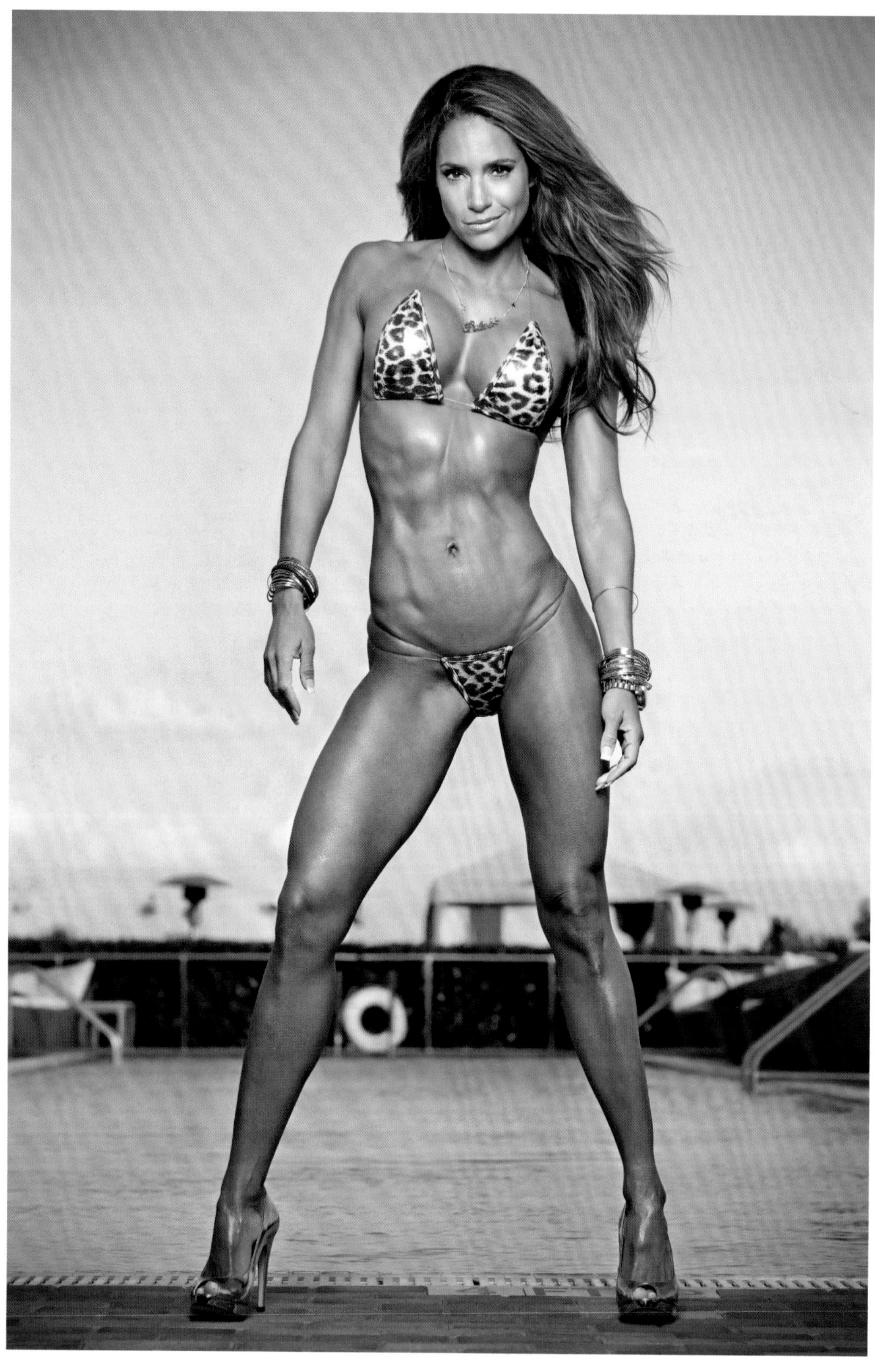

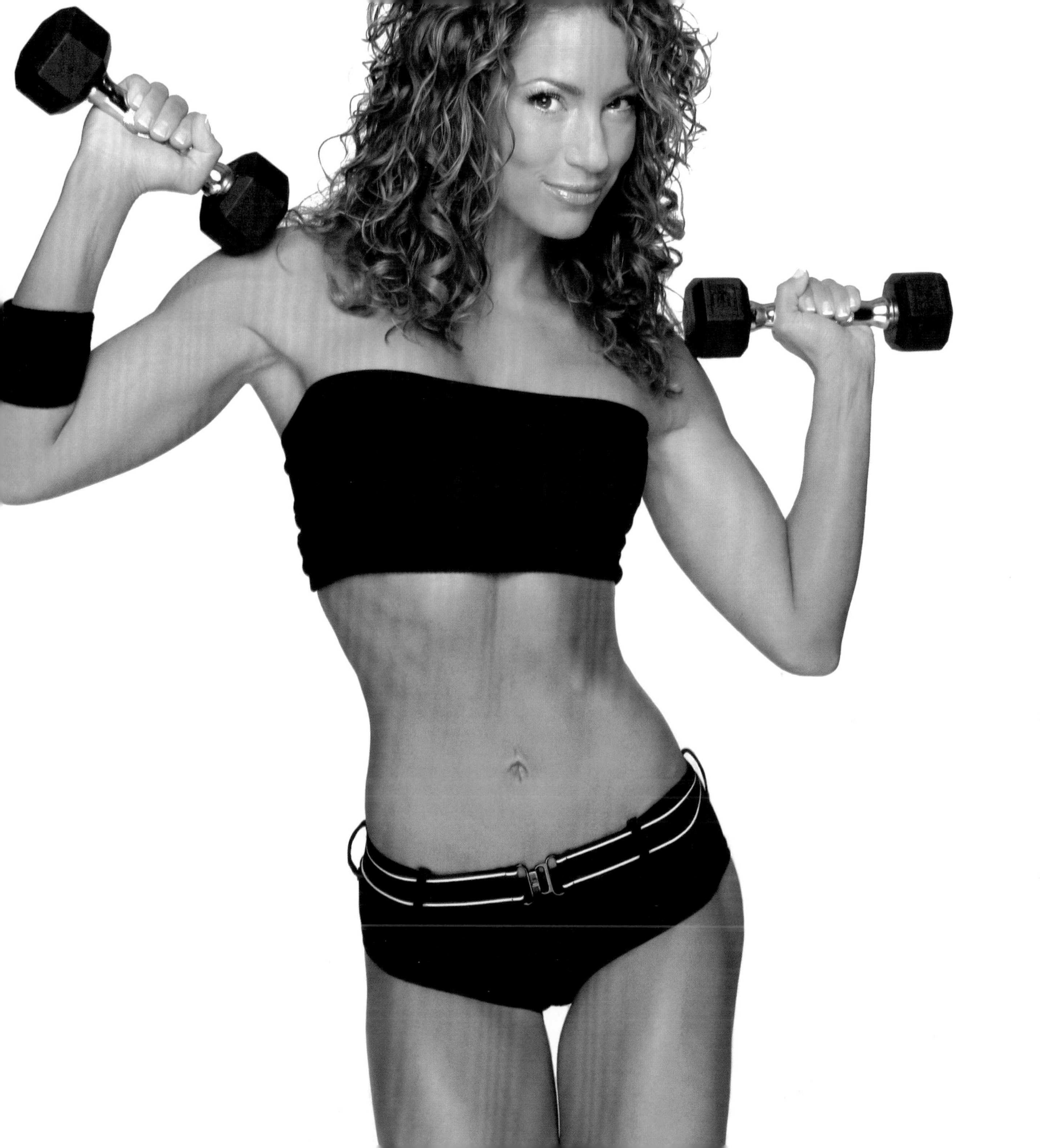

CHAPTER 14:

JNL-APPROVED!

JNL's Top List of Her Must-Haves & Favorite Things in Life!

"What's life without your favorite things?"

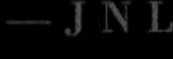

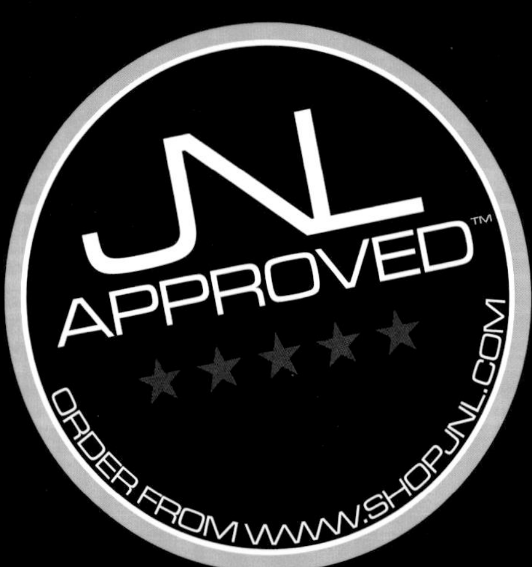

THE LIST OF JNL-APPROVED PRODUCTS

Being a super fitness model, highly sought-after keynote speaker and author, as well as an international weight-loss success story, I receive endless emails asking me what my favorite things are—the things I cannot live with and that I always use. Now I've got a complete list just for you.

Lean dessert protein by BSN. Being a modern-day multitasking woman and mother, I don't have time to julienne vegetables and mince green onion. So, I quickly whip up a lean dessert protein shake that saves me time and energy, and enables me to maintain my weight loss goals.

ATROPHEX by BSN: Being a busy mom, and CEO, I need endless amounts of energy, to keep me fueled throughout the day. I also love to get an extra burn in while training. This is why I rely upon BSN's super-posh energy management supplement Atro-Phex. It helps me to also shed water weight, it boosts my mood, and also helps me to have mental acuity and focus better.

N.O. XPLODE AND N.O. XPLODE NT: I always take a pre-workout igniter, and the best, hands-down, is BSN's NO Xplode. I take one scoop and stir it into some water in a small glass, drink it all at once, and then head to the gym or work out at home. It's the best supplement that I can trust to make sure I always get a great workout in.

EXERCISE DVDS. When I'm long on needing a workout and short on time, I love to pop in an exercise DVD and press "play". I love my entire library of six CD's from my Fabulously Fit Moms series. They are super challenging, and give results FAST! They are available at www.ShopJNL.com

ABCIRCLEPRO. This fantastic tool has helped me burn fat and calories, and chisel out my core without having to get on the floor and do another sit-up. It allows me to get in a quick three- to five-minute workout to keep my six-pack abs in check and stay camera ready. The AbCirclePro is available at www.JNLAbCirclePro.com . Make sure you upgrade to get the "bundle" which includes the fitness computer, plus the 3 additional exercise DVD's to keep you motivated!

DARK CHOCOLATE: You've got to get your anti-oxidants in somehow, right? I love extra dark chocolate, and my favorites are Godiva and Dove. Try a small square every other day to keep yourself sane and happy.

RED WINE: I love to relax with a glass of red wine at night, before my warm baths when I soak my muscles, and even before a massage, to help me wind down. Red wine helps reduce the risk of the number one killer of women, heart disease! So cheers to your health! My favorite wine is Estancia's Cabernet Sauvignon.

TRAINING GLOVES: I never train without them! I love the cushy Everlast ones that actually look like kick boxing gloves. They are super padded, have a great grip when you have to lift heavy, and come in cool fitness model colors, like hot pink, black, yellow, and also red!

SPEED ROPES: as all of you know, I love to jump rope in between my sets. I call this technique the "JNL Fusion Training," where I work in my cardio and conditioning in between my weight training, allowing me to get the best of both worlds at once: to burn fat, and build muscle. My favorite jump rope of all time is by Buddy Lee, who is a jump rope master and Olympic athlete. My favorite one is the Buddy Lee Master Jump Rope. It's available at www.BuddyLeeJumpRopes.com

FITNESS COMPETITION DESIGNS & ACTIVE WEAR: When I step on stage to compete, I always trust my really great friend Berns to create my masterpiece! She is the master designer and CEO of www.PassionFruitDesigns.com She also is a super brain when it comes to creating the active wear outfits from scratch that I wear monthly on my HSN appearances.

COACHING PROGRAMS ARE JNL-APPROVED! I always say that the correct information is priceless. During one of my latest key media appearances, the interviewer looked me straight in the eyes and asked, "How important is hiring a life coach and why is coaching important?" I was boggled by this question. The interviewer was questioning whether life coaching actually produces results. My answer is this: life coaching is absolutely essential. In this dog-eat-dog world, where it's pretty much survival of the fittest, you have to know what to do to get ahead of the pack, break away from all the wannabes, and set yourself up as a doer. Even the most successful athletes, the top strategic minds of tech empires, and the most amazing mixed martial artists in the UFC, rely upon life coaches to give them that cutting, winning edge [Ed1].

I can tell you right now that I would probably be light years ahead of where I am right now if I had truly understood the importance of life coaches ten years ago. If I had embraced my ability to hire a coach and not tried to do it the hard way, I would not have wasted so much time, money, and energy before I figured it out.

The problem is that a lot of people are close-minded; they're afraid to try to new techniques that actually have been proven to work, and they shun the metaphysical approach that the top coaches use. My point is this; to get results, you have to be highly coach-able. You've got to listen to the experts.

So many people have the right intentions but are using belief systems that were passed down to them. I hate to say it, but your parents' paradigms are not what's happening in today's multitasking, information-in-an-instant age. In this new era, you need to be equipped with the latest, most innovative way to produce results. One of my favorite books, *Who Moved My Cheese?*, puts it this way: you must adapt and be flexible because there is only one constant in life, and that's change. You must be able to work with change and focus on how to streamline your results. But who's going to give you those answers? Life coaches—people who have done it before.

Once you fully understand how important life coaching is, you'll realize why now is the time for you to implement what you know. I pride myself in providing a top-of-the-line coaching program, The Mind, Body and Soul Program, to help you lose weight and gain a new identity as a healthy, super-fit athlete; to help you de-clutter yourself mentally; to help you get rid of self-sabotaging behaviors; and help you create a business out of your own true passions. If you don't know what your passions are anymore, I will help you reawaken them.

You can access the complete coaching services I provide at JenniferNicoleLee.com. I have a complete menu of different coaching programs that are designed to help you find the one that's right for you.

- If you want to increase your productivity and efficiency, you can do a one-on-one coaching consultation with me at **CLUBJNL.COM**.
- If you want to look like a fitness model, you can go to **FITNESSMODELPROGRAM.COM AND WWW.THEFITNESSMODELDIET.COM**
- If you want to look like you just walked out of a bikini catalog, not as rock hard as a fitness model, you can go to **BIKINIMODELPROGRAM.COM**.
- If you want to reawaken your inner goddess, reconnect with your sensual side, and get your "sexy" back, you can do that with my innovative, unique, sensually reawakening program entitled **THESEXYBODYDIET.COM**.
- If you're looking for a complete four-week, twenty-eight-day guide to take you by the hand and tell you what to eat, how to train, and even equip you with motivational quotes, positive affirmations, and powerful visualization exercises, visit **GETFITNOWWITHJNL.COM**.
- If you're looking to really blast fast and rev your metabolism, you can visit **JNLCRACKTHECODE.COM**.
- If you have all the right intentions and are still not seeing results, I have an amazing e-Book, **101 THINGS NOT TO DO**, available at **101THINGSNOTTODO.COM**. The concept behind the book is that the things you're doing now, thinking they're healthy for you, are actually sabotaging your efforts.
- And if you want to improve the quality of your lifestyle in all areas, you can visit **MINDBODYANDSOULPROGRAM.COM**. So, as you can see, I have a program designed especially for you and your desired outcome.
- I developed a complete bedding line, with fitness, health, comfort & luxury all in mind! You must visit www.JNLFitHome.com to see my favorite pillows, sheets, and bedding.

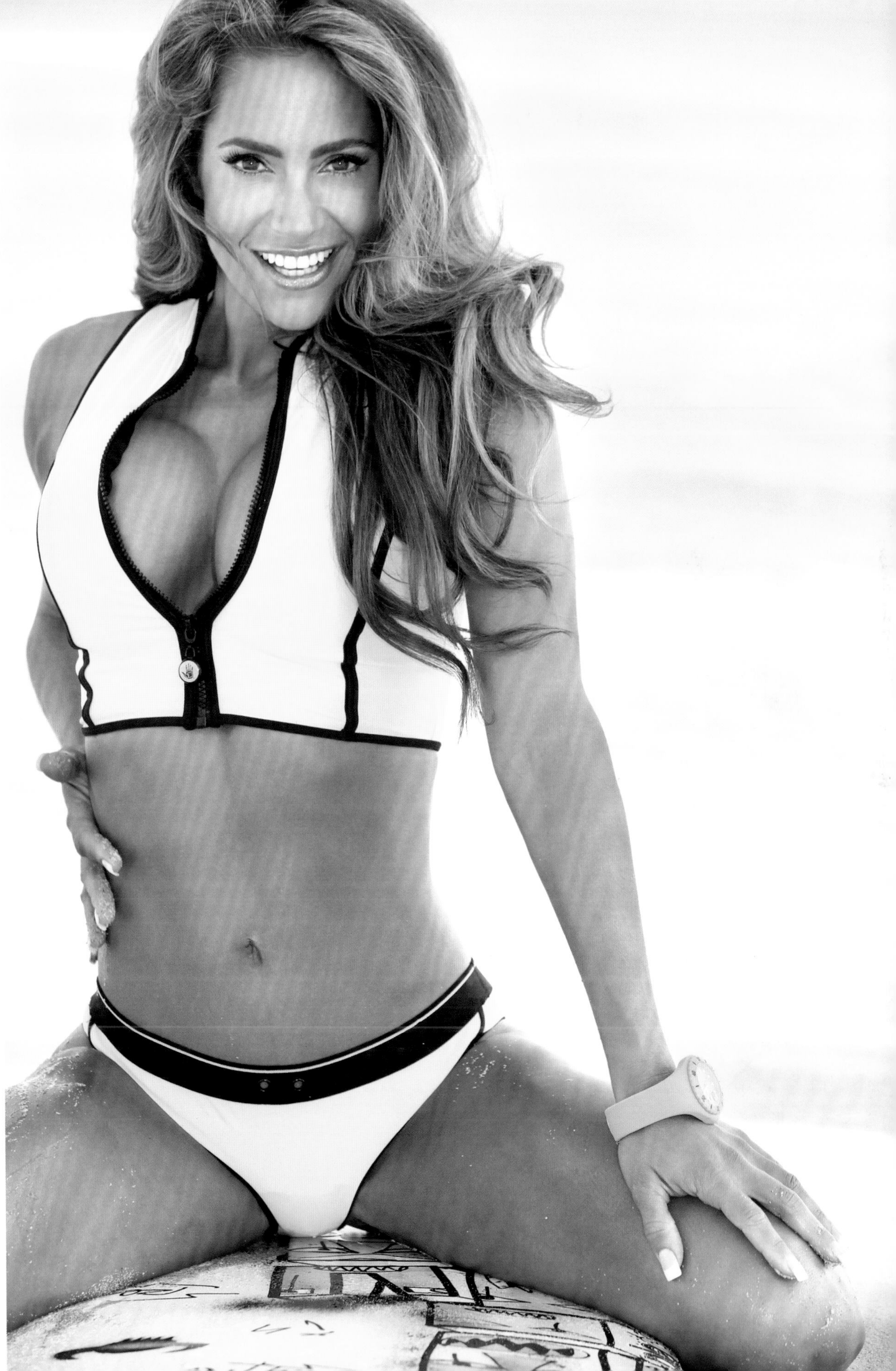

LAST THOUGHTS FROM YOUR FITNESS FRIEND, COACH AND MENTOR, JNL

Dearest Fitness Friend,

This program is one of the greatest gifts that you could have given yourself. Now, it's up to you to use it! It's like buying a book. Either you choose to read it or you allow it to collect dust in your library. It's not up to me what you do with the information that I am giving you; however, if you are reading this right now, it is highly unlikely that you are unmotivated, undirectable or uncoachable, or comfortably miserable. I know that you are determined, dedicated and committed to making your life's goals happen!

There is a choice in life. You can hope that things will happen, or you can make things happen! I urge you to choose the latter, just as I have done. I could have easily blended into the comfortable mediocrity that surrounded me when I was at my heaviest, after giving birth to my second son. I had no mentor, coach or real parental guide to show me the keys to success, but I did not allow any of those things to be my excuse. Rather, I took my life into my hands and got into the driver's seat of my own destiny, focused on being the best that I could be.

I have handed you the tools, techniques, success clues, and principles that will give YOU results in your life. It's up to YOU to utilize them, and to create and experience magic every day of your life!

If you have any intimate, personal comments, questions, or concerns that you need me to address/answer one-on-one with you, please feel free to contact me for a telephone and/or webcam consultation by applying at www.clubjnl.com.

Smile and Be Well,

JNL

ABOUT THE AUTHOR

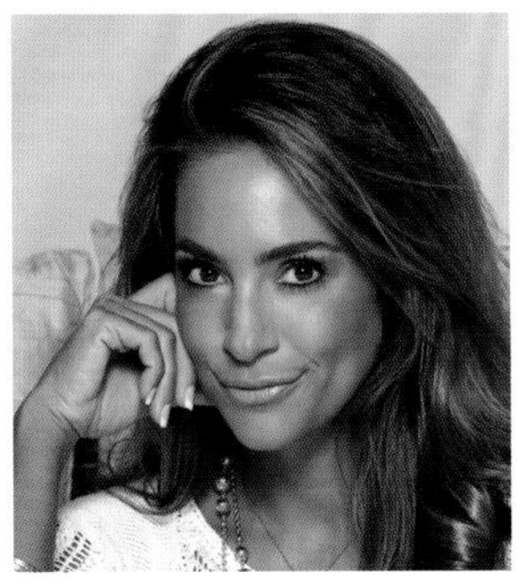

JENNIFER NICOLE LEE is one of the world's most accomplished entrepreneurial CEOs. Thanks to the popularity of her wildly successful infomercial appearances, she is a household name in over 90 different countries worldwide, with her fitness messages translated into over 20 different languages. She is a bestselling author, highly sought-after motivational keynote speaker, certified life coach, Team BSN athlete, and a specialist in Sports Nutrition and Supplementation, with a focus on anti-aging. Her inspirational weight loss success story has motivated millions to take action in their own lives. Her cutting-edge, yet timeless, lifestyle fitness expertise has been featured on *The Oprah Winfrey Show, The Big Idea with Donny Deutsch, E! Entertainment, Inside Edition, Fox & Friends, CBS Early Morning Show,* and WE Entertainment's *"Secret Lives of Women."* She has been featured in countless magazines and editorials, and is regarded as one of the world's top fitness celebrities, thanks to her remarkable health, vibrancy, youth, and glamour. JNL is a regular featured fitness expert and celebrity on the HSN Channel, sharing her favorite wellness, fitness, and lifestyle products. She is the CEO of JNL, Inc., a company she founded with this mission statement: "I will share and shine my light to help others realize and then achieve their lifestyle goals, as I believe that everyone deserves to increase the quality of their lives." Jennifer lives in Miami with her husband Edward and sons Jaden Byron and Dylan Edward.

You can visit Jennifer Nicole Lee at her website:

JENNIFERNICOLELEE.COM

JENNIFERNICOLELEE.BIZ

My Space: MYSPACE.COM/JENNIFERNICOLELEE

Twitter: TWITTER.COM/THEJNL

Ning: THEJNLNETWORK.COM

YouTube: YOUTUBE.COM/USER/THEJENNIFERNICOLELEE

Facebook: JNLFB.COM